NCRP REPORT No. 156

Development of a Biokinetic Model for Radionuclide-Contaminated Wounds and Procedures for Their Assessment, Dosimetry and Treatment

Recommendations of the
NATIONAL COUNCIL ON RADIATION
PROTECTION AND MEASUREMENTS

December 14, 2006

National Council on Radiation Protection and Measurements
7910 Woodmont Avenue, Suite 400 / Bethesda, MD 20814-3095

WN
650
N2775da
2007

LEGAL NOTICE

Disclaimer

Library of Congress Cataloging-in-Publication Data

National Council on Radiation Protection and Measurements.
   Development of a biokinetic model for radionuclide-contaminated wounds and procedures for their assessment, dosimetry, and treatment : recommendations of the National Council on Radiation Protection and Measurements, December 14, 2006.
      p. ; cm. — (NCRP report ; no. 156)
   "This report was prepared by Scientific Committee 57-17 on Radionuclide Dosimetry Model for Wounds."—Pref.
   Includes bibliographical references.
   ISBN-13: 978-0-929600-93-2
   ISBN-10: 0-929600-93-2
   1. Radiation injuries—Treatment—Mathematical models. 2. Radiation dosimetry—Mathematical models. 3. Radioisotopes—Toxicology—Mathematical models. 4. Wounds and injuries—Complications. 5. Skin—Effect of radiation on. I. National Council on Radiation Protection and Measurements. Scientific Committee 57-17 on Radionuclide Dosimetry Model for Wounds. II. Title. III. Series.
   [DNLM: 1. Radiation Injuries—therapy—Guideline. 2. Radiometry—methods—Guideline. 3. Models, Biological—Guideline. 4. Radioisotopes—adverse effects—Guideline. 5. Risk Assessment—methods—Guideline. 6. Wounds, Penetrating—therapy—Guideline. WN 650 N2775da 2007]
   RA569.N357 2007
   362.196'9897--dc22

                                                          2007033262

[For detailed information on the availability of NCRP publications see page 390.]

Preface

The National Council on Radiation Protection and Measurements (NCRP) and International Commission on Radiological Protection (ICRP) have both published reports on radiation dosimetry models for radioactive material entering the body by inhalation and ingestion (ICRP Publication 66, *Human Respiratory Tract Model for Radiological Protection*; ICRP Publication 67, *Age-Dependent Doses to Members of the Public from Intake of Radionuclides: Part 2. Ingestion Dose Coefficients*; NCRP Report No. 58, *A Handbook of Radioactivity Measurements Procedures*; and NCRP Report No. 125, *Deposition, Retention and Dosimetry of Inhaled Radioactive Substances*). Another potential route of entry into the body for radionuclides is through wounds. The incidence of radionuclide-contaminated wounds in individuals is relatively low, but >2,100 cases are reported in the scientific literature. The vast majority of the reported cases have occurred in facilities involved in the production, fabrication or maintenance of components for nuclear weapons, and the contaminants involved have been actinides (uranium, plutonium and americium). Contaminated wounds may also occur, albeit infrequently, in biological and radiopharmaceutical laboratories, as well as in certain areas of the nuclear power industry. More than 90 % of wounds have occurred in the arms and hands (primarily the fingers) and most of the wounds have involved punctures, with chemical burns accounting for the bulk of the others.

In the 1991 Persian Gulf War, another type of contaminated wound occurred in which military personnel were injured by radioactive depleted uranium fragments. The size of the fragments and nature and location of the wounds resulted in some fragments being surgically removed and some being left *in situ*. Neither the local dosimetry at the wound site nor the translocation of the radionuclide from the wound to internal organs has been systematically addressed by the formulation of biokinetic or local dosimetry models.

The uptake of radioactive material into the systemic circulation from a wound is variable, depending on the physical and chemical form of the radionuclide, depth of the wound and extent of injury, treatment administered, and time elapsed between injury and treatment. The highly variable nature of all these aspects of contaminated wounds makes a simple assessment of radiation dose to the exposed individual difficult to obtain and served as a major impetus in the development of the current Report.

As NCRP was in the early stages of forming a scientific committee to investigate the topic of radionuclide-contaminated wounds, ICRP was also about to establish a task group on the subject. In order to avoid redundancy of information or potential conflicts in recommendations between the two organizations, ICRP chose not to form a task group and instead requested that an ICRP member be utilized as a member of the NCRP scientific committee. ICRP also requested to be kept informed of report progress on a regular basis. Similarly, NCRP decided not to develop a revised model of the human alimentary tract, but to provide a representative to the ICRP task group developing that model. This cooperation has been advantageous to both organizations.

This Report was prepared by Scientific Committee 57-17 on Radionuclide Dosimetry Model for Wounds. Serving on Scientific Committee 57-17 were:

Bryce D. Breitenstein, Jr., *Chairman*
Long Beach, California

Members

Eric G. Daxon[*]
Battelle Memorial Institute
San Antonio, Texas

Raymond A. Guilmette
Los Alamos National
  Laboratory
Los Alamos, New Mexico

Patricia W. Durbin
Lawrence Berkeley National
  Laboratory
Berkeley, California

John J. Russell
Washington State University
Richland, Washington

Ronald E. Goans
MJW Corporation
Clinton, Tennessee

Richard E. Toohey
Oak Ridge Associated
  Universities
Oak Ridge, Tennessee

[*]Resigned from the Committee effective September 8, 1999.

Advisors

Fletcher F. Hahn
Lovelace Respiratory
 Research Institute
Albuquerque, New Mexico

Jean Piechowski
Centre d'Energie Atomique
Paris, France

Consultants

Robert W. Bistline
Abilene, Kansas

Thomas M. Koval
Rockville, Maryland

Richard A. Clark
State University of New York
Stony Brook, New York

Melissa A. McDiarmid
University of Maryland
Baltimore, Maryland

NCRP Secretariat
Bruce B. Boecker, *Staff Consultant* (2004–)
Thomas M. Koval, *Scientific Staff* (1997–2002)
Cindy L. O'Brien, *Managing Editor*
David A. Schauer, *Executive Director*

The Council wishes to express its appreciation to the Committee members for the time and effort devoted to the preparation of this Report. NCRP also gratefully acknowledges the financial support provided by the U.S. Department of Energy, U.S. Department of Homeland Security, U.S. Navy, and the Defense Threat Reduction Agency.

Thomas S. Tenforde
President

Contents

Executive Summary

The scientific literature contains case reports on >2,100 wounds contaminated with radionuclides. The vast majority of these reported wounds have occurred in the proximal and distal phalanges of workers in facilities that process plutonium. Since 1990 the use of depleted uranium (DU) in military munitions has resulted in combat wounds with DU shrapnel. In addition to contaminated wounds arising in industrial and military situations, medical use of radioactive material as a radiographic contrast agent [i.e., Thorotrast® (VanHeyden Company, Dresden-Radebeul, Germany), a colloidal suspension of thorium dioxide] has resulted in the development of granulomas (thorotrastomas) at injection sites, a type of foreign-body reaction complicated by the radiation delivered to the site.

By definition, a contaminated wound breaches the skin, which normally presents an effective barrier to the ingress of radioactive materials into the body. Skin is the largest organ of the human body, and its primary physiologic role is temperature regulation and maintaining homeostasis of body fluids and electrolytes. Human skin is a complex tissue, consisting of numerous distinct layers and types of cells. Immediately below the skin, the subcutis consists of loose connective tissue covering the muscle layer, with a variety of inorganic and organic chemicals and cells that affect the local retention and translocation of radionuclides introduced to it.

Although numerous biokinetic and dosimetric models for intakes of radionuclides by inhalation and ingestion have been published, a comparable consensus model for intake *via* contaminated wounds has not, even though the total amount of activity associated with a contaminated wound is typically much larger than that associated with worker exposures *via* inhalation or ingestion. Thus, in the mid-1990s the National Council on Radiation Protection and Measurements (NCRP) in collaboration with the International Commission on Radiological Protection (ICRP) established a scientific committee tasked with developing such a wound model.

Every contaminated wound presents the possibility of radionuclide uptake into the systemic circulation, with resulting doses to internal organs and tissues. Consequently, contaminated wounds

1

are almost always treated rapidly with excision of the wound site and administration of drugs to increase the excretion of radionuclides taken up into the systemic circulation, or to block their deposition in specific organs or tissues. Because of the paucity of data from humans who have had radionuclide-contaminated wounds but not had surgical or chemical decorporation, it was necessary to design and parameterize the wound biokinetic model using experimental animal data. For wound contamination with initially soluble radionuclides, data were found for 48 elements, which encompass all the groups of the periodic table except for the noble gases. The elements for which data were found and used in the wound model are shown in Figure ES.1. However, for colloids and particulate materials, much less information was available, mostly for uranium, plutonium, americium, and nuclear weapons test debris. Nevertheless, the data have been adequate to provide estimates of model parameters for relatively insoluble materials.

The NCRP wound model, shown in Figure ES.2, is a biokinetic model consisting of five compartments that comprise the wound site. Additionally, blood and lymph-node compartments receive radionuclides cleared from the wound site. The compartmental design was based on understanding of the physical and chemical properties of the deposited radioactive material, which can be soluble, a mixture of soluble and colloidal material, particulate or

Fig. ES.1. Periodic table of the elements; the 51 elements for which data were available from experimental animal studies are shaded.

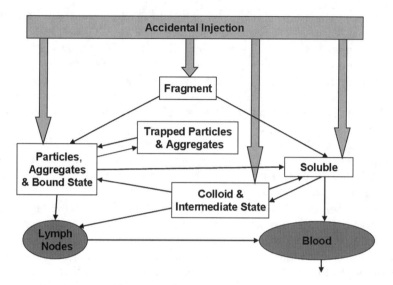

Fig. ES.2. NCRP wound model.

fragment. The intent was to provide a mechanistic basis for describing the biokinetics of radionuclides in wounds. Transfer of material between compartments is characterized using first-order rate constants, which empirically were found to be adequate for describing the data sets encountered to date.

Radionuclides introduced into the wound site as initially soluble materials enter the soluble compartment. Based on analysis of experimental data and aqueous chemistry considerations, two additional compartments were needed: (1) colloid and intermediate state (CIS) and (2) particles, aggregates and bound state (PABS). The initial partitioning of a radionuclide between the soluble and CIS compartments following injection is strongly influenced by aqueous solution chemistry, in particular, an element's tendency to hydrolyze at neutral pH. This affects its physicochemical state as well as its tendency as a charged molecule to bind locally to tissue molecules. For soluble materials, the principal clearance pathway from the wound site is *via* the blood. The amount of lymph-node clearance is dependent on the hydrolytic tendency of the material, which tends to produce more particulate characteristics.

Four default categories of soluble materials have been defined in the wound model: weak, moderate, strong and avid. Although these four categories were determined empirically based on wound retention times observed in the collected data from 70 experimental studies, the radioelements grouped roughly according to their tendencies for hydrolysis at the neutral pH of a wound site as well as the tendency to form stable complexes *in situ*. These tendencies increase with increasing oxidation state as $1^- < 1^+ < 2^+ < 3^+ < 4^+$. Thus, the weak category contains complex oxo- and chloro-anions, monovalent and divalent cations. The moderate category contains chemical analogs of members of the weak category but with unique chemical properties that confer longer wound-site retention. The strong category consists mainly of trivalent elements such as yttrium, lanthanum and gallium, trivalent lanthanides and actinides including small masses of plutonium, and the avid category consists of tetravalent zirconium, tin, thorium, plutonium, and pentavalent protactinium.

Fragments and particles are both solid materials, which may be essentially pure substances like plutonium or DU metal, or oxides, or solid materials contaminated with radionuclides. For the purposes of the wound model, the difference between particles and fragments is that the latter are too large to be phagocytized. Colloids are most commonly formed as hydrolysis products of radioactive metals, and also have particulate properties. These materials are introduced into the wound model by direct injection into the CIS, PABS, or fragment compartments for colloids, particles and fragments, respectively. In general, one of the principal differences in behavior between initially soluble and insoluble materials is that the latter materials, being particulate with low solubility rates, can have significant clearance from the wound to lymph nodes; soluble materials typically do not. Additionally, wounds can contain significant masses of materials, which may also elicit inflammatory reactions in the wound tissue. As such, biological sequestration and capsule formation may occur, which provides a biological barrier to clearance from the wound site. These phenomena led to the creation of the trapped particles and aggregates (TPA) compartment.

During the parameterization of the wound model for insoluble materials, it became evident that the CIS compartment was not needed for particles and fragments. This is because the transfer rates from PABS and fragment compartments are so small that there is virtually no likelihood of having high enough concentrations of radioactive material in the soluble compartment such that hydrolysis/polymerization reactions would be probable. Therefore, CIS is not used for particles and fragments, which simplifies the modeling.

One of the important applications of the NCRP wound model relates to the need to interpret bioassay data from U.S. soldiers who were wounded with DU fragments during the Persian Gulf War.

Because the human data from medical follow-up of the wounded soldiers were too sparse for modeling, reliance was again placed on the use of experimental animal data. Using indirect data to estimate wound-site retention in rats implanted with DU metal wafers, the DU was shown to be retained in the wound for very long times (~300 y). Notwithstanding this long retention, measurable amounts of DU are still predicted to be excreted, and urine bioassay could potentially be used for intake estimation (Appendix D).

An example of the application of the wound model to aid in the interpretation of bioassay data, particularly for supplementing data from *in situ* wound measurements of DU, has been provided in Appendix D. Here the wound model was coupled with the uranium systemic biokinetic model of ICRP Publication 69 (ICRP, 1995a) and used it to predict the urine excretion patterns for uranium (or DU) for the three most likely default categories: weak, particle and fragment. The urine patterns show that the greatest discrepancy in urine excretion rate occurs 1 d after exposure, in which the weak and particle fractions differ by more than three orders of magnitude, as do particle and fragment. Thus, knowing the physicochemical form of uranium or DU immediately after exposure will be very important in properly interpreting the urine excretion data. By ~100 d, the excretion rates tend to converge so that the differences become less important. Because the shapes of the urine excretion curves differ significantly, serial urine bioassays can be used to deduce which category of uranium in the wound is most reasonable. Similar predictions can be made for fecal excretion as well as uptake and retention in various systemic tissues and organs.

This Report provides guidance on appropriate bioassay measurements in cases of contaminated wounds and their interpretation. Equipment and methods for direct assessment of radioactive material in contaminated wounds are described, and tables of dose coefficients for skin (shallow) dose from surface contamination and local dose from embedded radioactive materials in a wound are provided. Dose coefficients and intake retention and excretion fractions have been derived for uranium by coupling the wound model with the ICRP systemic model for this element, and examples of their use are included. Development of these parameters for other radionuclides remain to be done; in the interim, tables of systemic dose from the complete uptake of various radioactive materials in a wound are also included by assuming that the radionuclide is intravenously (i.v.) injected in soluble form.

Finally, this Report provides detailed guidance on the medical management of contaminated wounds, using plutonium as an example. Treatment of life-threatening medical conditions always takes priority over radiological assessment and treatment. Once the patient is stabilized, decontamination should proceed in the order of open wounds, body orifices, and then intact skin. Wounds should be copiously irrigated, and any foreign material removed and saved for radioassay. Excision of contaminated tissue may be performed, depending on the risk to important structures such as tendons and nerves, and the wound closed. In the case of contamination with transuranic radionuclides, chelation therapy with calcium- or zinc-diethylene triamine pentaacetic acid (DTPA) should be initiated, along with collection of urine and fecal samples for bioassay. Because the effectiveness of DTPA therapy decreases with time since uptake, initiation of therapy need not wait for complete radiological characterization of the contaminating radionuclide.

Guidance on the medical management of contaminated wounds is available from the Radiation Emergency Assistance Center/ Training Site (REAC/TS), an emergency response asset of the U.S. Department of Energy (DOE) in Oak Ridge, Tennessee at any time by calling (865) 576-1005; basic information is available on the web at http://orise.orau.gov/reacts (ORISE, 2007). Another source of medical advice is the Medical Radiological Assistance Team at the Armed Forces Radiobiology Research Institute in Bethesda, Maryland [http://www.afrri.usuhs.mil (AFRRI, 2007)].

1. Introduction

1.1 Background

Radionuclide-contaminated wounds have potentially serious health consequences because a natural barrier to radionuclide penetration has been breached. As a result the contaminating radionuclide has direct access to blood and extracellular fluids, and ultimately, to internal tissues and organs. Radionuclide-contaminated wounds are unusual in the nuclear industry, but because of the processes involved, they have become more common in plutonium facilities (Ilyin, 2001). Contaminated wounds can occur in laboratories that handle concentrated pure radionuclide solutions, and wounds contaminated with mixed radionuclides can be expected to occur during decontamination and waste disposal activities. A new kind of contaminated wound emerged during the Persian Gulf conflict in which a population of soldiers was wounded with multiple small, sometimes inoperable fragments of low-specific-activity depleted uranium (DU) (OSAGWI, 2000). Occupational experience, particularly with plutonium, and the recent military experience with DU shrapnel showed that wound accidents can involve internal radionuclide contamination levels that are considerably greater than those resulting from accidents in which inhalation is the route of entry.

Several multicompartment models have been developed to describe the biokinetics of radionuclides in contaminated wounds (Falk *et al.*, 2006; Piechowski, 1995), but neither the local dosimetry at a wound site nor the translocation of a radionuclide from a wound to internal organs has been addressed from the point of view of formulating physiologically based biokinetic and local dosimetry models for contaminated wounds. The absence of generic, rather than incident-specific, models was the impetus for the current Report. It was recognized that the pattern of a given radionuclide entering the blood from a wound would vary widely among different wounds, making development of a generic wound model difficult, but it was also considered that a thorough examination of the data on radionuclide intake *via* wounds might demonstrate that the behavior of radionuclides deposited in wounds is no more variable than that of radionuclides entering the body *via* inhalation or ingestion.

7

Human data are rare for wounds contaminated with radionuclides other than the actinides (*e.g.*, Kelsey *et al.*, 1998). Even among the reported actinide contamination cases, wound kinetics cannot be characterized because many such reported accidents occurred before the development of radiation detection equipment optimized for a wound, and more importantly, most actinide-contaminated wounds are treated by excision and chelation therapy (Ilyin, 2001). Therefore, animal data must be used to predict the kinetics for wounds contaminated with the broad array of radionuclides that may be encountered in the laboratory, in industry, or with an explosive radiological dispersal device. Furthermore, only data from controlled animal experiments can adequately describe the influences of the chemical and physical properties (including mass) of a contaminant on its retention at a wound site.

Studies of the retention of radionuclides in simulated wounds in experimental animals have focused almost exclusively on deposited actinides (*e.g.*, Bistline *et al.*, 1972; Harrison *et al.*, 1978a; Johnson *et al.*, 1970a; 1970b; Stradling *et al.*, 1993). By far the largest and most varied body of experimental animal data concerned with radionuclide retention at a wound site is a byproduct of an extensive laboratory program that developed metabolic data in rats (tissue distribution and routes and rates of excretion) for a large number of previously unstudied or poorly understood elements (Durbin, 1960; 1962; Durbin *et al.*, 1957; Hamilton, 1947a; 1947b; 1948a; 1948b; 1949a; Scott *et al.*, 1947). Those studies provided much of the biological data first used to set radiation protection standards for internally-deposited radionuclides (ICRP, 1959; NBS, 1953).

In the development of a wound model for radionuclides, the prediction of the regional deposition and retention of radioactive materials at the wound site, the clearance of radioactive materials from the wound site, and the dosimetric and biological consequences of that regional deposition, retention and clearance are far from straightforward. Because there are no formally recognized wound models, it is the goal of NCRP to formulate a model that is metabolically sound and can be universally accepted.

The most common areas of the body to involve a wound contaminated with radioactive materials are the proximal and distal phalanges. This is reasonable since most wounds involve industrial or laboratory endeavors using either the hands or the proximal areas of the arms. A search of the health-physics literature and major U.S. and worldwide databases (Kathren, 1995; Ricks *et al.*, 2001) indicates that the most common radionuclides historically involved in wound cases in the United States have been [238,239]Pu, along with [241]Am and [235,238]U. The prevalence of these radionuclides in industrial wounds is of course related to nuclear weapons research and development, primarily in the major DOE research and production facilities.

A fundamental difficulty in developing a wound model is that medical considerations have generally (and properly) taken precedence over radiological considerations and usually the wound is initially decontaminated with various chemical agents, surgically debrided, or perturbed with internally-administered chelating agents (particularly in the case of the actinide elements). Therefore, it is relatively rare to be able to observe the undisturbed natural history and biokinetics of radioactive material encountered in the management of contaminated wounds.

1.2 Purpose and Scope

The present NCRP Report provides a summary of scientific data that describe the behavior of radionuclides injected intramuscularly (i.m.) or subcutaneously (s.c.) in animals. The Report uses these data to formulate a mathematical model to describe the deposition (i.e., initial activity present at the wound site), clearance (removal of activity from the wound site by biological processes), and dosimetry of radioactive substances present in wounds. The Report focuses on fundamental considerations of human anatomic structure and function in applying this model to wound deposition, retention, clearance and dosimetry for radioactive materials in humans. Although the mathematical treatment of deposition and retention presented herein is intended for radioactive contaminants, in many cases it may also be applicable to nonradioactive substances.

The result of this effort is an integrated mathematical model of deposition and clearance that is suitable for calculating radiation dose to skin, subcutis tissue, muscle, and other organs and tissues. The Report provides a framework for interpreting human exposures from wound counting and from bioassay results. It is intended to be used by scientists, physicians, and other personnel concerned with the effects of radioactive and chemically toxic substances and to estimate the absorbed dose to dermal and subdermal tissue. The mathematical model described in this Report is designed to predict the most likely mean values for the deposition and clearance parameters of various radionuclides in contaminated wounds. Variation in these patterns might be expected for individuals who may differ in size (i.e., percent adipose tissue) and in health status, and in responses to the medical treatment of the wound. Nevertheless, the mathematical model presented in this

Report is expected to be useful in interpreting health-physics data encountered in management of wounds. It should be noted that the development of systemic dose coefficients for intakes of radionuclides *via* contaminated wounds is beyond the scope of this Report.

An important characteristic of the wound model presented herein is information that is presented on particle deposition and clearance. This model, although simplified, allows a user to estimate initial particle deposition or dose at any time post-accident. Most of the experimental data in this Report were derived from studies with radioactive substances, but the wound model also applies to nonradioactive materials. However, dosimetry concerns for chemically toxic agents will pose different issues from those involving radioactive materials. The most frequently calculated radiation dose parameters are the energy deposition rate in tissue and the time-integrated total energy deposition. For wounds involving toxic chemicals, it may also be important to know peak exposure concentration, duration of exposure, cytotoxicity, and action of potential metabolic products.

This Report is divided into seven sections and six appendices. Section 1 presents a brief introduction to radionuclide-contaminated wounds and the scope of the Report. Section 2 describes the anatomy and physiology of human skin and s.c. tissues, with emphasis on the mechanisms that clear radionuclides from the wound site. Section 3 describes human experience with injected radioactive materials including industrial, military and iatrogenic cases. Section 4 describes the biokinetic model generated from the animal data. Section 5 describes exposure assessment and dosimetry and considers wound assessment, local dosimetry, and systemic dosimetry. Section 6 describes the medical management of patients who have been exposed to radioactive material *via* wounds. Section 7 presents a summary of the Report and its conclusions. The animal data on which the wound model is based are described in the first three Appendices. Appendix A describes experimental animal data in which soluble radionuclides have been administered, usually by s.c. or i.m. injection; Appendix B describes the animal data in which insoluble radionuclides were deposited in experimental wounds; and Appendix C describes the translocation of radionuclides from experimental wounds in animals. Appendix D presents some worked examples of the wound model's predictions for retention, clearance and dosimetry of uranium. Appendix E contains information on instrumentation and calibration for wound monitoring; and Appendix F contains a detailed discussion of the biological effects of wounds, including wound pathobiology, radiation effects, and foreign-body carcinogenesis.

2. Skin Biology

This Section provides a brief overview of the anatomy and physiology of intact human skin and describes the biological and chemical processes responsible for binding materials at a wound site or transporting them away from the site. Finally, the process of wound healing is also described.

2.1 Skin Anatomy

Skin anatomy and physiology have been described in NCRP Report No. 130, *Biological Effects and Exposure Limits for "Hot Particles"* (NCRP, 1999). The skin plays major roles in maintaining homeostasis of body fluids and electrolytes and in thermoregulation. It also provides a barrier against pathogens and senses the external environment. Figure 2.1 is a photomicrograph of human skin, showing its distinct layers of the epidermis, dermis and subcutis.

2.1.1 *The Epidermis*

The human epidermis has several well-defined layers. The outermost, the *stratum corneum*, or horny layer, consists mostly of dead cells, typically 15 to 20 layers thick. In the skin on the palms, fingertips, and soles of the feet, the *stratum lucidum*, a transparent layer of a few rows of dead cells lies beneath the stratum corneum. In the skin of the rest of the body, the *stratum granulosum* lies directly beneath the stratum corneum, and consists of four to five layers of cells in a transitional state from the viable cells beneath to the dead cells above. The cells in this layer contain dense granules in their cytoplasm. The bottommost layer consists of the *stratum spinosum*, post-mitotic cells with numerous desmosomes (*i.e.*, cell-to-cell contacts that bind the layer together). The stratum spinosum lies directly on a single layer of cells, the *stratum basale*, or basal layer, which consists of mitotic cells that give rise to the layers above. (The *stratum basale* is also known as the *stratum germinativum*.) The basal layer is separated from the dermis underneath by a basement membrane that is highly undulated, and forms ridges known as "rete pegs" extending into the epidermis (Marieb, 1992).

11

1. Epidermis

2. Papillary layer of the dermis

3. Reticular layer of the dermis

4. Subcutaneous layer

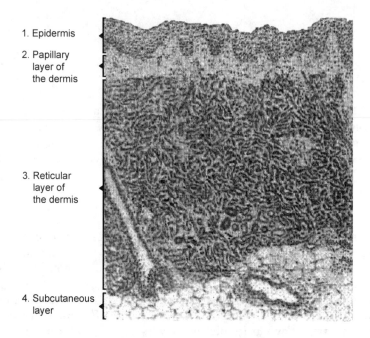

Fig. 2.1. Photomicrograph of human skin showing its organization into distinct layers. The epidermis (1) with the distinct undulations of the basal layer "rete pegs." The papillary dermis (2) with loosely arranged collagen fibers and a well-developed papillary vascular network, and the much thicker reticular dermis (3) with its thick structural collagen bundles. The bulbs of hair follicles impinge on the s.c. adipose layer (4) (NCRP, 1999).

2.1.2   The Dermis

The dermis has two layers, the papillary and the reticular. The papillary layer contains collagen fibers interwoven with elastin fibers. It is well-vascularized and is metabolically active, with the primary function of thermoregulation, and is well-supplied with sensory nerve endings. The reticular layer is the primary structural component of skin, consisting of collagen, elastin and reticular fibers.

2.1.3   The Subcutis

The subcutis (also called the hypodermis) is a variably thick layer of adipose and loose connective tissues that separates the skin from the underlying muscle mass. It contains the specialized structure of the skin appendages (*i.e.*, hair follicles and sebaceous glands, and in nonfurred animals, the sweat glands) (Ham, 1974). It is frequently the preferred site for injected materials, referred to as s.c. injection.

2.2 Binding and Transport of Injected Materials

2.2.1 *Loose Connective Tissue*

In striated muscle such as at an i.m.-injection site, a delicate network of loose connective tissue encloses the individual muscle fibers, and thicker layers surround the fiber bundles and muscle masses.

Loose connective tissue consists of an elastic meshwork of collagen and elastin fibers accompanied by a rich network of blood and lymph vessels, small scattered populations of macrophages, fibroblasts, mast cells, and variable numbers of fat cells; all contained in and supported by an amorphous semi-fluid gel. The solids of the gel phase are mainly the hydrated high-molecular-weight mucopolysaccharides, hyaluronic and chondroitin sulfuric acids. Both the structural proteins and the mucopolysaccharides of the loose connective tissue gel phase contain potential metal-binding sites, such as the carboxyl groups of mucopolysaccharides, and the carboxyl (aspartic and glutamic acid), hydroxyl (tyrosine), and sulfhydryl (cysteine) side chains of proteins (Dounce and Lan, 1949; Gurd and Wilcox, 1956; Ham, 1974; Luckey and Venugopal, 1977; Passow *et al.*, 1961; Pecoraro *et al.*, 1981; Rothstein and Clarkson, 1959; Taylor, 1973a; 1973b).

The deposition of foreign ions, including excess H^+, in tissue can induce a local inflammatory reaction, in which chemical mediators cause dilation of arterioles and venules and temporarily increase local blood flow and exudation of plasma between the endothelial cells and dilated venules. Inflammation is accompanied by the appearance in the affected tissue volume of substantial numbers of polymorphonuclear leukocytes and mononuclear leukocytes (monocytes) that have migrated through the walls of the venules. After entering the tissue, monocytes differentiate into macrophages, and these cells engulf debris left in the affected area including radionuclide-contaminated tissue constituents (Ham, 1974).

2.2.2 *Tissue Fluids and Their Contents*

2.2.2.1 *Extracellular Water.* The water of the gel phase (the tissue fluid) contains electrolytes and small molecules at about the same concentrations as plasma. Also present are low concentrations of leaked smaller plasma proteins, mainly albumin, but also the iron-transport protein, transferrin, a small glycoprotein that migrates electrophoretically with the β-globulins (Katz, 1970). Filterable solutes and water diffuse through the gel between the cells and capillaries. The nonfilterable proteins are returned to the blood by way of the lymph capillaries. The plasma membranes of cells are highly selective barriers to the influx of small molecules, ions and water (Ham, 1974; Passow et al., 1961). Thus, nuclides injected in soluble form in aqueous solution will be found initially only in the tissue fluid at the injection site. The structure of the connective tissue gel phase inhibits the movement of particles >0.2 μm in diameter, impeding transport of injected colloids or larger hydroxide aggregates formed at the injection site.

Total extracellular water [ECW (plasma plus tissue fluid)] of striated muscle is reported to be 0.14 to 0.17 mL g^{-1} of wet weight in male rats (Barratt and Walser, 1969) and 0.23 mL g^{-1} in female mice (Durbin et al., 1992). A value of 0.18 mL g^{-1} can be calculated for adult human muscle (ICRP, 1975). The total ECW of loose connective tissue is not well characterized. Reported values of ECW for the whole pelt of rats and mice are 0.22 and 0.48 mL g^{-1}, respectively (Durbin et al., 1992; Pierson et al., 1978). A value of 0.15 mL g^{-1} can be calculated for adult human skin (ICRP, 1975). Plasma accounts for ~10 % of the ECW of muscle, human skin, and rodent pelt (Durbin et al., 1992; Everett et al., 1956; ICRP, 1975), and the tissue fluid volumes of those tissues are, by difference, ~90 % of the respective total ECW values. Reasonable values for the tissue fluid volumes of muscle, human skin, and rodent pelt are 0.17, 0.14, and 0.32 mL g^{-1}, respectively.

2.2.2.2 *Inorganic Electrolytes.* The most abundant inorganic complexing species in tissue fluid is HCO_3^- (0.027 mol L^{-1}) (Gamble, 1954). Many multivalent cations form sparingly soluble carbonates, but only a few, most importantly the dioxo cations UO_2^{2+}, NpO_2^{2+}, and PuO_2^{2+}, form stable soluble bis- and tris-carbonate complexes at physiological pH. For those hexavalent actinides, complexation with tissue fluid bicarbonate is an important mechanism contributing to their clearance from a wound site. The concentrations of $H_2PO_4^-$ and SO_4^{2-} in tissue fluid are low (<0.001 mol L^{-1}), and because their 1:1 complexes with most multivalent cations are weak, those anions probably contribute little to clearance of metal ions from a wound.

2.2.2.3 *Organic Acids.* Tissue fluid contains low concentrations of several organic acids, among which citrate ion (~10^{-4} mol L^{-1}) is the most prominent (Altman and Katz, 1961; Neuman and Neuman, 1958). Citric acid is a multidentate alpha-hydroxy tricarboxylic acid with great affinities for "hard" metal ions (e.g., tungsten, cobalt and nickel) and its structure is ideal for metal coordination, because stable five-member rings can be formed. The stability constants (log-K) of 1:1 metal-citrate complexes with ions of Groups III (3, 13) and IV (4, 14) are correlated with their charge/radius ratios (e/r), and range from 5.6 for Cr^{3+} (e/r = 31 e nm^{-1}) to 15 for Pu^{4+} (e/r = 41.7 e nm^{-1}) (Martell and Smith, 1982; Smith and Martell, 1977; 1989). The stabilities of the M^{3+} and M^{4+} citrate complexes are all several orders of magnitude greater than that of calcium-citrate (log-K = 3.2), and multivalent cations are expected to compete successfully with Ca^{2+} for citrate ion in vivo. Plasma and tissue fluid contain other alpha-hydroxy acids (isocitric, malic, oxaloacetic) at much lower concentrations than citrate, and those acids may also form soluble complexes with and participate to a lesser degree in transport of multivalent cations in vivo.

A number of "hard" multivalent cationic nuclides have been introduced into mammalian plasma in vivo and in vitro. Those cations associate predominantly with plasma proteins (see below), but in all cases investigated a small, filterable low molecular weight fraction has been identified. For examples see Bruenger et al. (1971), Duffield and Taylor (1986), Durbin (1973), Popplewell and Boocock (1967), and Taylor (1973a; 1973b). The small fractions of Am^{3+}, Cm^{3+}, and Pu^{4+}, for example, are filtered by the kidneys into urine and have been identified as citrate complexes (Popplewell et al., 1975; Stradling et al., 1976). It is reasonable to consider that small amounts of other multivalent cations circulate and are excreted in urine as citrate complexes.

Locally injected citrate ion is capable of complexing Pu^{4+}, if it is administered immediately after the plutonium is deposited in an i.m. wound (Volf, 1975).

2.2.2.4 *Transferrin.* Apotransferrin (iron-free transferrin) binds a wide variety of di-, tri-, and tetravalent metal ions under idealized laboratory conditions (reviewed by Pecoraro et al., 1981). Association of several tri- and tetravalent cations with the transferrin of mammalian plasma has also been demonstrated in vivo in studies of plasma from nuclide-injected animals and in vitro by addition of nuclides to plasma from animals with normal levels of transferrin iron saturation (Beamish and Brown, 1974; Bruenger et al., 1971; Duffield and Taylor, 1986; Durbin, 1973; 2006; Popplewell and Boocok, 1967; Stevens et al., 1968; Stover et al., 1968; Taylor,

1973a; 1973b; 1998; Turner and Taylor, 1968). Transferrin was identified as the main carrier of Am^{3+} and Cf^{3+} in the plasma of animals, although those complexes are weak and do not survive separation procedures (Bruenger et al., 1971; Popplewell and Boocock, 1967; Turner and Taylor, 1968).

Each transferrin molecule possesses two similar, globular sialoprotein binding sites that are highly selective for encapsulating Fe^{3+} ($e/r = 46.5$ e nm^{-1}) in preference to other biologically essential metal ions. Iron binding at both sites involves deprotonation of two tyrosine moieties. Thus, in order for a foreign multivalent cation to occupy either binding site, its ionic radius must be small enough to fit into the iron-binding cavity, and it must also have sufficient charge density (as measured by e/r) to deprotonate the pairs of tyrosine phenols required for stable binding to the phenolic oxygens (Harris et al., 1981; Luk, 1971; Pecoraro et al., 1981).

Metal coordination with apotransferrin was investigated by spectrophotometric titration of the transferrin complexes with several metal ions with a broad range of electric charge and ionic radii. Two tyrosines were coordinated at each binding site by all of the transition metals investigated and the smaller lanthanides (each transferrin molecule bound two metal ions and released four tyrosine protons) (Figure 2.2). The larger metal ions were able to fit only into one of the iron-binding sites, and the number of coordinated tyrosines per transferrin molecule decreased from four to two, demonstrating the nonequivalence of the binding sites. Because of the size differences in the two sites, the larger Th^{4+} ion is bound stably at only one site and weakly at the other, while the smaller Zr^{4+} and Pu^{4+} ions are expected to be stably bound at both sites. Europium-3+ appears to be an indicator of the maximum size (0.095 nm) of a multivalent cation that can bind stably at both of the transferrin binding sites, and the larger La^{3+}, Am^{3+}, and Cm^{3+} ions are expected to bind stably at only one site.

Not all of the multivalent cations that have been shown to be tenaciously retained in a wound have been investigated for complexation with transferrin. However, there is sufficient evidence for the existence and stabilities in vivo of the transferrin complexes formed with many of their chemical analogues to be able to predict that transferrin is a good ligand for "hard" metal ions in general, and that the stabilities of those complexes will depend on e/r of the specific nuclide. Thus, transferrin can be considered to play an important role in the in vivo transport of all "hard" metal ions in tissue fluid and lymph as well as in plasma.

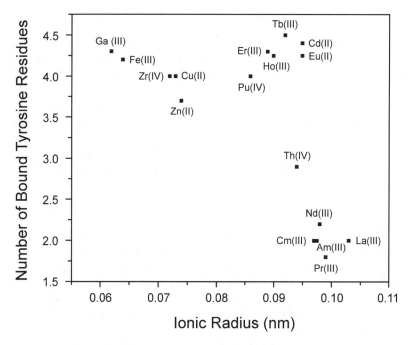

Fig. 2.2. Number of tyrosine moieties engaged in binding metal ions as related to metal ionic radii (VI coordination assumed) (Harris *et al.*, 1981; Pecoraro *et al.*, 1981). Not measured and shown are Zr(IV) and Pu(IV), which are small enough to fit into both iron-binding sites and displace four tyrosine protons, and La(III), Am(III), and Cm(III), which are too large to occupy the smaller binding site and probably displace only two tyrosine protons per transferrin molecule.

2.2.3 *Connective Tissue Macrophages*

When a particle makes a contact with the surface of a phagocytic cell, the cell membrane invaginates around it at the point of contact, engulfing and internalizing it in a vesicle (phagolysosome). Macrophages recognize and engulf solid particles with a size range from ~0.01 to 20 μm in diameter (Snipes, 1989). Larger particles of PuO_2, for example, are phagocytized by peritoneal and lung macrophages more efficiently and rapidly than smaller particles 0.08 to 0.75 μm in diameter (Sanders, 1967). One to 2 y after i.m. injection in rats, the small ThO_2 particles of Thorotrast® (0.005 to 0.01 μm diameter) were almost entirely contained within macrophages in the connective tissue between the muscle bundles, and readily detectable amounts had been transported to the local draining lymph nodes (Hahn *et al.*, 2002).[1] Very small particles of PuO_2 (~0.001 μm in diameter) i.m. injected in rats were rapidly translocated from the wound site, uptake in local lymph nodes was minor, and an important fraction was excreted into the urine. Those particles may have been too small to stimulate phagocytosis (Harrison *et al.*, 1978a).

Once inside the phagocyte, the initial phagolysosome fuses with one or more lysosomes to form a larger phagolysosome (Sbarra *et al.*, 1976). The lysosomes are rich in acid hydrolases, and the inner surface of the lysosome membrane secretes H^+, such that the pH inside the lysosome is 4.5 to 5.5, depending on species (Ganz and Lehrer, 1995). The phagolysosomes also maintain useful concentrations of the oxidants, peroxide, superoxide anions, and hydroxyl radicals (Hatch *et al.*, 1980; Kobzik *et al.*, 1990). This acidic, highly oxidative environment favors dissolution of many, but not all, metals and metal compounds (Helfinstine *et al.*, 1992; Kreyling and Scheuch, 2000). Within the lysosomes, organic matter is digested, and some inorganic materials are dissolved at the ambient pH. Indigestible residues such as polymerized metal hydroxides and oxides and minute metal and plastic fragments, remain within the phagocytes in secondary lysosomes (residual bodies); some phagocytes eventually contain many residual bodies. Phagocytes continue to ingest particles until toxic amounts of breakdown products accumulate in their cytoplasm, killing the cells. Residual bodies may also be extruded. In either case, the load of indigestible particles will be rephagocytized by a new population of macrophages, and the process will be repeated (Ham, 1974; Tessmer and Chang, 1967).

The association of insoluble metal hydroxide and oxide particles with macrophages is a possible mechanism for the very slow release of some high-specific-activity alpha-emitting nuclides from a wound in soluble form. Radiological "dissolution," that is, particle fragmentation with the breaking of chemical bonds by the recoiling daughter atoms of the alpha decays, may produce particles small enough to be dissolved at the reduced pH of the lysosomes (Fleischer and Raabe, 1977; NCRP, 2001a).

2.2.4 *Particle Transport by Macrophages*

It is not clear whether a particle as large as 20 μm can be transported by the macrophage that has engulfed it. Observations of

---

[1]Hahn, F.F. (2003). Personal communication (Lovelace Respiratory Research Institute, Albuquerque, New Mexico).

animals that chronically inhaled significant masses of aerosol particles showed that the clearance mechanisms acting in the parenchymal region of the lung could be overwhelmed by overloading the resident alveolar macrophage population (Lehnert and Morrow, 1985). Morrow (1988) hypothesized that the phenomenon of dust overloading was caused and perpetuated by the loss of mobility of the alveolar macrophages that had phagocytized many particles. In particular, he postulated that mobility ceases when ~60 % of the macrophage volume is occupied by phagocytized particles (Morrow, 1988). This has been supported at least in part by experimental data in rats instilled with 10 μm (Oberdorster, 1993) or 15 μm particles (Snipes and Clem, 1981), in which there was virtually no clearance of particles from the lung. Additionally, Mueller *et al.* (1990) showed that the migration *in vitro* of rat and dog alveolar macrophages decreased with increasing numbers of ingested particles, and ceased at high particle loadings. It is not known whether this mechanism also applies to interstitial macrophages, but it is logical to assume that it does, since the mechanism is probably linked both to energy consumption by the macrophage, which would not be specific to the different macrophage types, and to the inability of macrophages loaded with solid particles to move through tight spaces. It should be noted that loss of macrophage mobility due to particle ingestion does not imply concomitant loss of the ability of the cell to maintain acidic pH (~5) within its phagolysosomes. Particle dissolution *in vivo* driven by pH may still occur despite the inability of the macrophages to transport phagocytized particles to the lymphatics that drain the wound site.

2.3 Wound Healing

According to strict medical usage the animal experiments that involved i.m. or s.c. injection or deposition of radioactive materials are not wounds, because skin trauma was minimal. However, as used in radiation protection, any event in which radioactive material breaches the skin barrier is considered a "contaminated wound." For the purposes of this Report, "wound" is used in the broadest sense as an injury to the body in which the skin or other tissue is broken, cut, pierced, torn, scraped, burned, etc. Healing of mechanical breaches of the skin occurs in three stages: inflammation, reepithelialization, and formation of granulation tissue. A detailed description of wound healing and pathobiology is provided in Appendix F.

2.3.1 *Inflammation*

The initial injury causes blood vessel disruption with consequent bleeding, platelet aggregation and coagulation, which lead to formation of clots that plug the severed vessels, fill the discontinuities in the wounded tissue, and provide a provisional matrix for cell migration. Inflammatory polymorphonuclear leukocytes (neutrophils) are recruited to the wound, where they cleanse the area of foreign matter (if small enough), including bacteria. If indigestible foreign material is present, neutrophil recruitment continues, causing further tissue damage in the attempt to sterilize the environment. The monocytes and macrophages recruited to the site remove foreign particles and emit chemoattractant molecules that recruit fibroblasts to the site.

2.3.2 *Reepithelialization*

Within hours after an injury, epithelial cells from the skin of the intact margins of the wound move quickly to cover the clot and the damaged connective tissue and proliferate to repave the surface with viable new epithelium. This epidermal migration ultimately results in sloughing of an eschar (scab). This process continues for 2 to 3 d.

2.3.3 *Formation of Granulation Tissue*

New granulation tissue begins to invade the wound site ~4 d after the injury. During that time new collagen is laid down and new capillaries permeate the growing granulation tissue mass. By the second to third week of healing, the wound contracts by collagen remodeling and a scar is completed (Singer and Clark, 1999).

2.3.4 *Burns*

Healing of burns differs somewhat from that of mechanical injuries, and it depends on the degree of damage (first-, second- or third-degree burn). The most important characteristic of a burn is the depth of damage. This affects the amount of necrosis, capillary destruction (the microcirculation is key to burn recovery), edema, and inflammation, and how much tissue must be repaired. Once the acute phase of burn pathology has occurred, healing proceeds similarly to that of mechanical wounds. Reepithelialization begins at the intact margins of the burned area or from deeply positioned epithelial appendages such as those associated with sweat ducts, hair follicles, or sebaceous glands. If the burn is deep, those processes proceed slowly.

2.3.5 Foreign-Body Reactions

Foreign-body reactions can occur in both shallow (skin) and deep s.c. (or muscle) wounds when the contaminant is an indigestible colloid, particle suspension, or fragment. The reaction results from a chronic inflammatory response, creating either a granuloma or fibrotic capsule. In both cases, the local tissue attempts to surround the foreign material and isolate it from normal tissue; the result can be a completely encapsulated deposit. Such granulomas or capsules can last for years depending on the persistence *in vivo* of the deposited material. Both radioactive and nonradioactive materials that persist at a wound site can also cause progressively enlarging cysts and benign and malignant tumors at the site in experimental animals and humans (Brues *et al.*, 1965; 1966; 1968; Dahlgren, 1967a; da Horta, 1967b; Guilmette *et al.*, 1989; Hahn *et al.*, 2002; Lang *et al.*, 1993; Liebermann *et al.*, 1995; Lushbaugh and Langham, 1962; Lushbaugh *et al.*, 1967; van Kaick *et al.*, 1978).

3. Etiology of Radionuclide-Contaminated Wounds

Intact skin presents an effective barrier to noxious agents, and with few exceptions, only small fractions of contaminating radionuclides are absorbed through it. However, when the integrity of the skin is breached, the absorption of contaminating radionuclides can increase by two or three orders of magnitude. For example, Ilyin et al. (1975) showed that the transdermal absorption of ^{85}Sr in human volunteers increased by a factor of >200, if the skin were scratched before applying the solution, whereas the increase was a factor of ~15 in similar work with rats (Ilyin and Ivannikov, 1979). This difference indicates the need for the usual caution in direct application of animal data to humans.

Similarly, Ilyin et al. (1977) showed that the systemic absorption of ^{210}Po in rats was 40 times greater through abraded skin compared with intact skin, and 750 times greater when the ^{210}Po was introduced into cutaneous and muscular wounds. Consequently, any contaminated wound is potentially serious from the point of view of radionuclide uptake and internal dose. It should be noted, however, that the transdermal absorption of radionuclides is increased only slightly through burned skin, whether the result of chemical or thermal injury (Sections 4.3 and A.4; Ilyin, 2001).

3.1 Industrial Experience

In a review of contaminated skin wounds and burns, Ilyin (2001) noted that at least some data have been reported on >2,100 cases of cutaneous injury complicated by contamination with radioactive materials. Schofield (1964) reported 1,250 cases of radionuclide-contaminated injuries at Windscale; Hammond and Putzier (1964) described 900 cases of hand injury in plutonium workers, of which 300 included contamination; Jech et al. (1969) reported 230 wounds at the Hanford site, of which 136 were contaminated with plutonium; Ohlenschlager (1970) reported 148 cases of wounds contaminated with alpha emitters at Karlsruhe; Johnson and Lawrence (1974) described 137 contaminated injuries at Los Alamos; and Bazhin et al. (1994) described 286 skin injuries contaminated with alpha emitters at the Mayak Association in Russia. Numerous other reports have described single contaminated wound cases, and one case report filled an entire issue of *Health Physics* (Thompson, 1983).

Review of these cases produces the following conclusions (Ilyin, 2001):

- The vast majority of contaminated wounds have occurred in facilities involved in the production, fabrication or maintenance of components for nuclear weapons, and the contaminants involved have been actinides (uranium, plutonium and americium).
- More than 90 % of wounds have occurred in the hands and arms, primarily the fingers.
- Almost 90 % of wounds have involved mechanical damage, mostly punctures; chemical burns from acid solutions account for almost all the others, with relatively few thermal burns reported.

These conclusions indicate that to be most useful, a wound model should focus on puncture wounds contaminated with actinides, and such is the thrust of this Report. The model and procedures described will be generally applicable, however.

Because of the high radiotoxicity of the transuranics in particular, the vast majority of workers who have experienced wounds contaminated with these radionuclides have undergone prompt medical intervention to minimize systemic uptake of the radionuclide. These interventions include surface decontamination such as scrubbing with various agents, surgical debridement or excision of the wound site, and therapy with appropriate chelating or blocking agents to increase the excretion rate of absorbed radionuclides and consequently reduce the radiation dose delivered to internal organs and tissues. The uptake of activity into the systemic circulation from a wound site is highly variable, depending on the physical and chemical form of the radionuclide, the depth of the wound and extent of tissue injury, the treatment given, and the time elapsed between injury and treatment. For example, the effectiveness of wound excision varies with the depth of the wound and the time elapsed since the injury, but for most wounds, excision (often repeated) can remove >90 % of the initial activity from the wound site (Ilyin, 2001). In almost all cases of wounds contaminated with transuranics, the chelating agent zinc- or calcium-diethylene triamine pentaacetate acid (DTPA) is administered; it is effective for enhancing the excretion of soluble forms (*e.g.*, nitrates) of these radionuclides from the body, but is essentially ineffective in removing less-soluble forms such as oxides (Ilyin, 2001).

Because of these interventions, which may drastically alter the local and systemic biokinetics of radionuclides in a wound, there are few human case reports in the literature that can be used to develop a biokinetic model for contaminated wounds. Consequently, modeling must rely primarily on animal data.

3.2 Military Experience with Depleted Uranium

3.2.1 *Introduction*

Depleted uranium (DU, ~99.8 % ^{238}U by mass) is used by the United States and other nations in kinetic energy munitions that are designed to defeat armored vehicles. A kinetic energy munition, or round, uses a high-density rod, or penetrator, fired at high velocity to penetrate armor plate. Figure 3.1 is a cutaway view of a DU armor-piercing, fin stabilized, discarding sabot tank round, and Figure 3.2 is a picture of a DU kinetic energy penetrator in flight (OSAGWI, 2000). The body of the penetrator is solid DU (with some alloyed constituents), while its tip is made of plastic and is designed to increase the stability of the penetrator in flight. The pieces falling away are the sabot that stabilizes the DU penetrator in the gun barrel. Tungsten and tungsten alloys are also used as kinetic energy penetrators, but they are not as effective as DU because they tend to "mushroom" and become blunt as they penetrate the target's armor. In contrast, DU penetrators undergo adiabatic shear and actually self-sharpen as they penetrate. DU penetrators are also used in smaller caliber munitions fired from aircraft and armored personnel carriers.

When the DU penetrator strikes a target, small particles of DU break off and extremely high temperatures are generated which cause the small particles to ignite. Once the penetrator enters the vehicle it generates shards of DU and spall (fragments of the target's armor) that incapacitate the crew and vehicle. The DU dust generated by this process settles in and on the vehicle and also on the crew inside the vehicle. Soldiers riding on an armored vehicle when it is struck by a DU round, may also receive DU shrapnel wounds, and be exposed to DU dust.

3.2.2 *Persian Gulf War Experience*

The Persian Gulf War was the first time DU munitions were used in combat. During the land war, 21 U.S. vehicles (six Abrams

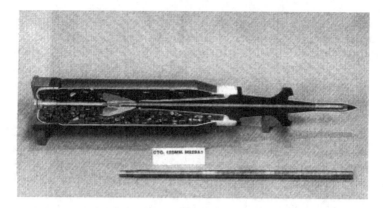

Fig. 3.1. Cutaway view of DU sabot round (OSAGWI, 2000).

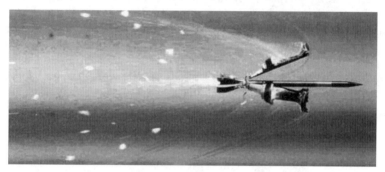

Fig. 3.2. DU penetrator in flight, discarding its sabot (OSAGWI, 2000).

tanks and 15 Bradley fighting vehicles) were struck by DU during friendly-fire incidents (*i.e.*, munitions fired by other U.S. forces). During these incidents there were 11 fatalities, and ~50 personnel were wounded severely enough to require medical attention (OSAGWI, 2000). Wounds suffered included burns, lacerations, broken bones, internal injuries, and retained fragments, some of which were DU. In addition to embedded fragments and wound contamination, personnel in or on these vehicles also had the potential for inhaling the DU particulates and aerosols generated during the penetration. Personnel entering a vehicle after it was struck by a DU penetrator could also have inhaled DU particulates.

Standard surgical criteria were used to determine whether embedded fragments should be removed, including the possibility of surgical damage to adjacent structures. In some instances, fragment removal was contraindicated because of their small size and the large number of fragments present or because of the patient's condition. Figure 3.3 is a radiograph of the calf of a veteran wounded in the Gulf War. In addition to severe lacerations, the patient suffered broken bones and other injuries. Direct radiation measurements over the wound sites and urinalysis confirmed that at least some of the fragments were DU.

Examination of the radiographs of two soldiers showed that each had multiple (from 10 to 30 fragments) imbedded fragments that ranged in size from 1 to >20 mm in diameter. Uranium bioassays taken over a year after the two soldiers were wounded showed that their urinary concentrations of uranium were 15 and 17 $\mu g\ L^{-1}$, respectively (Daxon, 1994). These levels are at least a factor of 100 below acute toxicity levels for the kidney but are at least a factor of 100 above natural excretion rates (0.04 to 0.4 $\mu g\ L^{-1}$) (ICRP, 1975). The slow uptake of uranium from embedded fragments is similar to a low-level chronic intake situation, in which the kidney burden slowly increases to an equilibrium level. For a potentially nephrotoxic kidney burden of 3 $\mu g\ U\ g^{-1}$ kidney, the Wrenn-Lipsztein-Bertelli model (Wrenn *et al.*, 1985; 1989) predicts a corresponding urine level of ~1,000 mg L^{-1}, still well above observed excretion rates in these individuals.

In 1992, the Office of the Army Surgeon General asked the Armed Forces Radiobiology Research Institute (AFRRI) to review

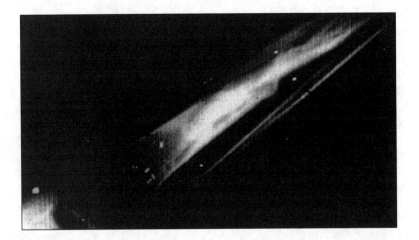

Fig. 3.3. Radiograph of the calf of a Gulf War veteran wounded by DU shrapnel (AEPI, 1995). The small opacities in soft tissue are DU fragments.

the potential health effects of these retained fragments. The AFRRI review did not recommend a change in fragment removal procedures but did recommend long-term follow-up and additional research. The U.S. Department of Veterans Affairs agreed to conduct the follow-up studies of personnel who were in friendly-fire incidents at the Baltimore Veterans Affairs Medical Center (VAMC). Animal research was initiated at AFRRI and also at the Lovelace Inhalation Toxicology Research Institute (now Lovelace Respiratory Research Institute) (Hahn *et al.*, 2002).

3.2.3 Summary of the U.S. Department of Veterans Affairs Follow-Up Program

In 1993, the U.S. government initiated the follow-up study of 33 Gulf War veterans who had been exposed to DU, many of whom contained embedded fragments of DU shrapnel in their bodies. The veterans underwent medical evaluation at the Baltimore VAMC, and were reexamined in 1997. Whole-body counts were performed at the Boston VAMC in an effort to quantify DU content in the body, and urine samples were analyzed for uranium. Histories were taken along with physical examinations, clinical laboratory tests, and psychiatric and neurocognitive assessments (McDiarmid *et al.*, 2000).

3.2.3.1 *Medical Surveillance and Results.* Medical examinations were performed on 29 DU-exposed veterans and 38 who had not been exposed. No clinically significant findings were noted in the exposed population, but subtle perturbations in the reproductive and nervous systems of those exposed veterans with retained embedded metal fragments were observed. Nearly 90 % of the DU-exposed and 71 % of the nonexposed veterans reported one or more active medical problems; for the exposed group, 76 % reported problems resulting from their combat injuries, while for the nonexposed group, nervous system problems were most frequently reported (52 %). No significant differences in hematologic parameters were noted between the two groups, although the high uranium group (those with urinary uranium concentrations >0.10 µg g^{-1} creatinine) showed a nonsignificant trend toward higher eosinophil counts. There were no differences between the high and low DU-exposed groups in any renal function parameters, which are of interest, as uranium is known to be nephrotoxic at high levels of intake. There was a statistical relationship between urine uranium levels and lowered performance on computerized tests of neurocognitive performance. Elevated urinary uranium excretion was statistically related to high prolactin levels, but no difference in semen parameters was noted between the high and low exposure groups. There was no difference in chromosome aberration frequency between the high and low exposure groups; sister chromatid exchanges were slightly higher in the low uranium exposure group, but not significantly (McDiarmid et al., 2000).

3.2.3.2 *Summary of Urine Bioassay and Whole-Body Counting Results.* Urinalysis for excreted uranium was performed on both 24 h urine samples and also on spot samples, using kinetic phosphorescence analysis with a detection limit of 60 ng L⁻¹. Urinary uranium results were expressed as microgram per gram creatinine, in accord with medical practice. These results can be converted to daily excretion rates by multiplying them by a factor of 1.7, as the mean value for daily creatinine excretion in males is 1.7 g (ICRP 1975), and then to microgram per liter by dividing by a factor of 1.4, as the daily urinary output of males is 1.4 L (ICRP, 1975) [more recent guidance from ICRP (2002b) gives the daily urinary output of males as 1.6 L].

In nonexposed veterans, the results ranged from 0.01 to 0.05 μg g⁻¹ creatinine, while in exposed veterans, levels ranged from 0.01 to 30.74 μg g⁻¹ creatinine; there was a high correlation between the results for 24 h samples and spot samples, and between results obtained in 1994 and in 1997. All values above 1 μg g⁻¹ creatinine occurred in nine veterans who had embedded shrapnel fragments. Six other veterans with embedded shrapnel fragments had urine concentrations below this level (Hooper et al., 1999; McDiarmid et al., 1999; 2000; 2001).

Whole-body counts for uranium were performed at the Boston VAMC in a flat-bed scanning geometry with two 10 × 10 × 45 cm thallium-activated sodium-iodide [NaI(Tl)] detectors, positioned one above and one below the bed. Counts were taken for 10 min as the detectors moved along the length of the body, resulting in seven distinct measurements. Calibration factors were obtained from measurements of a tissue equivalent phantom containing known amounts of DU pellets at various tissue depths and locations. A "uranium index" was calculated by averaging over the seven scan segments. The limit of detection for these measurements was ~70 mg DU.[2] Only nine veterans had body contents exceeding the detection limit, and all had been exposed to DU and exhibited elevated urinary DU excretion. Internal dose calculations based on

---

[2]McPhaul, K. (1998). Personal communication (University of Maryland School of Medicine, Baltimore, Maryland).

ICRP Publication 30 methodology (ICRP, 1979) resulted in values of committed effective dose equivalent incurred from DU absorbed systemically in a year that were <1 mSv for all but one case, whose committed effective dose equivalent was calculated to be just above that value at 1.1 mSv (McDiarmid *et al.*, 2000).

3.2.3.3 *Excretion of Uranium from Embedded Depleted Uranium Fragments.* Data were available from seven individuals who exceeded the detection limit for whole-body counting and also had elevated urinary uranium (Toohey, 2003a). Urinary excretion, in microgram DU per gram creatinine, was determined in 1997 and 1999. The body contents, in mg DU, were determined in 1997; it was assumed there were no significant decreases in total body content of DU in the interim. For the 1997 data, the mean excretion was (24 ± 28) µg DU g^{-1} creatinine, and for the 1999 data, the mean excretion was (11 ± 6) µg DU g^{-1} creatinine. However, there was no correlation of excretion with body content, as shown in the scatter diagram in Figure 3.4. For all 12 data points, the correlation coefficient was +0.20, but if the highest point is eliminated, the correlation coefficient drops to +0.03. For the 1997 data alone, the correlation coefficient is +0.13, and for the 1999 data alone, it is −0.06. Because the absorption and subsequent excretion of DU from embedded shrapnel is a function of particle surface area as well as particle composition and solubility, whereas the whole-body counting data measures total particle mass, a correlation between the two measurements should not be expected. However, it does appear that the excretion is decreasing with time, which may reflect encapsulation of embedded fragments and their increasing isolation from the systemic circulation. This decrease in excretion has been generally observed in the entire cohort (McDiarmid *et al.*, 2000; 2001; Squibb *et al.*, 2005).

3.2.4 *Embedded Radioactive Particles and Fragments*

Although information regarding the biological effects of embedded radioactive particles is scarce, several studies describe the effects of deposited plutonium compounds (Langham *et al.*, 1962). Lushbaugh *et al.* (1967) summarized the findings in eight radiation workers with plutonium-contaminated wounds and Carbaugh *et al.* (1989) and Lagerquist *et al.* (1972) reported on accidents involving americium- and plutonium-contaminated puncture wounds. The usefulness of these studies with respect to defining the long-term retention and effects of embedded radioactive particles and metal fragments is limited, however, because in these individuals the

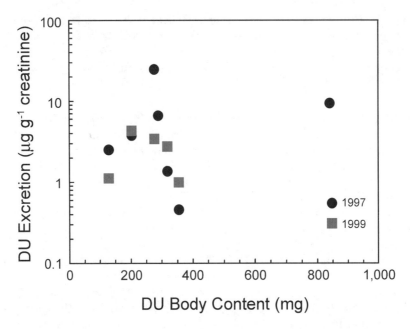

Fig. 3.4. Scatter diagram of daily urinary excretion of DU (microgram per gram creatinine) versus body content (milligrams) (Toohey, 2003a).

exposure duration was relatively short, the particle sizes were small, and in each case, the wounds were debrided to remove the embedded plutonium. These studies do suggest, however, that granuloma production in muscle and other tissues can occur subsequent to the embedding of fragments. Whether in the case of embedded DU fragments this encapsulation will be permanent or will undergo a degradation-regeneration cycle as suggested by Lushbaugh *et al.* (1967) for the plutonium cases they studied is uncertain. In their analysis of cases of injected plutonium, Lushbaugh *et al.* (1967) found that "... metallic plutonium implanted in the skin in minute amounts elicits a foreign-body reaction of the granulomatous type, which after subsiding in cellular activity becomes fibromatous." As time progressed, the collagen in the vicinity of the fragment lique-fied. Lushbaugh *et al.* (1967) speculated that the "pointed" nature of the granulomas they found and the fact that the granulomas became more superficial, suggested that the altered collagen might induce a cycle of inflammatory reaction followed by a reorganiza-tion and re-liquefaction of the collagen.

This scenario is partially substantiated by the clinical report written after a large DU fragment was removed from a patient 17 months after he was wounded. The surgeon noted that the fragment was contained in a fibrous capsule. When the capsule was punctured, ~1 to 2 mL of a black fluid "gushed forth" from the cystic space (Daxon, 1994). Unfortunately, neither the fluid nor the excised tissue was saved for analysis.

The experience of Cole *et al.* (1988) indicates that granuloma production in muscle and fatty tissue surrounding DU fragments will probably occur, as well as in all other tissue types that elicit similar cellular responses to foreign bodies. Cole *et al.* (1988) investigated a worker with a DU fragment embedded in the fatty tissue between the ribs and the skin as a result of an accident during machining. The 100 to 275 mg particle was surgically excised and found to be surrounded by what was described as a layer of tough fibrous tissue that was not readily removed from the particle. The total elapsed time between the accident and the surgical excision was eight months. The tissue removed was not examined histologically. It is still questionable whether such encapsulation is permanent or will undergo the degradation-regeneration cycle suggested by Lushbaugh *et al.* (1967) for the plutonium cases they studied. Similar behavior has been observed for thorotrastomas (Section 3.3). Although not considered to be malignant, thorotrastomas do increase in size with time, most likely due to migration of extravasated material and subsequent tissue reaction (Tauber, 1992).

Encapsulation could limit the chemical toxicity of the DU fragments by decreasing the rate of release of the metal, as has been observed for lead (Manton and Thal, 1986). Encapsulation can also result in the formation of pseudocysts. Pseudocysts were formed that contained fluid with very high concentrations of soluble lead and insoluble lead dioxide particles (Linden *et al.*, 1982; Manton and Thal, 1986), and with "black pigment ... firmly adherent ..." to portions of the inner wall of the capsule (Linden *et al.*, 1982). If these cysts should rupture, the rapid release of the fluid could cause periodic spikes in circulating lead levels and result in acute lead toxicity 5 to 40 y after the initial injury (Linden *et al.*, 1982; Manton and Thal, 1986; Viegas and Calhoun, 1986). Similar types of lesions may form around DU fragments. Intracapsular fluid may contain high concentrations of both soluble and insoluble DU. Tonry (1993) demonstrated that DU disks formed both a soluble fraction and black insoluble particulates when immersed in simulated lung fluid.

The radiation emitted by DU might affect the long-term integrity of the fibrous capsular wall of the pseudocyst and contribute to the potential for a breakdown of the encapsulation process, causing a release of uranium and producing latent toxicity. Analysis of eight workers with embedded ^{239}Pu fragments (Langham *et al.*, 1967; Lushbaugh and Langham, 1962) led to the conclusion that the high dose-rate radiation from ^{239}Pu caused a three-stage reaction; a granulomatous inflammatory process, followed by formation of a dense collagen encapsulation, which exhibited a final stage of degeneration and liquefaction. The process may then repeat itself, inducing a cycle of inflammatory reaction followed by reorganization and reliquefaction of the collagen. Similarly, Thorotrast®, which has a low dose rate that is comparable to that of DU (the dose rate from DU is four times that from Thorotrast®), produces these types of changes in tissues over a 5 to 10 y time span (Sections 3.3 and B.6.6) (Casper, 1967; Dahlgren, 1967b; da Horta, 1967b; Graham *et al.*, 1992; Stover, 1983; Swarm, 1967; Tauber, 1992; van Kaick *et al.*, 1978). Similar effects were observed in rats implanted with DU metal disks (Section C.3.8; Hahn *et al.*, 2002), and in rats and rabbits implanted with plutonium metal wire (Section B.6.3; Lisco and Kisieleski, 1953). In the latter case, the rate of encapsulation, breakdown and enlargement of the affected volume was faster, presumably driven by the higher absorbed dose rate from ^{239}Pu than from DU.

3.3 Medical Cases

Although contaminated wounds are infrequent occurrences in medical facilities, two situations deserve discussion. The first is a needle stick in a radiopharmaceutical laboratory. This situation may be treated exactly like any other puncture wound contaminated with a radionuclide. The other situation, which will be described in more detail, is injection of Thorotrast®, a colloidal suspension (solution of particulates) of thorium dioxide, which was used as a radiographic contrast medium for cerebral and limb angiography and for cholangiography. Although Thorotrast® worked well as a contrast medium because of its density, its colloidal nature led to its retention in the body *via* phagocytosis by tissues of the reticuloendothelial system (*i.e.*, liver, spleen, lymph nodes, and bone marrow), where it remained. Due to the long physical half-life of ^{232}Th (1.39×10^{10} y), all of these tissues received chronic irradiation (primarily alpha) from these deposits.

Numerous pathologic conditions, both benign and malignant (*e.g.*, blood dyscrasias and liver tumors), have been documented in patients following Thorotrast® injection (*e.g.*, Sugiyama *et al.*, 1986; Faber, 1985). Most of these conditions did not manifest until many years after injection, and latent periods of >20 y were common. Andersson *et al.* (1994) noted a median time of 35 y from the time of Thorotrast® injection to the diagnosis of a developing primary liver tumor.

Of the many Thorotrast®-induced pathological conditions suffered by these patients, the one relevant to this Report is the condition termed a thorotrastoma, or Thorotrast® granuloma. Thorotrast® was often administered by injection into the common carotid artery, however some of the solution often extravasated into the surrounding tissue and remained there for the life of the patient. The result of this constant alpha irradiation in the perivascular tissue areas was increased proliferation of fibroblasts and fibrosis, and induced masses of fibrous connective tissue (*i.e.*, a thorotrastoma often developed) (Polacarz *et al.*, 1992). Abscess formation within the thorotrastoma often developed over time. Although the vast majority of these fibrous growths were benign, they nevertheless increased slowly in size and could interfere with circulation and swallowing (Tauber, 1992). In addition, there are reports that neurofibrosarcomas, fibrosarcomas and undifferentiated sarcomas, and mucoepidermoid carcinomas developed in the tissue areas adjacent to the perivascular deposits of Thorotrast® (Barry and Rominger, 1964; Mori *et al.*, 2005). Stougaard *et al.* (1984) reported that ~10 % of the patients who received injections of Thorotrast® into the carotid artery developed thorotrastomas. Surgical removal of perivascular deposits of Thorotrast® or thorotrastomas has often led to such complications as arterial hemorrhage, delayed healing, and chronically suppurating fistulas (Liebermann *et al.*, 1995).

The U.S. Transuranium and Uranium Registries program (Kathren, 1995) has collected autopsy tissue samples and radiochemical data from two whole-body donors who had received i.v. injections of Thorotrast® and performed radiochemical analyses of their tissues. The first case, designated 1001, produced reports on clinical and autopsy findings, dosimetry, radiochemical analyses, and autoradiographic and molecular evaluations, which were collected in a single issue of *Health Physics* (Guilmette and Mays, 1992). Case 1001 developed a benign thorotrastoma at the injection site (Tauber, 1992). Tissue samples from 1001 were examined for alterations in proto-oncogene or tumor-suppressor gene structure. Alteration of the c-*fms* gene was observed in a blood sample from Case 1001. This gene specifies the cell surface receptor for macrophage colony-stimulating factor; the receptor is involved in the regulation of hematopoiesis (Collart *et al.*, 1992).

The second whole-body case, designated 1054, was presented by Russell *et al.* (1995). Case 1054 died from complications resulting from a large cholangiocarcinoma. However, there was no evidence of a thorotrastoma or remaining Thorotrast® deposits in the neck region near the injection site. Examination of a blood sample from a third U.S. Transuranium and Uranium Registries whole-body Thorotrast® case, designated 1053, did not find any alteration in two genes, *Rb* or *fms*, that are highly associated with leukemia. Case 1053 died from an acute subdural hematoma resulting from a fall, and the autopsy did not reveal any evidence of a thorotrastoma in or near the injection site.

Thorium, like other actinides, is primarily an alpha emitter (~90 % of the emissions), and the similarities between its subdermal and i.m. depositions with the resultant tissue responses and those in DU-induced wounds in military personnel are comparable. Although the administration of Thorotrast® for medical purposes is somewhat different from the accidental incorporation of alpha emitters such as plutonium *via* a puncture wound, cut or abrasion, the actual trauma and the pathological and physiological events that follow should be similar.

4. Generic Biokinetic Model for Radionuclides in Wounds

The NCRP wound biokinetic model, depicted schematically in Figure 4.1, consists of seven compartments. Five of these (fragment, soluble, CIS, PABS, and TPA) comprise the wound site, and two (blood and lymph nodes), can receive materials leaving the wound site. The five-compartment wound site is considered to be relatively tissue insensitive and, therefore, independent of the anatomic location of the wound. This is a simplification, but given that most wounds occur in the skin, subcutis (shallow connective tissues) or muscle, the assumption is a reasonable first approximation. Additionally, most of the experimental wound data relate to these tissues. Because of a lack of relevant data, the model does not differentiate between contaminated wounds arising from punctures, abrasions, lacerations or burns. It is recognized, however,

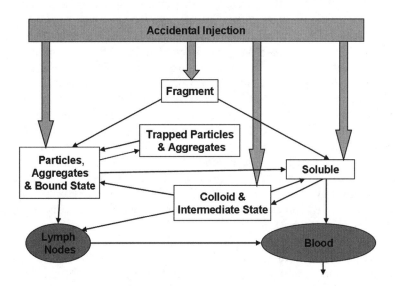

Fig. 4.1. General compartment model of the biokinetics of radionuclides and/or radioactive materials deposited in a wound.

that the degree of tissue injury will likely affect the biokinetics of the deposited radionuclide (Sections A.3, A.4, and 4.3).

The compartmental representations of the wound site are based on the physical and chemical properties of the deposited radioactive material. In this model, material introduced into a wound is described as being in solution, colloidal, particulate or fragments. These categories cover most forms of materials that have been encountered in the workplace and are suitable initial conditions for modeling. Transfer of the material between compartments is characterized using first-order kinetics. Empirically this approach has been adequate for describing the data sets encountered to date, and, therefore, more complex time-dependent transfer rate coefficients have not been used.

Fragments and particles are solids, and may include essentially pure materials, such as plutonium metal or oxides, mixtures such as metal alloys or mixed oxides, or solid materials contaminated on their surfaces with soluble radionuclides (*e.g.*, americium-contaminated pipette tips). Particles and fragments differ in that particles are much smaller. Particles may be the contaminating material, or they may arise from fragments (*e.g.*, from the corrosion in aqueous media of metals such as natural or DU) (Hahn *et al.*, 2002) or plutonium (Lisco and Kisieleski, 1953). An arbitrary upper size cutoff of 20 μm diameter has been applied to particles. This size corresponds roughly to the largest solid particle that can be phagocytized by tissue macrophages (Snipes, 1989).

Radionuclides introduced into a wound initially in soluble form, or that are transported from the fragment or PABS compartments as a result of dissolution *in vivo*, enter the soluble compartment. The analysis of wound retention data from experimental animals i.m. injected with a wide variety of radionuclides in solution made it apparent that three compartments were needed to describe the broad range of their biokinetic behaviors (Appendix A). Based on aqueous chemistry considerations, two compartments, CIS and PABS, are provided in the wound model. These compartments interact with the soluble compartment and provide the mathematical flexibility needed to describe the various wound retention patterns observed for the 48 radioelements described in this Report (Tables A.1 and A.2).

The initial partitioning of material containing a radionuclide between the soluble and CIS compartments is strongly influenced by its aqueous solution chemistry, in particular, by the element's tendency to hydrolyze at the neutral pH of the tissue fluid and plasma bathing the wound site (Gamble, 1954). An element's tendency to hydrolyze often determines its persistence at the wound site, not only because of the changed physical state from a dissolved solute to a solid phase, but also because of the great tendency of highly charged metal ions to bind locally to fixed tissue constituents (Appendices A and C). The more favorable the reactions with water and with ligating groups of fixed tissues, the more radionuclide will shift to the CIS, and the less radionuclide will be transported to blood in ionic form or as a soluble complex with circulating endogenous ligands. Because there is a likelihood that these chemical reactions are reversible, albeit slowly, bidirectional movement of the radionuclide is allowed between the soluble and CIS compartments.

The PABS compartment is envisaged to comprise not only particles, but also radionuclides that have been transformed beyond the CIS state, which was caused by the initial chemical reactions *in vivo*. These less mobile chemical states can include robust hydroxide precipitates and/or polymers, or chemical forms that bind stably *in situ* to wound tissue constituents. The result is that radionuclide in the PABS compartment is retained more tenaciously at the wound site. As in the case of CIS, material in the PABS compartment may be solubilized slowly. Additionally, because this material may have biologically recognizable particulate properties, it may also be transported to the regional draining lymph nodes by tissue macrophages that have phagocytized the particulate material.

The model allows fragments to be transformed *in situ* into particles or to dissolve into soluble species. Particles or aggregates of material containing radionuclide can dissolve or be transported *via* lymphatics from the wound site. The model also provides a compartment designated as TPA. This compartment was introduced primarily to accommodate the altering of particle and dissolution kinetics due to fibrous encapsulation of the deposited material, the so-called foreign-body reaction (Bischoff and Bryson, 1964; Brand *et al.*, 1976). The foreign-body reaction has been shown to be dependent on the amount and/or size of the embedded material as well as its composition. Although suspected, it is not known whether the additional tissue insult of irradiation also affects this process. With time, fragments are also likely to become encapsulated in fibrous connective tissue. The kinetics of radionuclide movement from a fragment are not as likely to be affected as that from particles, because the rates of corrosion of radioactive fragments to particles and of particle solubilization are already very slow. Therefore, a separate "trapped fragments" compartment was not included.

Although the structure adopted in this model is reasonable from phenomenologic and mechanistic perspectives, there are no data available of which NCRP is aware that allow these wound-site compartments to be evaluated independently. It is useful to note that, for any given form of the contaminating radionuclide, only a portion of the wound model is used, typically three compartments. This is illustrated in Figures 4.2, 4.3, 4.4, and 4.5 for soluble, colloid, particle and fragment forms, respectively. Therefore, the complexity of the model is less than it appears in the generic model. On the other hand, if the contaminating material consists of a mixture of forms, then all the relevant portions of the model will need to be used.

4.1 Implementation of the Wound Biokinetic Model

Fitting of individual radionuclide and composite data sets with the wound model was accomplished using the simulation and modeling software, SAAM II [SAAM Institute, Inc., Seattle, Washington (Barrett *et al.*, 1998)]. In most cases, the amount of data to be modeled was limited, making it necessary to constrain the fitting process such that a minimum number of parameters were fitted at any given time. This was particularly the case for movement of material into the lymph-node compartment, for which there were few data, particularly for the initially soluble radionuclides. In most cases, stable convergent solutions were obtained for the

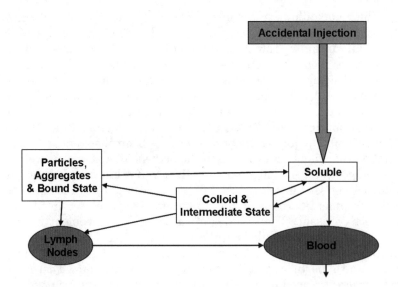

Fig. 4.2. Wound model for injection of soluble substances into the soluble compartment.

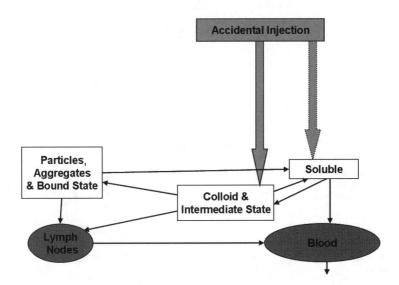

Fig. 4.3. Wound model for injection of colloids into the CIS compartment.

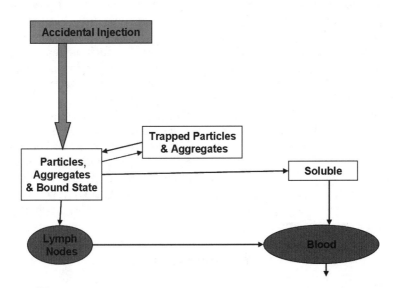

Fig. 4.4. Wound model for injection of particles into the PABS compartment.

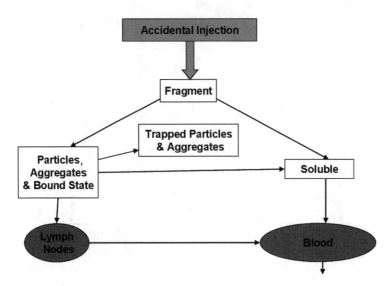

Fig. 4.5. Wound model for injection of fragments into the fragment compartment.

various individual or composite data sets. However, in some cases, the mathematical solutions were unstable to initial starting conditions. In these cases, expert judgment consistent with the chemical principles used in the original design of the model was used to select the most reasonable solution. Not surprisingly, because of the small data sets used, uncertainties in the fitted rate constants were often very large. Nevertheless, the fitted solutions describing the wound retention of radionuclides were always good representations of the data and, therefore, from a dosimetric perspective, useful. Additionally, the predicted behavior of the individual radionuclides within the various wound subcompartments was consistent with postulates of chemically driven behavior, and gave confidence that the underlying basis for the modeling was reasonable. Wherever the data sets described below were sufficiently large, the wound model was used along with the fitting software Origin® (OriginLab Corporation, Northampton, Massachusetts), to generate the wound retention equations and curves shown in Appendices A, B and C.

4.2 Modeling Results

The wound model was used to describe the behavior of radionuclides for which adequate amounts of wound retention data were available. In some cases, mainly because of the short physical half-lives of the radionuclides, wound retention data were available only for a few days. However, these data were useful when combined with those for other radionuclides with more substantial data sets, as was done in developing the default retention categories, weak (W), moderate (M), strong (S), and avid (A). Wound retention simulations are provided here to illustrate some of the properties of the model, fits for the four default categories, and descriptions of modeling colloids, particles and fragments.

4.2.1 *Modeling of Individual Radionuclides*

4.2.1.1 *Cesium-137.* Data from studies of i.m.-injected ^{137}CsCl in rats (Tables A.1 and A.2) were analyzed with the wound model using a three-compartment wound site (soluble, CIS, PABS). The results are shown graphically in Figure 4.6 together with the fitted transfer rates. In this case, the simple aqueous chemistry of monovalent cations indicated that the PABS compartment would play no role in the biokinetics. Therefore, the transfer rate from CIS to PABS was set to zero. Accordingly, the model transfer rates indicated that ≥90 % of the injected cations left the wound site directly from the soluble compartment to blood with a 0.4 h half-time. This value is comparable to that obtained for the weak category radionuclides (15 to 50 min), of which cesium is a member. It is likely that the longer-term retention of a few percent of the injected activity in the CIS compartment is due to an experimental artifact (Section A.1.1)

It should be noted that the data on human exposure to ^{137}Cs from the accident in Goiânia, Brazil indicated a long-term retention of ^{137}Cs in scar tissue at wound sites (Section 4.3.7), but this would not be expected to occur with i.m. or s.c. injection.

4.2.1.2 *Actinium-227.* Data from the study of i.m.-injected ^{227}AcCl$_3$ in rats (Tables A.1 and A.2) were analyzed with the wound model using the three-compartment wound site (soluble, CIS, PABS). The results are shown graphically in Figure 4.7 together with the fitted transfer rates. For this trivalent radionuclide, the model predicts that during the first 24 h following injection of the dissolved chloride, ~60 % of the actinium transferred from the soluble compartment is transported to blood (half-time 1.4 d) and the remaining 40 % to CIS. Of the total amount entering the CIS compartment, ~97 % is recirculated back to the soluble compartment, but at a much slower rate (0.023 d^{-1}). The remaining 3 % is trapped in the PABS compartment, where it is retained for a long time (half-time >7,000 d). Thus, for this case most of the radionuclide kinetics is

Transfer rates for wound-site retention of a soluble ^{134,137}Cs$^+$ tracer i.m. injected in rats.[a]

Pathway	Transfer Rate (d^{-1})
Soluble to blood	44
Soluble to CIS	3.5
CIS to soluble	0.067
CIS to PABS	0.0[b]

[a]Material injected into soluble compartment.
[b]Parameter value fixed.

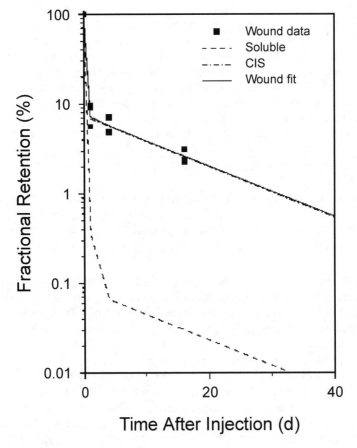

Fig. 4.6. Model fit of wound retention of i.m.-injected ^{134,137}Cs$^+$ in rats (data from Table A.2).

Transfer rates for wound-site retention of a soluble $^{227}Ac^{3+}$ tracer i.m. injected in rats.[a]

Pathway	Transfer Rate (d^{-1})
Soluble to blood	0.49
Soluble to CIS	0.35
CIS to soluble	0.023
CIS to PABS	0.00069
PABS to soluble	0.000010
PABS to lymph nodes	0.00002[b]

[a]Material injected into soluble compartment.
[b]Parameter value fixed.

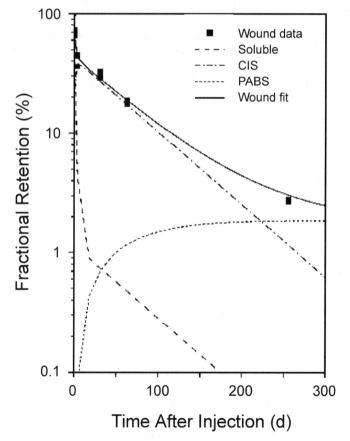

Fig. 4.7. Model fit of wound retention of i.m.-injected $^{227}Ac^{3+}$ in rats (data from Table A.2).

described by interaction between the soluble and CIS compartments, but the PABS compartment comes into play in predicting long-term retention for ~2 % of the deposited actinium. Although this latter quantity persists beyond the range of the data, it is within the bounds of the default parameters for the strongly-retained category, of which it is a member. Because the mass of ^{227}Ac injected was small (0.017 µg), there was no reason to invoke immobilization in the TPA compartment. Therefore, the transfer rate from PABS to TPA was set to zero. On the other hand, the lack of substantial mass does not negate the possibility that some of the actinium was being strongly fixed to tissue constituents at the wound site, which would provide a reasonable explanation for the 2 % long-term retention predicted by the model.

4.2.2 *Modeling of Default Categories of Soluble Radionuclides*

4.2.2.1 *Basic Data Set.* Appendix A presents brief descriptions of the experiments in which soluble radionuclides were i.m. injected, with only a few exceptions, in rats. The data for 54 radionuclides (isotopes of 50 elements) in dilute saline solution that were i.m. injected in rats are given in Table A.1 (experimental conditions and data sources) and Table A.2 (serially timed data for radionuclide retention at the wound site).

The solution chemistries of the study of radionuclides, most importantly their tendencies to hydrolyze and form stable complexes, were expected to dominate their retention in a deep i.m. puncture wound (Ilyin and Ivannikov, 1979; Morrow et al., 1968), as illustrated in Figure 4.8, in much the same manner as they influence dissolution and transport to blood of radionuclides deposited in the respiratory tract (ICRP, 1994a). Accordingly, the data for retention of the individual radionuclides are arranged in Tables A.1 and A.2 in the expected order of their increasing tendency to hydrolyze and/or form stable complexes at physiological pH, that is, in the order of their increasing positive electric charge (Ahrland, 1986; Cotton and Wilkinson, 1980; Latimer, 1952).

Concentration strongly influences cation hydrolysis and complexation and is, therefore, also expected to influence radionuclide retention in a puncture wound. In constructing the basic data set for the purpose of classifying wound retention of radionuclides in solution, those studies were excluded in which the mass of administered radionuclide was >5 µg. Five micrograms (11.4 kBq) is about the largest mass of $^{239}Pu^{4+}$ that can be i.m. injected in a rat in an appropriately small volume ($\leq$0.5 mL) of a weakly acidic solution (pH 1 to 1.5), while still avoiding hydrolysis of the Pu^{4+} in the

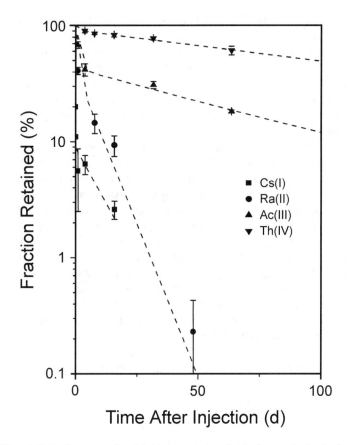

Fig. 4.8. Influence of oxidation state and tendency to hydrolyze at physiological pH on retention at an i.m. wound site in rats of small masses (≤5 µg) of four representative cationic radionuclides injected in saline solution: $^{137}Cs^+$ (1.8×10^{-2} µg) and $^{223}Ra^{2+}$ (2.9×10^{-5} µg) do not hydrolyze at pH 7.4 and form only weak complexes; $^{227}Ac^{3+}$ (10^{-2} µg) and $^{234}Th^{4+}$ (4.2×10^{-4} µg) hydrolyze at physiological pH and form stable complexes. (Data taken from Table A.2; dashed lines are multicomponent fits to the data.)

injection medium. For uniformity, a cutoff of 5 µg injected was applied to all of the study radionuclides, regardless of their chemical properties. With that limitation, data from 46 of 50 radioelements studied were considered suitable to use for classifying radionuclide retention in an i.m. wound.

4.2.2.2 *Radionuclide Retention Categories.* For the purpose of classification, radionuclide retention in an i.m. puncture wound was considered to be the combined result of the fraction of the injected radioactive material remaining at the wound site 1 d after deposition and the rate(s) at which the initially-retained fraction was subsequently cleared from the wound, as judged by the fraction retained at 16 or 64 d. The study radionuclides were assigned, on the basis of those criteria, to one of four quantitatively distinct wound retention classes, weakly, moderately, strongly or avidly retained.

Retention at the wound site after an i.m. injection in rats [percent of injected dosage (% ID), mean ± standard deviation (SD)] was calculated for each of the four retention categories at each post-injection interval by combining the data from all of the radionuclides assigned to that category at each interval. At each post-injection interval the differences between and among the wound content of the four retention categories are statistically significant [t-test, $p \leq 0.02$ (Mack, 1967)]. The mean wound retention of the radionuclides in the four wound retention categories is shown in Table 4.1 and Figure 4.9 for post-injection intervals from 1 to 64 d. The semilogarithmic curves shown in Figure 4.9, that describe wound retention for the four retention categories and their corresponding equations, were obtained by fitting the wound retention curve predicted by the wound model. The equations for retention $R(t)$ of small masses (≤ 5 µg) of soluble radionuclides i.m. injected in rats are of the form:

$$R(t) = \sum_i A_i e^{-\lambda_i t}, \tag{4.1}$$

where $R(t)$ is radionuclide retention at the wound site (% ID), A_i is the partition coefficient (i.e., the percent of the deposited amount retained for retention component i), λ_i is the retention rate constant for retention component i, and t is days after deposition.

4.2.2.2.1 *Weakly-retained radionuclides.* Retention of these 14 radionuclides at the wound site was ≤ 10 % of the injected dosage at 1 d, and thereafter rapid clearance reduced retention at the wound site to ≤ 3 % at 16 d. The wound retention data for these radionuclides are collected in Table A.3. This group includes seven anions ($^{131}I^-$, $^{71}GeO_3^{2-}$, $^{74}AsCl_5^{2-}$, $^{124}SbO_3^-$, $^{75}SeO_4^{2-}$, $^{95,96}TcCl_6^{2-}$, and $^{191}WO_4^{2-}$) and seven cations ($^{86}Rb^+$, $^{137}Cs^+$, $^{45}Ca^{2+}$, $^{90}Sr^{2+}$, $^{140}Ba^{2+}$, $^{64}Cu^{2+}$, and $^{230}UO_2^{2+}$). At the low molar concentrations injected, none of these chemical species, except for $^{230}UO_2^{2+}$, hydrolyze at physiological pH or form stable complexes with fixed tissue constituents, and the specific metallo-anions in this retention category

TABLE 4.1—*Retention of weakly, moderately, strongly and avidly-retained radionuclide groups at an i.m. wound site in rats; injected radionuclide plus carrier mass ≤5 μg.*

Retention Category	Percent of Injected Dosage Retained at Wound Site at Days After Injection, Mean ± SD for (n) Radionuclides[a,b]				
	1 d	4 d	14 – 16 d	28 – 32 d	60 – 64 d
Weak[c]	2.8 ± 2.0 (11)	2.5 ± 2.2 (10)	1.2 ± 1.2 (4)	—	—
Moderate[d]	31 ± 15 (6)	15 ± 7.0 (5)	8.6 ± 0.9 (5)	4.9 ± 2.2 (3)	3.9 ± 1.3 (2)
Strong[e]	66 ± 13 (20)	45 ± 12 (17)	36 ± 14 (15)	34 ± 8.8 (15)	19 ± 10 (10)
Avid[f]	86 ± 5.3 (3)	84 ± 5.8 (5)	82 ± 1.6 (3)	77 ± 2.9 (3)	62 ± 3.8 (3)

[a] $SD = \left[\sum \mathrm{dev}_i^2 \, (n-1)^{-1} \right]^{1/2}$ (Mack, 1967); (n) is the number of study radionuclides contributing data at time t, at all post-injection times and dev_i is the standard deviation of the experimental data for each radionuclide i, for $i = 1$ through n.

[b] Means for each retention category are significantly less than those for the next most retentive category, that is, weak < moderate < strong < avid (t-test, $p \leq 0.02$; Mack, 1967).

[c] Data for individual weakly-retained radionuclides from Table A.3.

[d] Data for individual moderately-retained radionuclides from Table A.4.

[e] Data for individual strongly-retained radionuclides from Table A.5.

[f] Data for individual avidly-retained radionuclides from Table A.6.

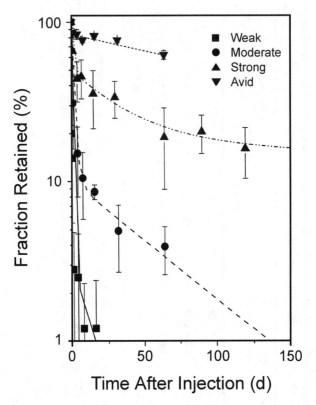

Fig. 4.9. Fractional radionuclide retention at an i.m.-injection site in rats (percent of amount deposited, mean ± SD) of 14 weakly-retained radionuclides, seven moderately-retained radionuclides, 21 strongly-retained radionuclides, and six avidly-retained radionuclides. The curves were obtained from the combined data for each wound retention category (Tables A.3 to A.6) by using the wound model and the Origin® software.

appear to have been stable to reduction to lower, more readily hydrolysable oxidation states. Retention in a deep puncture wound (% *ID*) of those representative weakly-retained radionuclides is described by the equation:

$$R(t)_{\text{weak}} = 53e^{-66t} + 44e^{-5.7t} + 3e^{-0.07t}. \quad (4.2)$$

This group of monovalent alkali metals, divalent alkaline earths, copper and uranyl ion, oxo- and chloro-anions, and monovalent anionic iodine forms the weakly-retained radionuclide category. The results of modeling the data from this category are shown in

Figure 4.10 along with associated fitted compartment transfer rates. The predominant characteristics of the weak radionuclides are the rapidity with which they leave the wound site and the amounts that are rapidly cleared. About 53 % is transferred from the wound site with a 15 min half-time, 44 % with a half-time of 2.9 h, and the remaining 3 % is cleared with a half-time of ~10 d (Equation 4.2). These features are reflected in the model by a >2:1 preference for transfer from the soluble compartment to blood compared with transfer from soluble to CIS. Additionally, the recirculation from CIS back to soluble is also relatively rapid, with a rate constant of 2.8 d^{-1}. The longer retained fraction of ~3 % is, according to the model, transferred to the PABS compartment. However, for these radionuclides, this may not be an accurate description of their physicochemical state. The rate of transfer out of the PABS to the soluble compartment has a half-life of ~9 d, which is considerably more rapid than the PABS-soluble transfer rates calculated for the other categories of radionuclides (see below). For the weakly-retained radionuclides, the small long-retained fraction may reflect weak binding to tissue constituents, but it may also be due to the technical artifact discussed in Appendix A.1.1., that is, an over-estimate of retention due to the failure to account for a small amount of the injected radionuclide in the skin and tissues of the paw of the injected leg. However, the retained fraction described by the data cannot be neglected, as it accounts for ~85 % of the radiation dose to the wound site. It would be useful if this issue could be clarified by new data, even though the dose to systemic organs is usually of greater interest.

4.2.2.2.2 *Moderately-retained radionuclides.* Retention of these seven dissimilar radionuclides ranged from 11 to 55 % at 1 d, and subsequently moderate rates of clearance reduced retention at the wound site to ≤5 % at 64 d. The wound retention data for these moderately-retained radionuclides are collected in Table A.4. These radionuclides are chemical analogues of members of the weakly-retained category, and none is expected to hydrolyze *in vivo*. Their greater and more prolonged retention, compared with their weakly-retained analogues, appears to have a variety of causes. Silver-110 ($^{110}Ag^+$) forms insoluble chlorides and carbonates and binds to free sulfhydryl groups of proteins, $^{223}Ra^{2+}$ forms insoluble carbonates, sulfates, and phosphates, and binds more strongly to proteins than the lighter weight alkaline earth elements. The highly oxidized metals deposited as complex anions ($^{48}VO_3^-$, $^{105}RhCl_6^{3-}$, $^{127m}TeO_4^{2-}$, $^{191,193}PtCl_4^{2-}$, and $^{188}OsO_5^{2-}$) may have been reduced to lower states that hydrolyze and/or form complexes with

Transfer rates for wound-site retention of initially soluble
weakly-retained radionuclides i.m. injected in rats.[a]

Pathway	Transfer Rate (d⁻¹)
Soluble to blood	45
Soluble to CIS	21
CIS to soluble	2.8
CIS to PABS	0.26
PABS to soluble	0.08
PABS to lymph nodes	0.00002[b]

[a]Material injected into soluble compartment.
[b]Parameter value fixed.

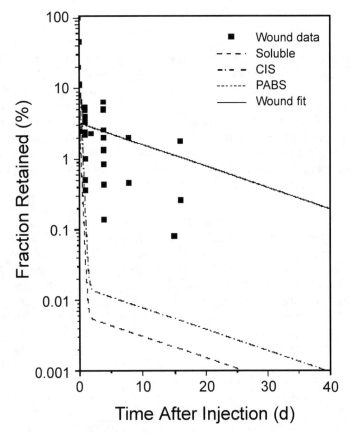

Fig. 4.10. Model fit of wound retention of weak category radionuclides
i.m. injected in rats (data from Table A.3).

tissue proteins. Retention in a deep puncture wound (% *ID*) of these moderately-retained radionuclides is described by the equation:

$$R(t)_{\text{moderate}} = 55e^{-47t} + 35e^{-0.43t} + 10e^{-0.017t}. \tag{4.3}$$

The results of modeling the data from this group of radionuclides are shown in Figure 4.11 along with the associated fitted transfer rates. There are similarities between the weak and moderate categories in that both exhibit rapid clearance of about half of the deposited radionuclide. For the moderate group, ~55 % of the injected dose is cleared with a half-time of 21 min, but the remainder clears more slowly than for the weak group; 35 % is cleared with a half-time of 1.6 d and 10 % is cleared with a half-time of 41 d (Equation 4.3). The model simulations indicate that partitioning of these soluble radionuclides between blood and the CIS is ~4:3, and the recirculation from the CIS back to the soluble compartment has a rate constant of 0.40 d^{-1}. About 14 % of the radionuclide entering the CIS compartment is transported to the PABS, from which it is transported back to the soluble compartment at a rate of 0.018 d^{-1} (40 d half-time). The short-term clearance of the moderate category is similar to that of the weak category, indicating that there is little tendency for an important fraction of the moderate category radionuclides to be retained at the wound site. The principal difference between the weak and moderate categories is the slower rate of movement of radionuclides out of CIS for the latter. The longer-term retention of moderate group radionuclides after the initial rapid clearance indicates that there may be greater competitive complexation with endogenous ligands within the wound site, compared with that for the weak group radionuclides. The integrated retention for the moderate group is ~12 times greater than that for the weak group radionuclides. Therefore, assuming identical radiation decay characteristics, the dose to the wound site per unit of moderate group radionuclides deposited would also be 12 times greater.

4.2.2.2.3 *Strongly-retained radionuclides.* Wound retention of these 21 radionuclides was 32 to 85 % at 1 d, and subsequent slow clearance reduced retention to 8 to 40 % at 64 d. The wound retention data for these radionuclides are collected in Table A.5. This group includes one anion (^{106}RuCl$_5^{2-}$) and 20 cations (^{7}Be^{2+}, ^{51}Cr^{3+}, ^{67}Ga^{3+}, ^{88}Y^{3+}, ^{95}Nb^{3+}, ^{114m}In^{3+}, ^{140}La^{3+}, ^{143}Ce^{3+}, ^{143}Pr^{3+}, ^{147}Nd^{3+}, ^{147}Pm^{3+}, ^{154,155}Eu^{3+}, ^{160}Tb^{3+}, ^{170}Tm^{3+}, ^{227}Ac^{3+}, ^{241}Am^{3+}, ^{242,244}Cm^{3+}, ^{210}Po^{4+}, ^{238}Pu^{4+}, and ≤3.2 μg of ^{239}Pu^{4+}). A major fraction of the

Transfer rates for wound-site retention of initially soluble
moderately-retained radionuclides i.m. injected in rats.[a]

Pathway	Transfer Rate (d^{-1})
Soluble to blood	44
Soluble to CIS	31
CIS to soluble	0.40
CIS to PABS	0.065
PABS to soluble	0.018
PABS to lymph nodes	0.00002[b]

[a]Material injected into soluble compartment.
[b]Parameter value fixed.

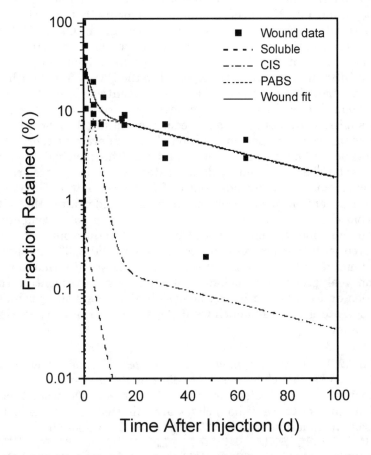

Fig. 4.11. Model fit of wound retention of moderate category radionuclides i.m. injected into rats (data from Table A.4).

highly oxidized $^{106}RuCl_5^{2-}$ appeared to have been reduced to a lower, hydrolysable oxidation state. The injected amounts of the isotopes of ytterbium, niobium, lanthanum, and the trivalent lanthanides and actinides were so small that their local concentrations in the tissue fluid at the wound site were all <0.1 μmol L^{-1}, and they would not be expected to precipitate as hydroxides. However, in neutral solution, even at very low concentrations, these trivalent cations form microcolloids despite the fact that their solubility products, K_{sp}, are not exceeded [$K_{sp} = (M^{n+}) (OH^-)^n$] (Luckey and Venogopal, 1977; Schubert and Conn, 1949; Schwietzer, 1956). The ion products of five other cations (isotopes of beryllium, chromium, gallium, indium, and polonium) even at the low concentrations injected, were close to their respective values of K_{sp}, and were likely to have hydrolyzed at the wound site. The K_{sp} for Pu(OH)$_4$ is so small (~10^{-52}) that even microgram amounts are expected to hydrolyze at pH 7.4. All of these multivalent cations are also expected to form stable complexes with the constituents of the connective tissue gel phase and with tissue proteins (Appendix C). Retention in a deep puncture wound (% ID) of strongly-retained radionuclides is described by the equation:

$$R(t)_{strong} = 50e^{-1.1t} + 32e^{-0.029t} + 18e^{-0.00086t}. \qquad (4.4)$$

This group of radionuclides is the largest of the four categories, and includes for the most part trivalent radionuclides [lanthanides, actinides, Groups IIIA (13) and IIIB (3), chromium, niobium] as well as divalent beryllium, tetravalent polonium and small deposited masses (≤5 μg) of plutonium. The results of modeling the data from this group of radionuclides are shown in Figure 4.12 along with the associated fitted transfer rates. For these radionuclides, there appears to be significant competition between hydrolysis and binding to fixed tissue ligands, versus binding to soluble circulating endogenous ligands. This is reflected in the significantly slower initial clearance rate for the strong group radionuclides {i.e., 50 % of the material that leaves the soluble compartment is cleared to blood with a 16 h half-time, and the remainder is retained longer [i.e., 32 % clears with a half-time of 24 d and 18 % with a half-time of 770 d (Equation 4.4)]}. Thus, initially soluble strong category radionuclides are approximately equally partitioned between transport to blood and immobilization in CIS. The radionuclide in the CIS is partitioned between recirculation to the soluble compartment and conversion to PABS at a ratio of ~2.5:1. Additionally, the rate of transfer of the strong group radionuclides from the CIS back

Transfer rates for wound-site retention of initially soluble strongly-retained radionuclides i.m. injected in rats.[a]

Pathway	Transfer Rate (d^{-1})
Soluble to blood	0.67
Soluble to CIS	0.60
CIS to soluble	0.024
CIS to PABS	0.0097
PABS to soluble	0.0012
PABS to lymph nodes	0.00002[b]

[a]Material injected into soluble compartment.
[b]Parameter value fixed.

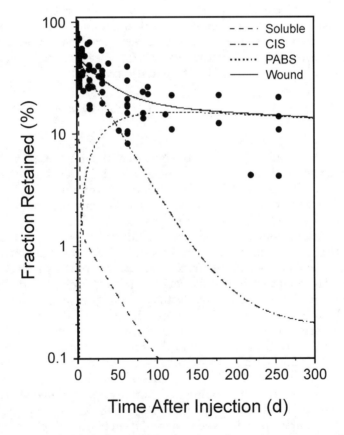

Fig. 4.12. Model fit of wound retention of strong category radionuclides i.m. injected in rats (data from Table A.5).

to soluble is ~5 % of that for the moderately-retained radionuclides. The integrated retention for the strong group is ~30 times that for the moderate group and 380 times that for the weak group. Thus, these radionuclides are of significantly greater concern from the perspective of potential radiation dose to the wound site, and correspondingly slower translocation to blood and systemic deposition sites.

4.2.2.2.4 *Avidly-retained radionuclides.* Retention of this group of six radionuclides (isotopes of five elements) was ≥80 % at 1 d, early clearance was about one-half of that for the strongly-retained radionuclides, and the wound site contained ≥50 % at 64 d. The wound retention data for these radionuclides are collected in Table A.6. This group includes $^{46}Sc^{3+}$, $^{95}Zr^{4+}$, $^{113}Sn^{4+}$, $^{233}Pa^{5+}$, and $^{228,234}Th^{4+}$. At pH 7.4, the small Sc^{3+} ion hydrolyzes readily and forms complexes as stable as those of a tetravalent cation. Even at the low molar concentrations injected, the ion products of these cations at physiological pH are much greater than their respective values of K_{sp}. All were in solution in the injection media, but would have hydrolyzed and/or formed stable complexes with fixed tissue constituents at the wound site. Retention in a deep puncture wound (% *ID*) of the avidly-retained radionuclides is described by the equation:

$$R(t)_{\text{avid}} = 19e^{37t} + 81e^{-0.001t}. \qquad (4.5)$$

All of the experiments that provided wound data for the avidly-retained radionuclides were terminated at $t \leq 64$ d; consequently, their longer-term retention behavior is ill-defined. It is reasonable to predict that late wound clearance of the avidly-retained radionuclides is similar to or slower than that of the strongly-retained group, for which the last defined slope constant is 0.00086 d^{-1}.

This small group of radionuclides consists of trivalent scandium, tetravalent zirconium, tin and thorium, and pentavalent protactinium. The results of modeling the data from these radionuclides are shown in Figure 4.13 along with the associated fitted transfer rates. The distinguishing characteristic of this group is the relatively small fraction of deposited radionuclide that rapidly leaves the wound site (*i.e.*, only ~10 % during the first day). The data set for these radionuclides is small and, to the detriment of the modeling, does not extend beyond 64 d after injection. This deficiency prevented determining a long-retained component, as was done for the strong group, for which the data extended to 256 d. Thus, model simulation together with expert judgment was used to

Transfer rates for wound-site retention of initially soluble avidly-retained
radionuclides i.m. injected in rats.[a]

Pathway	Transfer Rate (d^{-1})
Soluble to blood	7.0
Soluble to CIS	30
CIS to soluble	0.03
CIS to PABS	10
PABS to soluble	0.005
PABS to lymph nodes	0.00002[b]

[a]Material injected into soluble compartment.
[b]Parameter value fixed.

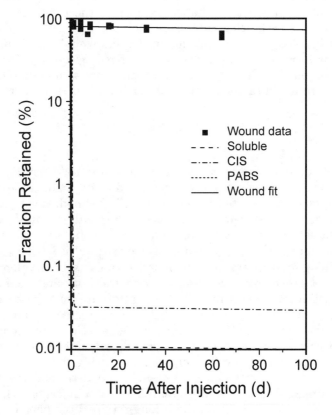

Fig. 4.13. Model fit of wound retention of avid category radionuclides
i.m. injected in rats (data from Table A.6).

obtain a set of transfer rates that produced a wound retention function equivalent with that of Equation 4.5. The results indicate that 19 % of the injected radionuclide is transported initially from the wound site with about a 0.5 h half-time and the remaining 81 % is cleared with about a 700 d half-time (Equation 4.5). According to the modeling, about four times more radionuclide is converted to the CIS state than is transferred to blood. This probably reflects the significant tendency of these radionuclides to hydrolyze and/or bind to fixed tissue ligands versus complexation with soluble circulating endogenous ligands. Upon transfer to CIS, the radionuclide is modeled to transfer relatively rapidly (~1.7 h half time) and virtually quantitatively to PABS. Movement from PABS to soluble is within a factor of four of that for the strong group and they overlap within the uncertainties of the analyses. The difference in these transfer rates is probably due to the fact that all of the avid radionuclides were administered in tracer quantities (*i.e.*, masses «1 µg), which was not always the case with the strong group radionuclides. Reduced mass decreases the likelihood of forming precipitates or polymers as a result of hydrolysis, but probably favors binding of the avid radionuclides to local tissue constituents. Thus, the lack of long-term experimental data for the avid group, and the very small injected masses contribute to the uncertainty in modeling this group. It can be concluded that the principal difference between the strong and avid groups would be the smaller rapidly cleared fraction for the avid group, which is expected to be highly mass-dependent. On the other hand, long-term retention times for the two groups would be expected to be similar, as are shown in the respective models.

4.2.2.3 *Conditions that Alter Retention of Soluble Radionuclides in Wounds.* The "base case" retention of soluble radionuclides in deep puncture wounds was derived from experiments in which rats were i.m. injected with a small volume of a dilute simple salt solution containing ≤5 µg of radionuclide plus stable carrier. Other experimental evidence described in Appendix A demonstrates that:

- Wound retention is usually enhanced and prolonged by increasing the local concentration (mass) of a dissolved radionuclide plus carrier (Section A.5.1), effectively shifting it to a more slowly-clearing category (*e.g.*, from strongly to avidly retained).
- Wound retention can be enhanced and prolonged by reduction *in situ* of a radionuclide in a highly oxidized state to a lower oxidation state with a greater tendency to hydrolyze

and form stable complexes; for example, the moderate rather than the weak retention behavior of $^{48}VO_3^-$, $^{105}RhCl_6^{3-}$, and $^{185}OsO_5^{2-}$.

- Clearance is greatly enhanced and accelerated, if the radionuclide is deposited in a wound in the form of a complex sufficiently stable to compete, at least temporarily, with hydrolysis (Appendix A.5.2).
- Retention of the individual radionuclides in a soluble mixture deposited in a deep puncture wound (*e.g.*, i.m. injection of a mildly acidic solution of mixed fission products), appears to depend on their individual chemical properties and to be largely independent of the retention behavior of the other radionuclides present (Appendix A.1.4.6).
- Retention at the wound site may be enhanced if the skin is damaged by abrasion or thermal, chemical or radiation burn (Section 4.3)

4.2.2.4 *Summary for Soluble Radionuclides.* Four quantitatively distinct categories of retention of dissolved radionuclides deposited in deep puncture wounds were defined empirically by the behavior of small masses (≤ 5 µg) of 47 individual radionuclides i.m. injected in rats. The identities and properties of the radioelements included in each retention category support the initial premise that retention of an initially soluble radionuclide in a wound is determined largely by its solution chemistry at physiological pH. With few exceptions, the weakly-retained radionuclides are anions and monovalent and divalent cations; the strongly-retained radionuclides are mainly trivalent cations, but that group also includes Be^{2+}, the lower oxidation states of ruthenium, and very small masses of Po^{4+} and Pu^{4+}; the avidly-retained radionuclides are all tetra- or pentavalent cations. The moderately-retained radionuclides appear to be special cases of complex metallo-anions and cations of low charge, for which more prolonged retention was caused by processes such as reduction to a lower, more hydrolysable oxidation state or complexation with tissue constituents.

The wound retention of each radionuclide category could be described by a negative multiexponential equation representing the average behavior of its constituent radionuclides (Equations 4.2 to 4.5). For convenience, rounded default values of the parameters of those equations are collected in Table 4.2. The trends of those parameters demonstrate that initial clearance of soluble radionuclides from a deep puncture wound becomes less and slower and long-term retention at the wound site becomes greater and more protracted as the radionuclide retention category shifts from

TABLE 4.2—*Default parameters of multiexponential equations for puncture wound retention of small masses (≤5 μg) of soluble radionuclides injected in rats.*[a,b]

Radionuclide Retention Class	Default Parameters for Wound Retention Equations								Source
	A_1 (%)	λ_1 (d^{-1})	A_2 (%)	λ_2 (d^{-1})	A_3 (%)	λ_3 (d^{-1})	A_4 (%)	λ_4 (d^{-1})	
Weak	55	55	40	6.0	5.0	0.1			Equation 4.2
Moderate	55	55	35	0.5	10	0.02			Equation 4.3
Strong			50	1.0	30	0.03	20	0.001	Equation 4.4
Avid			19	37			81	0.001[c]	Equation 4.5

[a] Wound retention equations of the form $R(t) = \sum_i A_i e^{-\lambda_i t}$, where $R(t)$ is percent of injected amount retained at the wound site and t is days after injection.

[b] Rounded values of parameters of the source equations.

[c] All experiments providing data for retention of avid category radionuclides were terminated at ≤64 d. A default value, 0.001 d^{-1}, is that obtained for the longer-studied strong category radionuclides.

weak to avid. The default parameters predict that 2 d after deposition in a deep puncture wound of weakly, moderately, strongly or avidly-retained radionuclides, the fraction retained at the wound site will be on average 5, 10, 50, and 80 % of the amount deposited, respectively, and that by 30 d, the retained fractions will have been reduced to 0.25, 5, 32, and ~78 %, respectively.

The intercompartmental transfer rates derived for the wound model to describe the behavior of small masses of soluble radionuclides i.m. injected in rats are shown in Table 4.3.

4.3 Retention of Soluble Radionuclides in Other Types of Wounds: Quantitative Comparison with Intramuscular Data

In addition to deep puncture wounding simulated by an i.m. injection, several radionuclides in solution have been applied to different kinds of wounds and to the intact and damaged skin of rats

TABLE 4.3—*Transfer rates obtained using the wound model for retention of small masses of radionuclides in solution i.m. injected in rats.*[a]

Pathway	Intercompartmental Transfer Rates (d^{-1}) for Radionuclide Wound Retention Categories[b]			
	Weak	Moderate	Strong	Avid
Soluble to blood	45	44	0.67	7.0
Soluble to CIS	21	31	0.60	30
CIS to soluble	2.8	0.4	0.024	0.03
CIS to PABS	0.26	0.065	0.0097	10
CIS to lymph nodes[c]	2×10^{-5}	2×10^{-5}	2×10^{-5}	2×10^{-5}
PABS to soluble	0.08	0.018	0.0012	0.005
PABS to lymph nodes[c]	2×10^{-5}	2×10^{-5}	2×10^{-5}	2×10^{-5}

[a]Injected radionuclide mass ≤5 μg.
[b]Input into soluble compartment of wound model (Figure 4.2).
[c]The transfer rates from CIS to lymph nodes and PABS to lymph nodes were fixed at 2×10^{-5} d^{-1}.

and mice. These include s.c. injection and application to shallow lacerations and abrasions and to thermally and acid-burned skin. These experiments are described in Appendix A, and the data for radionuclide retention at the site of the wounding or skin damage or application to the skin are collected in Tables A.9 to A.13. The results obtained at 1 d after radionuclide application or injection is summarized in Table 4.4. To accommodate data for individual radionuclides with a range of properties after applications involving a range of damage to the skin barrier in one table, the data in Table 4.4 are expressed as fraction absorbed, that is, 100 % minus the retained fraction.

In general, absorption of a given radionuclide from wounds or skin contamination is in the order: puncture wound > laceration ≈ abrasion > burned skin ≈ intact skin.

4.3.1 *Subcutaneous Injection*

Short-term studies (1 to 7 d) were conducted of the retention of 10 cationic radionuclides in solution at a s.c. wound site in rats. The experimental conditions and wound retention data are collected in Table A.9. Except for $^{111}Ag^+$, which may not have been in solution when injected, the amounts and residence times of these representative cations in a s.c. wound increased with increasing positive charge on the ion and its tendencies to hydrolyze and/or bind to protein, in agreement with the trend observed for the larger set of i.m.-injected radionuclides (Table 4.1).

Retention of s.c.-injected radionuclides in a wound can be compared with their retention after an i.m. injection (Tables A.7 and A.2). Retention of s.c.-injected $^{137}Cs^+$, $^{140}Ba^{2+}$, and $^{144}Ce^{3+}$ at 1 d, estimated from the metabolic data of Moskalev (1961b; 1961c; 1961d), and that of $^{228}Th^{4+}$ at 7 d, measured by Stradling et al. (1995a), agree reasonably well with their respective retentions at 1 and 7 d after an i.m. injection. In rats, absorption of $^{241}Am^{3+}$ at 1 d or $^{239}Pu^{4+}$ at 7 d after s.c. injection was more efficient (retention less) than after an i.m. injection. That difference was attributed to faster tissue fluid flow in the subcutis compared with muscle (Harrison et al., 1978a; Lewis, 1969; Lewis and Yates, 1972).

Practically, it is reasonable to assume that in human wound cases radionuclide retention in contaminated muscle and s.c. tissue will be similar.

4.3.2 *Lacerated Skin*

Eight radionuclides in solution were applied to the cut surfaces of incisions made through the skin into the underlying muscle of rats. Measurements of retention at the undisturbed wound site

TABLE 4.4—*Absorption at 1 d of some representative radionuclides in solution introduced into various types of wounds in rats and mice.*[a]

Radionuclide	Absorption at 1 d After Application or Injection (percent of administered amount)					
	Intact Skin[b]	Damaged Skin		Puncture Wounds		
		Abrasions[c]	Lacerations[d]	s.c. Injection[e]	i.m. Injection[f]	
[131]I[-]	2.5	80	93	—	99	
[137]Cs[+]	2.1	92	95	98	92	
[85]Sr[2+]	2.4	35	49	—	—	
[140]Ba[2+]	—	—	—	95	96	
[144]Ce[3+]	0.15	3.0	2.0	9.0	28	
[241]Am[3+]	0.014	6.0	6.0	44	15	
[210]Po[4+]	0.013	0.5	10	—	26	
[239]Pu[4+]	0.017	—	0.7	—	22	

[a]Data are expressed as absorption into the body to emphasize the small amounts of the radionuclides penetrating the intact skin.
[b]Data from Table A.11.
[c]Data from Table A.12.
[d]Data from Table A.10.
[e]Data from Table A.9
[f]Data from Table A.2.

were made for 1 to 7 d. The individual studies are described in Section A.3, and the data and sources are given in Table A.10. The trend of absorption of the study radionuclides is generally the same as was found for the same radionuclides deposited in deep puncture wounds (Table 4.4). Weakly-retained monovalent $^{137}Cs^+$ and anionic $^{131}I^-$ were absorbed from an incision at about the same rate as from a puncture wound. Smaller fractions of the applied multivalent cations were absorbed from a laceration than from a puncture wound; for example, absorption of $^{85}Sr^{2+}$ from a skin incision in rats was only about one-half of that expected from a puncture wound (Table A.2). Absorption at 1 d of two trivalent and two tetravalent cations from an undisturbed skin incision ranged from 3 % ($^{239}Pu^{4+}$) to 25 % ($^{210}Po^{4+}$) of that of a puncture wound.

The early absorption (in 24 h) of radionuclides from an untreated skin incision can be approximated as default fractions of the early absorption from a puncture wound of the same or chemically similar radionuclides, as follows: weakly retained, 1.0; moderately retained, 0.5; strongly retained, 0.2; avidly retained, 0.05. If the concentration of the radionuclide plus carrier in the contaminating solution is greater than the 10 to 100 µmol L^{-1} solutions that were used to contaminate the experimental wounds, it is expected that for multivalent cationic radionuclides, the fractional absorption will be less than the default fractions given above.

4.3.3 Abraded Skin

Seven radionuclides in solution were applied to small areas of scratched or scraped (abraded) skin of rats or mice, and radionuclide retention at the undisturbed application site was measured at several intervals during 1 d. The individual studies are described in Appendix A.4.2, and the data and sources are given in Table A.12. The general trend of radionuclide absorption from the abraded skin is the same as was observed for those same radionuclides applied to skin incisions or deposited in puncture wounds (Table 4.4). The amounts of the individual radionuclides absorbed from an undisturbed skin abrasion are nearly the same as from a deeper cut (laceration). Therefore, the default fractions of early radionuclide absorption from a puncture wound, suggested for application to contaminated lacerations (Section 4.3.2), can reasonably be applied to the case of contaminated abraded skin.

4.3.4 Intact Skin

Seven radionuclides in solution were applied to small areas of the shaved skin of rats. Absorption at 1 d is shown in Table 4.4. The individual studies are described in Appendix A.4.1, and the data and sources are given in Tables A.11 and A.13. Because there may have been technical problems in the early studies of the absorption of $^{239}Pu^{4+}$ through the skin of rats, only the more recent results for percutaneous absorption of $^{239}Pu(NO_3)_4$ in dilute HNO_3 applied to rat skin are included in Tables 4.4, A.11, and A.13 (Appendix A.4). The data in Table 4.4 show that fractional absorption of radionuclides applied to intact skin depends on aqueous solubility, tendency to hydrolyze at physiological pH, and tendency to bind to protein, and that radionuclide absorption through the skin is in the same order as absorption of these same radionuclides from damaged skin or from a puncture wound.

Early absorption through intact skin of radionuclides that are anions or cations of low electric charge ($\leq 2+$) is ~2.5 % of the amount applied, while absorption of readily hydrolyzed cationic radionuclides of higher charge ($\geq 3+$) is, on average, 0.05 % of the amount applied. Reasonable default values for transcutaneous absorption of radionuclides expressed as fractions of their early absorption from a puncture wound are, as follows: weakly and moderately retained, 0.025; strongly and avidly retained, 0.002.

4.3.5 *Thermally-Burned Skin*

Absorption of several chemically dissimilar radionuclides applied to the skin of rats immediately after infliction of Grade I to III thermal burns was, within the range of experimental error, not different from that through intact skin. However, the twofold increase in absorption of $^{144}Ce^{3+}$ through rat skin that had been burned 36 h earlier with a ultraviolet lamp could be attributed to disruption of the skin barrier (Table A.11).

4.3.6 *Acid-Burned Skin*

Absorption of $^{241}Am(NO_3)_3$, $^{210}Po(NO_3)_4$, or $^{239}Pu(NO_3)_4$ applied to shaved rat skin in 0.03 to 10 mol L^{-1} HNO_3 was determined (Appendix A.4.4). The experimental conditions and radionuclide absorption at 1 and 3 d are given in Table A.13 in the order of increasing HNO_3 concentration of the solutions applied to the skin. The skin of the rats in the baseline studies, for example, $^{239}Pu(NO_3)_4$ in 0.1 mol L^{-1} HNO_3, could not be considered undamaged, but the barrier to absorption appeared to remain intact. The baseline values of fractional absorption of the study radionuclides at 1 d are given in Table 4.4. When applied in 0.5 to 1 mol L^{-1} HNO_3, absorption of those radionuclides was, on average, five times their baseline values. When applied in solutions of ≥ 2.5 mol L^{-1} HNO_3, absorption of $^{241}Am^{3+}$ was somewhat greater than its baseline value, while absorption of $^{210}Po^{4+}$ and $^{239}Pu^{4+}$ was similar to or less than their baseline values. There was a clear trend, most prominent for $^{241}Am^{3+}$, towards continued absorption from the acid-burned skin, and the absorbed fractions of all three radionuclides were, on average, five times greater at 3 d than at 1 d.

4.3.7 *Radiation-Burned Skin*

Follow-up on the victims of the ^{137}Cs radiation accident in Goiânia, Brazil indicated that ^{137}Cs was detectable up to 3 y post-exposure in scar tissue in the skin of persons who received radiation burns from direct contact with high-activity particles of $^{137}CsCl$ (Lipsztein *et al.*, 1998). This long-term retention in scar tissue is not included in the current wound model, but should be borne in mind in case of similar incidents, as it could have a significant effect on both local and systemic dose calculations.

4.4 Modeling of Radioactive Colloids and Particles

Modeling the retention and translocation of radioelements deposited in wound sites as initially insoluble materials is more difficult than for soluble materials, because there are few suitable data sets from which model parameter estimates can be obtained. The consequence of this lack of data for deposited colloids, precipitates, particles and fragments is that it is impractical to consider developing default groupings of radionuclides based on their chemical properties, such as was done with the radionuclides injected in initially soluble forms.

Most of the data available for modeling involve exposure of animals to a variety of physicochemical forms of plutonium and a more limited number of solid forms of uranium (Appendix B). Data from studies in which colloidal or particulate plutonium were s.c. implanted into dog paws have been used to develop a working set of fitted model parameter values. Additional comparative modeling was also done by using data from rodents and rabbits in which variable amounts (up to 250 µg) of colloidal plutonium were i.m. injected. These results provide the basis for defining default biokinetic behaviors of relatively insoluble forms of radionuclides in wounds.

There are two phenomenologic/mechanistic aspects of modeling the biokinetics of colloids, particles, aggregates and fragments in a wound site that differ from the phenomena associated with wound sites contaminated with initially soluble radionuclides. First, the presence of biologically recognizable particulate material in a wound site has the potential to elicit a foreign-body reaction not associated with the deposition of soluble substances. This reaction usually begins with a localized inflammatory reaction, influx of neutrophils and mobile tissue macrophages, and later the development of fibrous connective tissue around the particle/fragment deposition site. With time, fibrous connective tissue can form a complete capsule, separating the foreign material from normal tissue. These phenomena are described in Section 2.3.5 and Appendix F.

Second, because most of the radioactive materials likely to contaminate a wound as colloids, particles, aggregates or fragments are sparingly soluble in water at neutral pH, it is reasonable to assume the following: after deposition of colloids, particles, aggregates or fragments containing a radionuclide, the rate of dissolution and transfer from the wound site will be small enough that the probability of initially solubilized ions being converted into less-soluble forms in CIS is likewise small. Therefore, atoms that are released from the PABS into the soluble compartment are assumed to proceed only to blood, at a rate determined empirically from the data. This simplification (i.e., setting the transfer rate from soluble to CIS equal to zero), allows the model as defined in Figure 4.1 to function for particles, aggregates and fragments without the need for two separate and competing pathways for soluble and insoluble materials (i.e., the soluble, CIS, and PABS compartments for the former, and the fragments, PABS, TPA, and soluble compartments for the latter).

In the following sections, results of modeling several data sets, most relating to plutonium-contaminated wounds, are presented. The primary data, taken from the Colorado State University dog studies, include plutonium introduced in nitrate form but likely to have been at least partially a plutonium colloid, as air-oxidized micrometer-sized particles, and as high-fired plutonium oxide submicrometer particles. A collection of studies in which rats were i.m. injected with colloidal plutonium hydroxide is also modeled, as is a separate study in which colloidal plutonium hydroxide was i.m. injected into rabbits. Tetravalent plutonium was used in all of the above studies.

Insoluble radioactive materials that have been deposited in experimental wounds in animals include aqueous suspensions of colloidal hydroxides, hydroxide polymers, and particulates of crystalline solids; dry particles; metal fragments; and actinide-contaminated minispheres of fused soil and structural materials. Except for i.m.-implanted suspensions of insoluble particles of some representative metal oxides and phosphates (Appendix B.2; Morrow *et al.*, 1968), the radioactive materials and contaminated solids studies are various chemical and physical forms of actinide elements, most often plutonium and uranium. Appendix B summarizes the experimental conditions and the wound retention data of those animal studies. Wound retention can be described for three categories of insoluble radioactive materials based on their physical and chemical forms: colloidal and polymeric hydroxides, small solid particles, and metal fragments and particles too large to be phagocytized.

4.4.1 *Wound Retention of $^{239}Pu^{4+}$ Hydroxide Colloids and Polymers Injected Intramuscularly in Rats and Rabbits and Subcutaneously in Dogs*

The wound retention data from the experiments involving colloidal $^{239}Pu^{4+}$ in wounds are given in Table B.1 for the rats and rabbits and in Tables B.2 and B.3 for the beagle dogs. All of those studies were originally intended as investigations of the biokinetics of i.m. or s.c.-injected Pu^{4+} or retention in puncture wounds of Pu^{4+} in solution. However, as discussed in Appendices A.1.1.4 to A.1.1.6, the solubility product of $Pu(OH)_4$ was exceeded in the injection media used ($\geq 10^{-6}$ mol L^{-1} plutonium, pH > 2), and the plutonium in each preparation was probably at least partially a suspension of colloidal hydrolysis products.

Retention of Pu^{4+} introduced into a deep puncture wound as a mixture of colloidal hydrolysis products differs quantitatively from that of a comparable mass of Pu^{4+} in solution, in that retention is greater and more prolonged. For example, a larger fraction of 2.9 μg of colloidal $^{239}Pu^{4+}$ at pH 2.4 s.c. injected in the dog paw (Figure B.4) is cleared more slowly than 1.6 to 3.2 μg of $^{239}Pu^{4+}$ in 0.1 mol L^{-1} HNO_3 i.m. injected in rats (Table A.2; Figure A.1).

No individual study of the i.m. injection of 16 to 240 μg of colloidal $^{239}Pu^{4+}$ hydroxide in rats provided sufficient data to define both the early and later phases of plutonium retention at the wound site. However, the results of the five similar studies agreed reasonably well (Table B.1), and they were combined for analysis.

The data from each study or group of studies of deposited colloidal Pu^{4+} hydroxides in animals, namely 2.9 to 52 μg plutonium s.c. injected in dog paws (Appendix B.1.1.6; Figures B.3, B.4, and 4.14; Bistline, 1973), 16 to 240 μg plutonium i.m. injected in rats (Appendices B.1.1.1 to B.1.1.3; Figures B.1, 4.15, and 4.16; Lafuma *et al.*, 1971; Morin *et al.*, 1972; 1973a; Nenot *et al.*, 1972a; Scott *et al,*. 1948a), and 57 or 105 mg plutonium i.m. injected in rabbits (Appendix B.1.1.4; Figures B.2, 4.17, and 4.18; Taylor, 1969), were analyzed separately with the wound model. Four multiexponential

Transfer rates for wound site retention of ^{239}Pu s.c. introduced as partially colloidal nitrate into the forepaws of dogs.[a]

Pathway	Transfer Rate (d^{-1})
Soluble to blood	0.47
Soluble to CIS	2.64
CIS to soluble	0.025
CIS to PABS	0.049
PABS to soluble	0.0014
PABS to lymph nodes	0.00042
CIS to lymph nodes	0.0019
Lymph nodes to blood	0.029

[a]Material injected into soluble compartment.

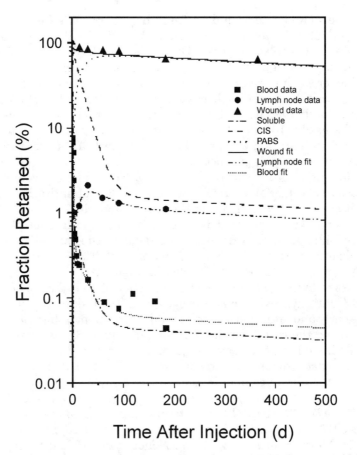

Fig. 4.14. Model fit of retention of plutonium [≥15 µg of partially colloidal ^{239}Pu(NO$_3$)$_4$] s.c. injected in dogs (wound and lymph-node data from Table B.2; blood data from Table B.3).

Transfer rates for wound-site retention of plutonium i.m. injected in colloidal form into rats.[a]

Pathway	Transfer Rate (d^{-1})
Soluble to blood	1.0
Soluble to CIS	86
CIS to soluble	0.58
CIS to PABS	0.016
PABS to soluble	0.00
PABS to lymph nodes	0.00002[b]
CIS to lymph nodes	0.00002[b]
Lymph nodes to blood	0.00001[b]

[a]Material injected into soluble compartment.
[b]Parameter value fixed.

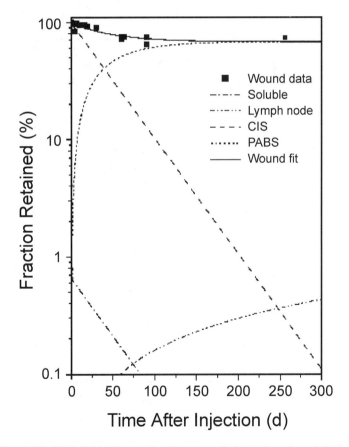

Fig. 4.15. Model fit of wound retention of plutonium i.m. injected as colloidal plutonium hydroxide (16 to 240 μg) into rats [data from Table B.1; ICRP (1994a) default lymph-node transfer rates used].

Transfer rates for wound-site retention of plutonium i.m. injected in colloidal form into rats; dog lymph-node transfer rates applied.[a]

Pathway	Transfer Rate (d^{-1})
Soluble to blood	0.062
Soluble to CIS	4.3
CIS to soluble	0.35
CIS to PABS	0.019
PABS to soluble	0.00
PABS to lymph nodes	0.00042[b]
CIS to lymph nodes	0.0019[b]
Lymph nodes to blood	0.029[b]

[a]Material injected into soluble compartment.
[b]Parameter value fixed.

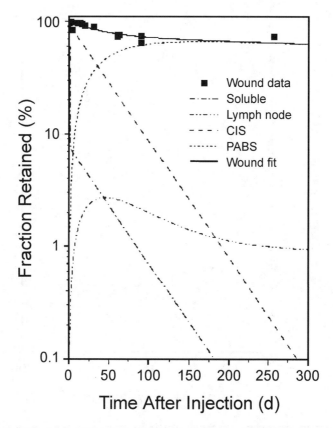

Fig. 4.16. Model fit of wound retention of colloidal plutonium i.m. injected into rats. Alternate approach using lymph-node transfer rates derived from study of plutonium colloid in dogs (Figure 4.14, wound data from Table B.1).

Transfer rates for the wound-site retention of plutonium i.m. injected in colloidal form into rabbits.[a]

Pathway	Transfer Rate (d^{-1})
Soluble to blood	0.058
Soluble to CIS	0.00
CIS to soluble	0.022
CIS to PABS	0.029
PABS to soluble	0.00
CIS to lymph nodes	0.00002[b]
PABS to lymph nodes	0.00002[b]
Lymph nodes to blood	0.00001[b]

[a]Material injected into CIS compartment.
[b]Parameter value fixed.

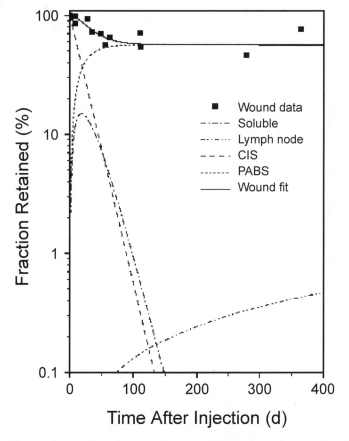

Fig. 4.17. Model fit of wound retention of plutonium i.m. injected as colloidal plutonium hydroxide into rabbits (57 or 105 µg; data from Table B.1).

Transfer rates for wound-site retention of colloidal plutonium i.m. injected into rabbits; dog lymph-node transfer rates applied.[a]

Pathway	Transfer Rate (d^{-1})
Soluble to blood	0.052
Soluble to CIS	0.00087
CIS to soluble	0.022
CIS to PABS	0.039
PABS to soluble	0.00
PABS to lymph nodes	0.00042[b]
CIS to lymph nodes	0.0019[b]
Lymph nodes to blood	0.029[b]

[a]Material injected into CIS compartment.
[b]Parameter value fixed.

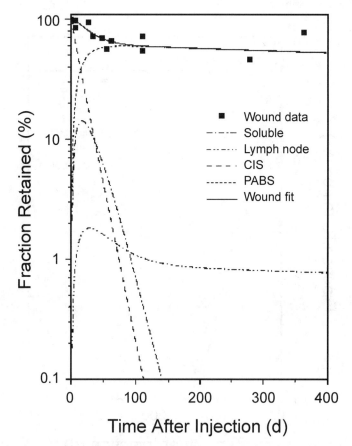

Fig. 4.18. Model fit of wound retention of plutonium i.m. injected as colloidal plutonium hydroxide into rabbits. Alternative approach using lymph-node transfer rates derived from study of plutonium colloid in dogs (Figure 4.14).

equations were obtained describing retention of the plutonium deposited at the wound site, and their parameters are collected in Table 4.5.

The initial clearance rates, λ_1, and the fractions of the deposited colloidal Pu^{4+}, A_1, cleared at those rates are problematic, because both λ_1 and A_1 are strongly influenced by the availability of early kinetic data. Only the studies in dogs provide early kinetic data in the form of serial blood sampling that was initiated within 2 h after the plutonium injection. The first rate constants, λ_1, provided by the dog studies are probably the best representation of the clearance of colloidal plutonium from a puncture wound during the first hours after the injection.

In the study using rabbits, wound plutonium retention was defined by radioanalysis of the i.m.-injected legs, and the first sample was taken at 1 d. The initial rate constant of the wound plutonium retention equation obtained in that study represents the average rate of clearance during the first 24 h after the injection. Variability of the wound plutonium retention among the small number of individual rabbits adds to the overall uncertainty of the parameters of the retention equation (Equation B.2a).

The first measurements of wound plutonium retention (radioanalysis of the i.m.-injected legs) in the rat studies, made at 1 to 4 d, and the scatter in the data of the combined studies obscure the earliest phase of wound plutonium retention in rats i.m. injected with 16 to 240 µg of colloidal Pu^{4+} hydroxide. The fraction cleared during the first day probably did not exceed 5 % of the deposited amount, and the initial rate of clearance was likely to have been similar to that found for rabbits i.m. injected with similarly large amounts of plutonium.

The initial phase of clearance of plutonium from the i.m. wound site could not be defined for the rats injected with 6.6 to 7.2 µg of a prepared $^{239}Pu^{4+}$ hydroxide polymer, because the preparation was a mixture of polymerized plutonium hydroxide and soluble plutonium citrate (Bahzin *et al.*, 1984; Appendix B.1.1.5). The fraction of the polymerized plutonium in the preparation cleared on the first day was likely to have been small.

The parameters of the wound plutonium retention equations shown in Table 4.5 demonstrate the dependence of early clearance on the amount of colloidal Pu^{4+} deposited. Large deposited masses that produce higher local concentrations of readily hydrolyzable or already hydrolyzed Pu^{4+} support more rapid formation of more and larger aggregates and cross-linked polymers, which are progressively more difficult to dissolve. A substantial fraction of a small mass of colloidal Pu^{4+} (2.9 µg) s.c. injected in the dog paw was

TABLE 4.5—*Parameters of multiexponential wound retention equations for suspensions of $^{239}Pu^{4+}$ hydroxides i.m. or s.c. deposited in rats, rabbits or dogs.*^{a,b,c}

Study Conditions					Parameters of Wound Retention Equations^a						
Plutonium Mass (µg)	pH of Medium	Study Length (d)	Animal	Injection Mode	A_1 (%)	λ_1 (d^{-1})	A_2 (%)	λ_2 (d^{-1})	A_3 (%)	λ_3 (d^{-1})	Equation Number
2.9	2.4	0.08 – 365	Dog	s.c.	23	26	8.0	0.05	69	7.6×10^{-4}	B.8
15 – 52	2.4	0.08 – 185	Dog	s.c.	15	3.1	8.0	0.056	77	7.3×10^{-4}	B.9
57, 105	~7	1 – 365	Rabbit	i.m.	5	1.3	31	0.022	64	1.2×10^{-4}	B.2a
16 – 240	1.5 – 2.5	1 – 256	Rat	i.m.	~3^d	~0.9^d	28	0.022	69	8×10^{-5}	B.1
Retention of ≥15 µg of colloidal $^{239}Pu^{4+}$; three studies combined					5	1.8	22	0.036	73	4.7×10^{-4}	4.6

^{a}Retention equations of the form $R(t) = \sum_i A_i e^{-\lambda_i t}$ were obtained from data analysis using the wound model and Origin$^®$ software. $R(0) = 100\%$.

^{b}Colloidal $^{239}Pu^{4+}$ hydroxide species formed in injection media (Appendix B.1.1.3).

^{c}Wound model analysis using lymph-node transfer rates obtained for dogs s.c. injected with 15 to 52 µg of plutonium

^{d}Initial fastest-clearing component estimated and subtracted from the two components shown in Equation B.1.

initially rapidly cleared to blood. A smaller fraction of the larger mass of colloidal Pu^{4+} (15 to 52 mg) similarly injected in dogs was initially cleared more slowly, but the amounts and rates of clearance of the longest-retained fraction were similar. Only small fractions of the largest mass of colloidal Pu^{4+} ($\geq$16 µg in rats and rabbits) were cleared with half-times $\leq$1 d, substantial fractions were cleared at moderate rates (half-times ~30 d), and the longest retained fractions were cleared at rates about one-tenth of that observed for the smallest mass of colloidal Pu^{4+} (2.9 µg) deposited in the dog paws.

The three rate constants of the wound plutonium retention equations shown in Table 4.5, λ_1, λ_2, λ_3, and the initial, fastest-clearing fraction of the deposited plutonium, A_1, are highly negatively correlated with the mass of colloidal Pu^{4+} deposited. The partition coefficient of the second term A_2, is positively correlated with the deposited mass of colloidal Pu^{4+}, while that of the slowest-clearing fraction, A_3, is less dependent on the mass of colloidal Pu^{4+} deposited. Linear regression was used to analyze the trends of the individual retention equation parameters and to predict equations describing plutonium retention in a puncture wound after deposition of colloidal Pu^{4+}. The predicted equations for retention of 1 or 16 µg of colloidal Pu^{4+} were almost the same as those obtained from the wound model analysis of the blood data for the dogs injected with 2.9 µg [Equation B.8 (blood data only)] or $\geq$15 µg [Equation B.9 (wound, lymph-node, and blood data)] of colloidal Pu^{4+}, respectively.

Retention of the larger amounts of colloidal Pu^{4+} (16 to 240 µg) deposited in a deep puncture wound was also approximated by using the wound model to reanalyze the combined wound plutonium data for the rats, rabbits and dogs injected with $\geq$15 µg. The plutonium retention curve for the combined wound data is shown in Figure 4.19, compared to the retention curves obtained for the individual contributing studies of retention of colloidal Pu^{4+} in the rats, dogs and rabbits. The equation of the combined wound retention curve ($\% \, ID$) is:

$$R(t)_{\geq 15 \text{ µg}} = 5e^{-1.8t} + 22e^{-0.036t} + 73e^{-0.00047t}, \qquad (4.6)$$

where t is days after plutonium deposition.

4.4.1.1 *Modeling Colloidal Plutonium Nitrate Injected Subcutaneously in Dogs.* The reanalyzed data used for this modeling are described in Appendix B.1. The results of modeling these data

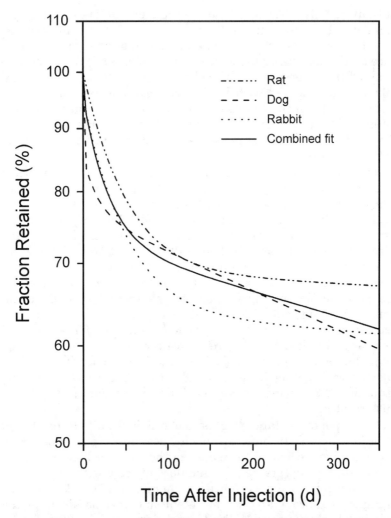

Fig. 4.19. Comparison of retention of ≥15 μg of colloidal Pu^{4+} in a deep puncture wound in rats (Figure B.1; Equation B.1), dogs (Figure B.3; Equation B.9), and rabbits (Figure B.2; Equation B.2a), each calculated from the model, with that calculated by the model from the three species combined.

are presented in Figure 4.14. Three data sets were available: wound site, lymph nodes draining the wound site, and blood. Both lymph-node and blood data were important for defining the relative partitioning of plutonium clearance from the wound site between clearance, presumably as particles, to lymph nodes and clearance by dissolution to the soluble compartment and transfer to blood. As described in detail in Appendix B.1, the original state of the plutonium in the injection solution was not known, but the records indicate that the plutonium (15 to 52 μg plutonium, pH 2.4) was at least partially in a colloidal hydroxide form when it was injected into the dog forepaw. Because the state of the injection solution was undetermined and probably consisted of a mixture of colloidal and soluble plutonium, the material was introduced initially into the soluble compartment of the wound model. Initially after injection, ~10 to 15 % of the plutonium left the wound site; most of this plutonium was detected in the blood. Concomitantly, the bulk of the remaining plutonium was in CIS, peaking at 1 d and decreasing thereafter. This initial partitioning between CIS and blood is reflected in the relative magnitudes of the transfer rates from soluble to CIS and soluble to blood, with approximately six times more plutonium transferring to CIS compared to blood. Of the plutonium in CIS, ~33 % was redistributed back to blood, 65 % was converted to the longer-retained PABS, and 2 % was transferred to lymph nodes. After ~10 d, most of the plutonium in the wound site was modeled to be in PABS, where it was retained for the duration of the study and accounted for the long-term retention at the wound site.

The modeling results also suggested that the colloidal form of plutonium used in this study was somewhat soluble in the long term. The movement of plutonium out of PABS to the soluble compartment was about three times greater than the movement of plutonium to lymph nodes. It is also interesting to note that the dissolution of plutonium from CIS to soluble, characterized by its transfer rate constant (0.025 d^{-1}), was similar to that from lymph nodes to blood (0.029 d^{-1}). This suggests that the transformation of the colloidal and/or polymeric forms of plutonium to a soluble form occurred in the lymph nodes in a manner similar to the presumably more labile form of plutonium resident in CIS. Note that the transfer rate of plutonium in PABS to soluble was ~0.05 of that for CIS and lymph nodes, suggesting that the shift from CIS to PABS was consistent with transformation of the colloid and/or polymer to a chemically less-soluble form. Although this discussion of the chemistry of the plutonium in this study is hypothetical and may apply solely to the results of this study, it is nevertheless within the bounds of published behaviors of plutonium hydroxy complexes, whose rates of polymerization and depolymerization depend strongly on how they were initially created in terms of solution pH, plutonium concentration, temperature and time of storage, and presence of competing complexing agents such as citrate (Cleveland, 1970; Lindenbaum and Westfall, 1965).

4.4.1.2 *Modeling Colloidal Plutonium Hydroxide Injected Intra-muscularly in Rats.* The wound retention of >5 µg of plutonium i.m. injected as colloidal hydroxide of indeterminate characteristics is shown for rats (combined data from several studies) along with the model fits in Figure 4.15. As in the case of the dogs injected with plutonium nitrate/colloid, the plutonium of undetermined physico-chemical state used in the rat studies was introduced into the soluble compartment of the wound model. Transfer of plutonium from the soluble compartment proceeds rapidly (12 min half-time), with the shift of ~99 % of the plutonium to CIS. Thereafter, clearance from CIS partitions between recirculation of ~98 % of the contents of CIS to soluble, from which 1 % proceeds to blood, and movement of ~2 % of the contents of CIS to PABS. This suggested rapid recycling of material between soluble and CIS compartments is not logical and is probably a modeling artifact. On the other hand, given the uncertain chemical state of the plutonium, it is possible that some of the hydroxylated forms of plutonium may be amenable to competitive complexation by endogenous ligands, resulting in shifts between so-called soluble and colloidal forms. However, it does not appear reasonable that this recycling mechanism would apply to so much of the plutonium (98 %). In any case, the underlying modeling substructure does not affect the good fit to the long-term retention of plutonium within the wound itself (Figure 4.15).

A part of the uncertainty associated with modeling the movement of plutonium within the soluble, CIS, and PABS compartments is due to the lack of data on transfer of plutonium to blood and lymph nodes. In particular, the lack of lymph-node data necessitated imposing assumed lymph-node transfer rates from CIS and PABS. The assumed rate from each compartment to lymph nodes was taken to be 2×10^{-5}, the value used for clearance of particles from the alveolar-interstitial region of the lung to the associated lymph nodes draining the parenchymal lung (ICRP, 1994a).

An alternative approach to assuming that clearance to lymph nodes is similar to that modeled for the lung parenchyma is to assume that the transfer rates determined from the modeling of the movement of plutonium colloid in the dog (Section 4.4.2) are similar for plutonium in the rat. This approach was applied to the rat data, with the results shown in Figure 4.16. The notable differences between this and the previous fit are: (1) the slower kinetics of exchange between the soluble compartment and blood (0.062 versus 1 d^{-1}) and CIS (4.3 versus 86 d^{-1}) compartments, (2) the slower return from CIS to soluble (0.35 versus 0.58 d^{-1}), and (3) the greater uptake in lymph nodes because of the larger transfer to lymph nodes from CIS (0.0019 versus 0.00002 d^{-1}) and PABS (0.00042 versus 0.00002 d^{-1}). Also employed in this modeling exercise was the transfer rate of plutonium from lymph nodes to blood of 0.029 versus the original assumption of 0.00001 d^{-1}. The effects on lymph-node uptake and retention can be seen in Figure 4.16, in which the uptake peaks at ~3 % at 30 d; for the preceding fit using the lung default transfer rates (Figure 4.15), the lymph-node values increase slowly but steadily so that 0.4 % is predicted to be in lymph nodes by 300 d after injection. The lymph-node data from Harrison *et al.* (1978b), in which rats were i.m. injected with 3.2 µg ^{239}Pu nitrate, showed ~2 % of the amount injected in lymph nodes one week after injection, which is more consistent with the model results in which the lymph-node transfer rates obtained from the dog study were used.

4.4.1.3 *Modeling Colloidal Plutonium Hydroxide Injected Intramuscularly in Rabbits.* The study of Taylor (1969) involved i.m. injection of a freshly prepared, neutralized solution of ^{239}Pu(NO$_3$)$_4$, which almost certainly was a colloidal suspension of plutonium hydroxide (Appendix B.1.1.4). Accordingly, it was considered more appropriate to introduce this plutonium preparation directly into the CIS rather than the soluble compartment. The plutonium initially present in the CIS compartment partitions almost equally between the soluble (43 %) and PABS (56 %) compartments, and with a half-time of ~28 d. These transfer rates out of CIS are similar to those modeled for colloidal plutonium in the dog. The effect of these transfers is that most of the long-retained plutonium ends up in PABS within ~50 d. It is also interesting to note that no recirculation from soluble to CIS is predicted, so that plutonium reaching the soluble compartment can only transfer to blood.

Similarly to the alternative modeling done with colloidal plutonium in rats (Section 4.4.1.2), the transfer rates from CIS and PABS to lymph nodes obtained from the dog study with colloidal plutonium were used to model the rabbit data. Unlike the analogous modeling done with the rats, there were few significant differences in the transfer rates for the wound-associated compartments. For this latter case, the soluble-CIS pathway was opened, but at a very slow rate (0.00087 d^{-1}). As expected, there is a difference in the uptake and retention of plutonium in the lymph nodes, with an early peak at ~20 d occurring due to transfer from CIS to lymph nodes, followed by a long-retained amount at about half the peak value, which is replenished mainly from plutonium in PABS. Without lymph-node data, the choice between modeling approaches is not clear. Nevertheless, the consistency of plutonium uptake and retention in lymph nodes based on the modeling results obtained using the dog data are logically more consistent.

4.4.1.4 *Summary of Modeling Colloidal Plutonium.* It was assumed that in cases of i.m. or s.c.-injected colloidal Pu^{4+}, some of the plutonium leaving the wound site would be transferred to the major draining lymph nodes. In three studies that lacked lymph-node data, dogs injected with 2.9 µg and rats and rabbits injected with 16 to 240 µg of colloidal Pu^{4+}, the transfer rates (CIS to lymph nodes, PABS to lymph nodes, lymph nodes to blood) that were obtained for the dogs injected with ≥15 µg of colloidal Pu^{4+} were introduced as fixed parameter values.

In three of the four studies involving injected colloidal Pu^{4+}, model solutions were obtained assuming that the plutonium had been introduced into the soluble compartment. In the case of the rabbits, the injection medium was reportedly neutral, and the best model solution was obtained by assuming the plutonium was introduced into the CIS compartment of the wound model (Figures 4.17 and 4.18). In the case of the rats, a satisfactory model solution (not shown) could also be obtained by assuming that hydrolysis of the injection media was well advanced and introducing it into the CIS compartment.

In performing the model calculations, it was found that the transfer rates, PABS to soluble, for both the rats and rabbits were vanishingly small ($<10^{-8}$ d^{-1}), and those transfer rates were fixed at zero.

The conditions of the animal experiments that involved deposition of colloidal Pu^{4+} in a simulated puncture wound differed substantially. The Pu^{4+} preparations were introduced into a muscle mass with a small connective tissue component in the i.m.-injected rats and rabbits, and into a mass of loose connective tissue in the s.c.-injected dog paws. The degree of hydrolysis of the Pu^{4+} may have ranged from incompletely formed hydrolysis products (2.9 µg Pu^{4+}, pH 2.4, one group of dogs) to fully-formed $Pu(OH)_4$, (57 or 105 µg Pu^{4+}, pH ~7, rabbits). Even so, their wound retention curves (Figure 4.19) and their wound retention equations (Equations B.1, B.2a, B.8, and B.9) are similar. Their wound model transfer rates have common features; the most prominent is the quantitative description of the tendency to undergo chemically and/or physiologically driven changes within the wound that render the plutonium more insoluble and progressively less mobile. The chemical changes from soluble to the CIS state are rapid, while resolubilization of the plutonium in the CIS state, CIS to soluble, is considerably slower. The transition to the less accessible PABS state, CIS to

PABS, occurs more slowly, but resolubilization of plutonium in the PABS state and transfer of aggregated plutonium to lymph nodes, PABS to lymph nodes, are so slow that within 2.5 to 4 months nearly all of the plutonium retained in the wound can be considered to be trapped and immobilized in the PABS state.

Over the range of 2.9 to 240 µg of colloidal $^{239}Pu^{4+}$, the rate of transfer from the soluble state to blood is inversely dependent on the mass of deposited plutonium in the wound and on the state of aggregation of the colloid in the injection medium. Mass dependent behavior is less apparent or absent for any subsequent changes that may occur within the wound. The rates of transition from soluble to the relatively insoluble CIS state and the rates of solubilization of the colloidal Pu^{4+}, CIS to soluble, vary among the Pu^{4+} dosages, animals, and experimental conditions, while the rates of transition from the CIS state to entrapment as aggregates and/or otherwise bound forms in the PABS state are comparable across the four studies, on average, 0.039 ± 0.014 d^{-1}.

The rates of transfer of the plutonium to lymph nodes from both CIS and PABS states are slow, as is the rate of resolubilization of Pu^{4+} trapped in the PABS state, PABS to soluble. Combined, those three transfer rates (PABS to soluble, CIS to lymph nodes, PABS to lymph nodes) determine the slow late clearance of colloidal Pu^{4+} from a wound. The transfer rates of colloidal Pu^{4+} into lymph nodes, which could be calculated by the wound model only for the dogs s.c. injected with ≥ 15 µg of plutonium, were imposed as fixed parameter values for modeling wound and/or blood data from the three other cases involving injected colloidal Pu^{4+}. Consequently, in those cases the net long-term exit rate from the wound has been constrained, perhaps artificially, to occur only *via* transfer to lymph nodes.

The relative transfers of plutonium to more insoluble states (soluble to CIS) (CIS to soluble)$^{-1}$, and (CIS to PABS) (CIS to soluble)$^{-1}$, and the relative retention versus release of sequestered plutonium, (CIS to PABS) (PABS to soluble and/or lymph nodes)$^{-1}$, favor progressive immobilization of plutonium and its prolonged retention in the wound. The relative transfers of 2.9 µg of colloidal Pu^{4+} can be compared directly with those obtained for ≤ 5 µg of a strongly-retained dissolved radionuclide (Table 4.3). The relative transfers, (soluble to CIS) (soluble to blood)$^{-1}$, which reflect the initial partitioning of the radionuclide between less- and more-soluble chemical forms, is five times greater for colloidal Pu^{4+}. The relative tendency for resolubilization of a radionuclide in the CIS state, (CIS to soluble) (soluble to CIS)$^{-1}$, for the colloidal Pu^{4+} is only 2 % of that for a small mass of strongly-retained radionuclide. Further immobilization of the deposited radionuclide relative to resolubilization, (CIS to PABS) (CIS to soluble)$^{-1}$, for the colloidal Pu^{4+} is five times greater, while the relative tendency for release of the colloidal Pu^{4+} from the PABS state by dissolution, (PABS to soluble) (CIS to PABS)$^{-1}$, is <10 % of that for a small mass of a strongly-retained radionuclide.

The wound model parameters developed from the s.c. injection of 2.9 µg of potentially colloidal Pu^{4+} in the dog paw (Table 4.6) can reasonably be applied to cases of deposition of 5 mg of colloidal Pu^{4+} in a wound.

The animal studies in which larger amounts of colloidal Pu^{4+} were deposited in simulated wounds (i.m. or s.c. injection; three species; mass range, 15 to 240 µg of colloidal Pu^{4+}; chemical status of the plutonium probably varying from mixtures of incomplete hydrolysis products to fully-formed plutonium hydroxide) encompass a broad range of experimental conditions. Combined, they may be regarded as representative of a deep puncture wound with >8 µg of colloidal Pu^{4+} suspended in a weakly acidic, alkaline or neutral solution. The wound model parameters developed from their combined wound plutonium data (Table 4.6) can reasonably be applied to cases of wound deposition of larger amounts of colloidal Pu^{4+}.

4.4.2 *Wound Retention of $^{239}PuO_2$ Particles Injected Subcutaneously in Dogs*

4.4.2.1 *Air-Oxidized $^{239}PuO_2$ Particles Injected Subcutaneously in Dogs.* The data set available from the study of the wound retention of plutonium s.c. injected into the forepaws of dogs in the form of air-oxidized $^{239}PuO_2$ particles (7 µm average physical diameter) contained adequate data to allow different modeling approaches. Although there were no tissue data available at early times after injection (<10 d), blood plutonium was measured from 1 d onward. Details of the treatment of data used here are given in Appendix B.1.3.

In the first modeling approach, the plutonium in the systemic compartments was calculated by summing the plutonium contents in the tissues associated with accumulation of soluble plutonium (all but the wound site and lymph nodes) plus estimates of plutonium excreted in urine and feces. Expressed in this way, the systemic compartment integrates all of the plutonium that clears to the blood. As such, it does not truly represent the time-dependent tissue content, but allows the model to partition the clearance of plutonium from the wound site between mechanical clearance to lymph nodes and dissolution/absorption to blood. The model fits to the three data sets, wound, lymph nodes and systemic, are shown in Figure 4.20 along with the associated transfer rates.

TABLE 4.6—Transfer rates of wound model for retention in experimental deep puncture wounds of plutonium deposited as colloidal $^{239}Pu^{4+}$ hydrolysis products.[a]

^{239}Pu (µg)	2.9	15 – 52	16 – 240	57, 105	15 – 240[b]
Animal	Dog	Dog	Rat	Rabbit	Combined Species
Injection mode	s.c.	s.c.	i.m.	i.m.	i.m., s.c.
Input to model	Soluble	Soluble	Soluble	CIS	Soluble
Intercompartmental Transfer Rates (d^{-1})					
Soluble to blood	6.3	0.47	0.062	0.052	0.27
Soluble to CIS	34	2.0	4.3	8.7×10^{-4}	3.2
CIS to soluble	0.025	0.025	0.35	0.022	0.19
CIS to PABS	0.048	0.049	0.019	0.039	0.034
PABS to soluble	1×10^{-5}	1.4×10^{-3}	0.00	0.00	0.00
CIS to lymph nodes	1.9×10^{-3} [c]	1.9×10^{-3}	1.9×10^{-3} [c]	1.9×10^{-3} [c]	1.9×10^{-3} [c]
PABS to lymph nodes	4.2×10^{-4} [c]	4.2×10^{-4}	4.2×10^{-4} [c]	4.2×10^{-4} [c]	4.2×10^{-4} [c]
Lymph nodes to blood	0.029 [c]	0.029	0.029 [c]	0.029 [c]	0.029 [c]
Blood to systemic	0.9[d]	0.9[e]	—[e]	—[e]	—[e]

[a]Wound model data: dog, 15 to 52 µg plutonium, Figure 4.14; rat, Figure 4.15; rabbit, Figure 4.17.
[b]Combined wound retention data for rats, rabbits and dogs injected with ≥15 µg of colloidal ^{239}Pu^{4+}.
[c]Parameter value fixed, based on transfer rate for dogs s.c. injected with 15 to 52 µg of colloidal ^{239}Pu^{4+}.
[d]Parameter value fixed, based on blood plutonium clearance from dogs (Appendix B.1.6.3).
[e]With no outlet, blood is subsumed in the systemic compartment.

Transfer rates for wound-site retention of plutonium as air-oxidized
$^{239}PuO_2$ particles s.c. introduced into the forepaws of dogs.[a]

Pathway	Transfer Rate (d^{-1})
Soluble to blood	0.052
Soluble to CIS	0.0[b]
PABS to TPA	0.047
TPA to PABS	0.0034
PABS to soluble	0.00048
PABS to lymph nodes	0.0045
Lymph nodes to blood	0.00001

[a]Material injected into PABS compartment.
[b]Parameter value fixed.

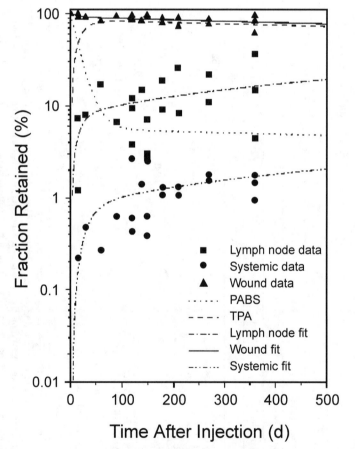

Fig. 4.20. Model fit of wound retention of plutonium in dogs s.c.
implanted with air-oxidized $^{239}PuO_2$ particles (wound, lymph-node, and
systemic data used from Table B.4).

Because the plutonium used in this study was prepared as solid micrometer-sized oxide particles, the particle portion of the model (PABS, TPA, soluble; Figure 4.4) was used to describe the wound site retention. Initially the $^{239}PuO_2$ was introduced into the PABS compartment. The relative transport out of PABS was 90 % to TPA, 9 % to lymph nodes, and 1 % to soluble. The rates of transport were not rapid, the fastest rate being that from PABS to TPA (15 d half-time). These rates are comparable to the movement of colloidal plutonium from the CIS compartment in dogs, rats and rabbits. However, for the latter two cases, the magnitudes of the transfer rates are affected by the lack of early data (*i.e.*, without such short-term data), the model is not able to define rapid transfer rates, even if rapid transfer from the wound site occurs. Nevertheless, the modeling results provide reasonably good fits to the wound site, lymph node, and systemic data. Even though the air-oxidized $^{239}PuO_2$ particles were prepared at low temperatures, they were relatively insoluble *in vivo*. The transfer rate from PABS to soluble, a measure of solubility, was $\sim 5 \times 10^{-4}$ d^{-1}, and that from lymph nodes to blood was 1×10^{-5} d^{-1}. This is about one-third of the inferred solubilization rate for colloidal plutonium s.c. injected in dogs (PABS to soluble rate of 1.4×10^{-3}), and it probably accounts for the somewhat longer wound-site retention of air-oxidized plutonium oxide particles versus colloidal plutonium hydroxide in the dog.

In the second modeling approach, the systemic data were replaced with blood plutonium data (Appendix C.4.5.1), which together with the wound site and lymph-node plutonium data allowed the model to partition the transport of plutonium from the wound site between lymph nodes and blood. The model results are shown in Figure 4.21 together with the associated transfer rates.

Several differences are noted in the results from the two modeling approaches. First, when the blood plutonium data are used, the transfer rate from soluble to blood is ~8,000 times more rapid than obtained with the systemic plutonium data. This is attributable partially to the availability of early blood data and partially to the different shapes of the uptake curves for blood and systemic plutonium. For the blood, the highest plutonium level was measured at 1 d, decreasing thereafter in a biphasic manner. In contrast, the systemic plutonium data increased biphasically, with a decreased uptake rate after ~50 d. Second, when the blood plutonium data are used, the rate at which plutonium transfers from PABS to TPA is 20 % of that when the systemic plutonium data are modeled. As will be noted subsequently, the latter kinetic agrees much better with the results of modeling the high-fired plutonium oxide data.

Transfer rates for wound-site retention of plutonium s.c. injected into the forepaws of dogs as air-oxidized $^{239}PuO_2$ particles.[a]

Pathway	Transfer Rate (d^{-1})
Blood to systemic	2.2
Soluble to blood	420
Soluble to CIS	0.0[b]
PABS to TPA	0.01
TPA to PABS	0.00053
PABS to soluble	0.00042
PABS to lymph nodes	0.0018
Lymph nodes to blood	0.0017

[a]Material injected into PABS compartment.
[b]Parameter value fixed.

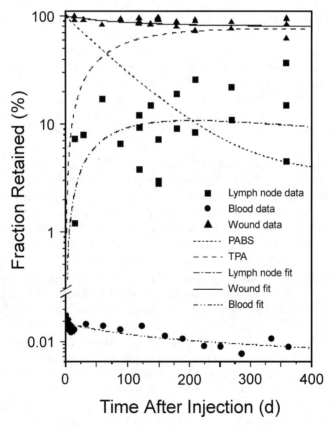

Fig. 4.21. Model fit of retention of plutonium in dogs s.c. implanted with air-oxidized $^{239}PuO_2$. Blood data used in lieu of systemic data; data from Tables B.4 and C.2.

Third, although the variability in the lymph-node plutonium data is substantial, it appears that the fit obtained using the systemic plutonium data better represent the trend in those data. Thus, the transfer rates derived from modeling the systemic data are considered overall a better representation of the transport of the air-oxidized plutonium oxide in the wound site and elsewhere.

4.4.2.2 *High-Fired* $^{239}PuO_2$ *Particles Injected Subcutaneously in Dogs.* The data set available from the study of s.c.-injected high-fired plutonium oxide particles (0.7 μm average physical diameter) in dogs was limited to data on wound site retention, uptake and retention of plutonium in the lymph nodes draining the wound site, and blood data (Appendix C.3.5.2). As with the air-oxidized plutonium particles, the plutonium was initially introduced into the PABS compartment, and the particle portion of the model was used (PABS, TPA, soluble). The results of the modeling are shown in Figure 4.22.

The wound-site plutonium retention is satisfactorily described, as are the uptake and retention of plutonium in lymph nodes and the blood plutonium content. Inclusion of the blood plutonium data was very important because it allowed the model to partition the plutonium leaving the wound site between the mechanical clearance to lymph nodes and dissolution/absorption pathways. Clearly, the solubility of these high-fired plutonium particles was less than that of the air-oxidized $^{239}PuO_2$ particles (PABS-soluble rate of 7.1×10^{-6} compared with 4.8×10^{-4} for air-oxidized plutonium), leading presumably to less plutonium transport to blood and less translocation to tissues for these high-fired particles.

There are similarities in the clearance rates to lymph nodes of the high-fired and air-oxidized $^{239}PuO_2$ particles, despite the differences in their solubilities and the fact that their particle sizes differed by a factor of 10 [0.7 μm geometric mean diameter (GMD) for the high-fired particles, 7 μm GMD for the air-oxidized particles]. The transfer rates from PABS to TPA were within a factor of two of each other, when comparing the high-fired particles with the wound model results obtained using the systemic plutonium data from the air-oxidized $^{239}PuO_2$; the high-fired $^{239}PuO_2$ particles were transferred faster. The transfer rate from PABS to TPA for the wound model results obtained using the blood data from the air-oxidized plutonium study was ~10 % of that for the high-fired plutonium. The transfer rates from PABS to lymph nodes were similar for the different sized particles using the systemic plutonium data for the air-oxidized $^{239}PuO_2$, but differed by about a factor of two when the blood plutonium data were used for the air-oxidized

Transfer rates for wound-site retention of plutonium as high-fired $^{239}PuO_2$ particles s.c. injected into the forepaws of dogs.[a]

Pathway	Transfer Rate (d^{-1})
Soluble to blood	100
Soluble to CIS	0.0[b]
PABS to TPA	0.11
TPA to PABS	0.012
PABS to soluble	7.1×10^{-6}
PABS to lymph nodes	0.0062
Lymph nodes to blood	0.00001[b]

[a]Material injected into PABS compartment.
[b]Parameter value fixed.

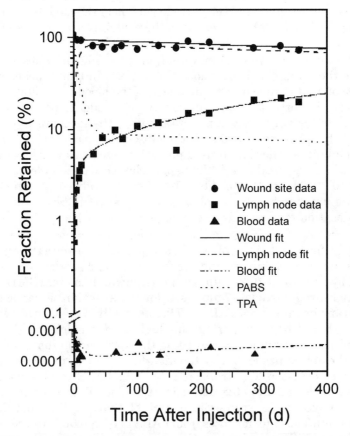

Fig. 4.22. Model simulation of wound retention of plutonium in dogs s.c. injected with high-fired $^{239}PuO_2$ particles (wound, lymph-node, and blood data from Tables B.5 and C.3).

particles. Both the first comparisons are well within the uncertainties of the parameters. Thus, assuming that the fits obtained using the systemic plutonium data for the air-oxidized particles are appropriate, then it appears that the rates of movement of micrometer and submicrometer-sized particles from the wound site to lymph nodes are similar for the different sized particles, at least when s.c. implanted in the dog.

Referring to the transfer of plutonium from the soluble to blood compartments, there is about a factor of 2,000 difference in the rates between the high-fired and air-oxidized $^{239}PuO_2$ particles using the fit to the systemic plutonium data for the air-oxidized particles, and a factor of five when the blood data are used. Although most of the difference in the former case can be attributed to the lack of early systemic data for the air-oxidized plutonium, this is not the case when the blood plutonium data for the air-oxidized $^{239}PuO_2$ particles were used. It is believed that the soluble to blood transfer rates derived using the blood plutonium data for both the air-oxidized and high-fired plutonium particles more accurately describe the transfers of plutonium from the wound site to blood.

4.4.2.3 *Summary for* $^{239}PuO_2$ *Particles Injected Subcutaneously in Dogs.* The major features of the wound retention of the s.c.-injected $^{239}PuO_2$ particles, regardless of their size or refractoriness, are:

- relatively rapid immobilization of the particles within the wound site (PABS to TPA), presumably caused by the local tissue response;
- very slow release of the trapped $^{239}PuO_2$ particles to solubilization or transfer to lymph nodes (TPA to PABS);
- accumulation of an important fraction of the s.c.-injected $^{239}PuO_2$ particles in the regional lymph nodes, but at a rate only ~10 % as fast as the rate of immobilization of the particles at the wound site (PABS to TPA), with the result that long-term transfer to the lymph nodes is greatly impeded;
- very little solubilization of the plutonium within the PABS compartment (PABS to soluble) at a rate ~1 % of the transfer rate, PABS to TPA;
- very slow solubilization of the particles accumulated in the lymph nodes (lymph nodes to blood).

The long-term trend towards prolonged retention of the major fraction of the deposited particles at the wound site is represented by a rate of transfer for PABS to TPA ~10 times faster than either the rate of return to the PABS state (TPA to PABS) or transfer to the regional lymph nodes (PABS to lymph nodes).

4.4.3 Analysis of the Retention of Other Insoluble Radioactive Particles in Wounds

4.4.3.1 *Radiolabeled Metal Oxide and Phosphate Particles Injected Intramuscularly or Subcutaneously in Rats.* Fine particles of eight metal oxides and phosphates that are insoluble in pure water were prepared with photon-emitting radiolabels. Aqueous suspensions (pH ~7) of those particles were i.m. or s.c. injected in the legs of rats, and retention of the radiolabel at the injection site was determined by detection of the photon emissions *in vivo*. Solubility in blood serum was determined by ultrafiltration (Appendix B.2; Table B.7; Morrow *et al.*, 1968).

The rates of clearance of the radiolabels from the wound site were positively correlated with their solubility in blood serum. Less than 1 % of the three chemically well-defined particle preparations dissolved during 2 h of incubation in blood serum. Their rates of clearance from the wound site, which were determined from 1 to 100 d, were $<3.5 \times 10^{-3}$ d^{-1} (Table B.7). Although those oxide and phosphate particles are insoluble in pure water (Weast, 1973), and only sparingly soluble in serum, their metal ions form stable complexes with citrate ion and with transferrin. All, $^{65}Zn_3(PO_4)_2$ in particular, are soluble to some degree in dilute acid, and would be expected to dissolve slowly within macrophage lysosomes (pH ~5.5) in the order: $Zn_3(PO_4)_2 > Cr_2O_3 > Fe_2O_3$.

4.4.3.2 $^{235}UO_2$ *Particles Deposited Intramuscularly in Rats and Rabbits.* Aqueous suspensions of fine particles of $^{235}UO_2$ were deposited by i.m. injection into the leg muscle of rats and one rabbit. Retention of the $^{235}UO_2$ was determined by detection of the weak photon emissions *in vivo* (Appendix B.3.1; Beiter *et al.*, 1975). The reconstructed wound uranium retention data (Table B.8) were sufficient for analysis with the wound model. The parameters of the resulting wound uranium retention equations (Equations B.18 and B.19) are shown in Table 4.7.

Although the mass of $^{235}UO_2$ i.m. deposited in the rabbit (16 mg) was four times larger than that deposited in the rats (4 mg), wound uranium retention in both species was nearly the same. In contrast with the wound retention patterns of the other insoluble oxide and phosphate particles tested, ~25 % of the deposited $^{235}UO_2$ was cleared from the wound sites at rates faster than 0.032 d^{-1} (half-time ~22 d). The last defined wound clearance rates for the $^{235}UO_2$ particles, 1.6×10^{-3} and 2.4×10^{-3} d^{-1} (Table 4.7), are similar to those obtained for the smaller deposited masses of other insoluble metal oxide or phosphate particles.

Even though $^{235}UO_2$ is nearly insoluble in serum (Morrow *et al.*, 1964), dissolution of some uranium may be expected soon after deposition of fine $^{235}UO_2$ particles in a wound, caused by oxidation of UO_2 to soluble UO_2^{2+} and complexation with bicarbonate ion in continuously flowing tissue fluid. Later, UO_2 particles confined within macrophages are shielded from contact with tissue fluid, and UO_2^{2+} formed within macrophage lysosomes can be trapped as crystalline $(UO_2)_3(PO_4)_2$ needles (Henge-Napoli *et al.*, 1994).

4.4.3.3 *Mixed Oxide Nuclear Fuel Particles Injected Intramuscularly in Rats.* Aqueous suspensions of mixed oxide (MOX) nuclear fuel particles (400 μg, ~5 μm GMD) were i.m. injected in the hind legs of rats. The rats were killed at 8 d, and the uranium, americium and plutonium in the cumulated urine and feces, injected leg, selected tissues, and residual carcass were determined (Appendix B.4.1; Paquet *et al.*, 2003). The fractions of the radionuclides cleared from the wound site in 8 d and the best estimates of their clearance rates (corrected for the retained fraction) are shown in Table 4.7.

A much larger fraction (64 %) of the deposited uranium oxide component of the MOX particles (presumably UO_2) was cleared from the wound site to blood at a markedly faster rate than was observed for pure $^{235}UO_2$. The initial clearance rate of the uranium component of MOX and the amount cleared at that rate closely resemble the initial clearance pattern of $^{235}UO_2$ (Appendix B.3.1; Beiter *et al.*, 1975). An important fraction (20 %) of the ^{241}Am contaminant of MOX (presumably AmO_2) was also cleared rapidly from the wound site (corrected half-time 4 d). In contrast, only a small fraction of the PuO_2 component of the MOX particles cleared in 8 d, but at a corrected rate of 0.25 d^{-1}, which is two to five times faster than the initial clearance rates observed for pure PuO_2 particles of similar size.

4.4.4 *Summary for Insoluble Radionuclides*

Table 4.7 contains sets of default parameters developed to describe retention of insoluble radioactive particles of transition

TABLE 4.7—Parameters of multiexponential wound retention equations for insoluble radioactive metal oxide or phosphate particles in aqueous suspension i.m. or s.c. deposited in rats or rabbits or s.c. in dogs.[a,b]

Deposited Material	Study Conditions				A_1 (%)	λ_1 (d^{-1})	A_2 (%)	λ_2 (d^{-1})
	Mass (μg)	Size[c] (μm)	Animal/Implant Mode	Length (d)				
Zn-Zn$_3$(PO$_4$)$_2$ [d]	≥16	~0.5	Rat/i.m.	100				$<3.5 \times 10^{-3}$
Cr-Cr$_2$O$_3$ [d]	≥16	~0.5	Rat/i.m.	100				$<3.5 \times 10^{-3}$
Fe-Fe$_2$O$_3$ [d]	≥16	~0.5	Rat/s.c.	100				$<1.4 \times 10^{-3}$
^{235}UO$_2$ [e]	4×10^3	1.0	Rat/i.m.	100	48	0.023	52	~0
^{235}UO$_2$ [e]	1.7×10^4	1.0	Rabbit/i.m.	100	37	0.027	63	~0
^{239}PuO$_2$-air oxidized[f]	13–512	7.0	Dog/s.c.	365	8.5	0.05	91.5	3×10^{-4}
^{239}PuO$_2$-heated[f]	~325	0.7	Dog/s.c.	365	4.3	0.13	95.7	6×10^{-4}
MOX-PuO$_2$ [g]	130	~5	Rat/i.m.	8	3.1	0.25		
MOX-AmO$_2$	<0.4		Rat/i.m.	8	20	0.17		
MOX-UO$_2$	370		Rat/i.m.	8	64	0.22		
^{235}UO$_3$ [e]	4×10^3	2.4	Rat/i.m.	70	52	0.16	48	0.017

Transition Metal Oxides and Phosphates

	Default Wound Retention Parameters			
	(10)	(0.06)	(90)	2×10^{-3}
UO_2	42	0.025	58	~0
PuO_2	6	0.09	94	4.5×10^{-4}

[a] Retention equations of the form $R(t) = \sum_i A_i e^{-\lambda_i t}$, $R(0) = 100\%$.

[b] Insoluble in pure water at room temperature (Weast, 1973).
[c] Best estimates of mean geometric median diameter.
[d] Radiolabeled oxides and phosphates (Appendix B.2).
[e] $^{235}UO_2$ and $^{235}UO_3$ (Appendix B.3.1; Equations B.18 and B.19).
[f] Air-oxidized $^{239}PuO_2$ particles (Appendix B.1.3; Equation B.10); high-fired $^{239}PuO_2$ particles (Appendix B.1.4; Equation B.14).
[g] Components of MOX fuel (Appendix B.4.1).

metals (*e.g.*, oxides and phosphates) and oxides of uranium and plutonium deposited in deep puncture wounds.

The set of default wound retention parameters shown in Table 4.7 for the fine insoluble particles of transitional metal oxides and phosphates includes an initial term that was not defined by Morrow *et al.* (1968). The *in vivo* measurements of retention of the deposited radioactive material in the injected rat legs were started 1 d after deposition of the particles, and regression analysis was used to fit one exponential term to all the data collected from 1 d to the end of the measurements. Those procedures were likely to have overlooked small fractions cleared early at faster rates. The wound retention patterns obtained for the similarly small particles of $^{235}UO_2$ and $^{239}PuO_2$ strongly indicated the existence of an initial small, rapidly-clearing component. Therefore, a small, fast-clearing component (10 % of the deposited amount) was introduced into the wound retention equation for insoluble metal oxide and phosphate particles. The wound retention equation defined by the default parameters for such particles (Table 4.7) should be useful for analysis of cases in which fine radioactive particles with similar chemical properties are deposited in a wound. What is not known are the fractions of the material that clear as particles to lymph nodes, or are transferred to blood by dissolution/ absorption; unfortunately, these parameters are clearly important for dosimetry.

The default wound retention parameters shown in Table 4.7 for deposited particles of $^{239}PuO_2$ should be applicable to cases of wounds contaminated with particles of similarly refractory materials, particles for which little dissolution *in vivo* is expected at the wound site, and wound clearance is likely to be almost entirely *via* transfer of phagocytized particles to local lymph nodes.

Particles of UO_2 deposited in a puncture wound are considered to be a special case, because of the tendency of U^{4+} to be slowly oxidized to U^{6+} *in vivo* at physiological pH, and because the concentration of HCO_3^- in tissue fluid is sufficient to facilitate complexation and clearance to blood of UO_2^{2+} formed *in vivo*.

The late clearance behavior of fine insoluble particles deposited in a puncture wound is well correlated with their solubility *in vivo* in serum and with their slow clearance from the respiratory tract (Morrow *et al.*, 1968). Some additional guidance about the appropriate set of default wound retention parameters to apply to a case of radioactive particles deposited in a wound can be found in publications by ICRP (1994b; 2002a) and NCRP (1997).

4.4.5 *Application of the Wound Model to Animal Data for Retention of Fine, Insoluble Radioactive Particles Deposited in Wounds*

The wound model was used to analyze kinetic data from animal studies of retention of $^{235}UO_2$ and $^{239}PuO_2$ particles in aqueous suspension deposited in simulated wounds. The insoluble particles were introduced into the PABS compartment of the wound model. The CIS compartment was ignored, because dissolution of the particles was expected to be so slow that the small amounts of solubilized metal would be complexed by circulating bioligands and hydrolysis and transition to the CIS state would be avoided. The sets of intercompartmental transfer rates obtained from those analyses are collected in Table 4.8.

4.4.5.1 *Particles of $^{239}PuO_2$ Injected Subcutaneously in Dog Paws.* In two experiments, aqueous suspensions of small particles of $^{239}PuO_2$ were deposited s.c. in the paws of dogs. One study, in which 7 µm air-oxidized $^{239}PuO_2$ particles were deposited, provided kinetic data from 15 to 365 d for plutonium retention in the wound and accumulation of plutonium in the major draining lymph nodes and in the tissues and cumulative excretion (systemic) and for blood plutonium from 1 to 365 d (Appendix B.1.3; Tables B.4 and C.2; Johnson, 1969). The second study, in which 0.7 µm heat-treated (high-fired) $^{239}PuO_2$ particles were deposited, provided kinetic data from 1 to 365 d for retention of plutonium in the wound, accumulation of plutonium in the lymph nodes, and the plutonium concentration in serial blood samples (Appendix B.4; Tables B.5 and C.3; Bistline, 1973). Both studies provided sufficient kinetic data for analysis using the wound model (Figures B.5, 4.20, 4.21, B.6, and 4.22). The parameters of the resulting wound plutonium retention Equations B.10 and B.14 are shown in Table 4.7.

The patterns of plutonium retention in the s.c. wound site following deposition of a large mass of $^{239}PuO_2$ particles are similar in the two studies, even though the air-oxidized particles were 10 times larger, and somewhat less refractory to dissolution in acid than the heat-treated $^{239}PuO_2$ particles.

In both studies, a small fraction (4.3 to 8.5 %) of the deposited plutonium was cleared from the wound site with half-times of 5 and 14 d, respectively, while the remainder was released slowly at rates ranging from 3×10^{-4} to 6×10^{-4} d^{-1}. The last defined rates of wound clearance of particles of chromium, iron, or uranium oxide or zinc phosphate, all of which are soluble in dilute acid, were, on average, $2.5 \pm 1 \times 10^{-3}$ d^{-1}, about five times faster than the average rate of clearance of the more refractory particles of $^{239}PuO_2$.

TABLE 4.8—*Transfer rates of wound model for retention of insoluble particles of $^{235}UO_2$ and $^{239}PuO_2$ deposited as aqueous suspensions in experimental deep puncture wounds; model input into PABS compartment.*[a]

Particles	$^{235}UO_2$		$^{239}PuO_2$		
Treatment History	Air Oxidized		Air Oxidized		High-Fired
Mass (µg)	4×10^3	1.6×10^4	94 ± 116		~323
Particle Size (µm)	~1.0		7.0		0.7
Animal and Injection	Rat, i.m.[b]	Rabbit, i.m.[b]	Dog, s.c.[c]	Dog, s.c.[d]	Dog, s.c.[d]
Intercompartmental Transfer Rates (d⁻¹)					
Soluble to blood	3.1[e]	3.1[e]	0.052	500	100
PABS to soluble	0.01	0.0092	4.8×10^{-4}	2.4×10^{-4}	7.1×10^{-6}
PABS to TPA	0.013	0.018	0.047	0.033	0.11
TPA to PABS	0.00	0.00	0.0034	0.0036	0.012
PABS to lymph nodes	0.001[e]	0.001[e]	0.0045	0.0036	0.0062
Lymph nodes to blood	0.029[e]	0.029[e]	1×10^{-5}	8×10^{-4}	1×10^{-5} [e]
Blood to systemic	0 [e,f]	0 [e,f]	0 [e,f]	0.9[e]	0.9[e]

[a]Wound model, Section 4.
[b]Wound data only [Table B.8; Figures 4.15 (rats) and 4.17)].
[c]Wound, lymph-node, and systemic data (Table B.4; Figure 4.20).
[d]Wound, lymph-node, and blood data (air-oxidized $^{239}PuO_2$ Tables B.4 and C.2, Figure 4.21; high-fired $^{239}PuO_2$ Tables B.5 and C.3, Figure 4.22).
[e]Fixed parameter value (see text).
[f]With no outlet, blood is subsumed in systemic compartment.

4.4.5.2 *Particles of* $^{235}UO_2$. Retention at the wound site when $^{235}UO_2$ particles were i.m. injected in rats and a rabbit was measured only for 100 d, and kinetic data are available only for uranium in the wound (injected leg). It was not possible, using only the wound uranium retention data, to discriminate between the processes that account for clearance of the ^{235}U from the wound site: dissolution of the $^{235}UO_2$ particles within the wound, PABS to soluble, and mechanical clearance of phagocytized $^{235}UO_2$ particles, PABS to lymph nodes. There is inferential evidence for loss of uranium from the wound by both processes. Accumulation in the contralateral (uninjected) legs of the rats of a small, but measurable, fraction of the ^{235}U i.m. deposited as $^{235}UO_2$ particles supports some $^{235}UO_2$ dissolution (Beiter *et al.*, 1975). Inhaled $^{235}UO_2$ particles accumulated within macrophages in the pulmonary lymph nodes of rats and dogs (Leach *et al.*, 1970), and black particles (presumably UO_2) were seen in the lymph nodes draining the site of i.m.-implanted DU metal wafers (Appendix B.6.4). It was reasonable to assume that some of the i.m.-injected $^{235}UO_2$ particles would be transported by macrophages to regional lymph nodes.

The following fixed parameter values were adopted for modeling wound retention of the i.m.-injected $^{235}UO_2$ particles. The transfer rate, soluble to blood, was fixed at 3.1 d^{-1}, based on the rate of clearance of UO_2^{2+} from an i.m.-injection site in rats (Table A.2). The transfer rate, PABS to lymph nodes, was fixed at 0.001 d^{-1} to allow for slower mechanical clearance to lymph nodes of the much larger masses of $^{235}UO_2$ deposited than the amounts of $^{239}PuO_2$ particles s.c. injected in the dogs. The rate of solubilization of $^{235}UO_2$ particles in the lymph nodes, lymph nodes to blood, was set at 0.029 d^{-1}, based on the rate of dissolution of aggregated colloidal Pu^{4+} in dogs (Figure 4.14). It should be noted that transfer from lymph nodes to blood does not affect the fit to the wound uranium data, but it contributes to prediction of the time course of accumulation of UO_2 in regional lymph nodes. Combined, those three fixed parameters provided the best fits to the wound uranium data for both the rats and the rabbit.

The results of modeling the wound uranium retention data for i.m.-injected $^{235}UO_2$ particles, constrained by the fixed parameter values discussed above, indicate a nearly equal competition between dissolution of the particles (PABS to soluble) and their sequestration (PABS to TPA). The zero value obtained for the transfer rate, TPA to PABS, suggests that the processes acting to immobilize the $^{235}UO_2$ particles at the wound site were not reversible at a measurable rate, at least based on the data from this brief, 100 d study. Combined, the results predict that there will be little additional loss of uranium (no more than 5 to 10 %) from the wound site at times >100 d after the initial deposition. The transfer rates shown in Table 4.8 for wound uranium retention after an i.m. injection of $^{235}UO_2$ particles may be specific to the large mass of UO_2 deposited, and faster clearance of the uranium from the wound site might reasonably be expected if a smaller mass of UO_2 particles were deposited. Recognize that there is considerable uncertainty in modeling these data because of the small number of animals, short duration of measurements, large implanted uranium masses, and variability in the *in vivo* measurements.

4.5 Retention of Radioactive Solids in Wounds

Three animal studies have been conducted of the retention and effects at the wound site of implanted radioactive solid fragments too large to be phagocytized. The implanted materials included thin wafers of DU metal (Hahn *et al.*, 2002), fragments of plutonium metal wire (Lisco and Kisieleski, 1953), and minispheres of local nuclear weapons test fallout containing or contaminated with americium and plutonium (Harrison *et al.*, 1990; 1993).

4.5.1 *Depleted Uranium Metal Fragments Implanted Intramuscularly in Rats*

Urinary excretion of uranium was measured periodically throughout the lifespans of six rats that were each implanted with four wafers of DU metal ($5 \times 5 \times 1.5$ mm, 2.6 ± 0.1 g total uranium), two in the muscle of each thigh. The time-dependent changes in the status of the DU implants and the implant sites were monitored radiographically. At death, 530 ± 166 d after the implants, the uranium content in kidneys and eviscerated carcass (implant sites removed) was measured, and several soft tissues and the implant sites were examined visually and histopathologically (Appendices B.3.4, B.6.4, and C.3.8; Hahn, 2000; Hahn *et al.*, 2002).

The daily urinary uranium excretion of the six individual rats increased steeply from zero to peak values (3×10^{-3} to 10×10^{-3} % of the implanted DU per day) at ~90 d and declined slowly thereafter (Guilmette *et al.*, 2005). The cumulative urinary uranium excretion of each rat was calculated by serially summing the measured urinary uranium excretion during the regular collection intervals and that calculated by linear interpolation to account for excretion during the intervals between collections. Urinary uranium represented ~90 % of the uranium solubilized and cleared from the wound site, while the remaining 10 % was retained in the kidneys and carcass (mainly bone). Total uranium absorbed at any time after the implant was assumed to be equal to 1.1 times the cumulative uranium excretion (Appendix B.3.4.2). Cumulative uranium absorption (systemic uranium) calculated for the individual rats is shown in Table 4.9. The parameters of the corresponding wound uranium retention equations obtained using the wound model, are shown in Table 4.10.

Corrosion and disintegration of the edges and surfaces of the DU wafers were visible in x rays as early as 21 d after the implants. By 365 d, the corroded DU wafers were encapsulated within dense mineralizing fibrous tissue. The capsules, as much as 0.5 mm thick, adhered tightly to the corroded surfaces of the DU wafers. Shards of black radiopaque material, presumably corroded fragments of DU, granular particles (some <4 μm in diameter), and particle-laden macrophages were imbedded in the fibrous tissue of the capsules.

The uranium content of the regional lymph nodes was not measured, but at death, they appeared gray in color, and histopathological sections revealed phagocytized particles of black hydrous UO_2. The wound model calculations suggested that ~0.023 % of the implanted uranium may have been associated with the local lymph nodes at that time.

By 662 d after the DU wafers were implanted, uranium absorption was calculated to be 0.96 ± 0.55 % of the amounts of DU deposited. Wound uranium retention at 662 d, calculated as 100 % minus the sum of the systemic fraction (uranium solubilized and absorbed into blood) and the fraction attributed to uptake in lymph nodes, is 99.02 ± 0.55 % of the amounts implanted.

By the end of the first year the partially fragmented and corroded DU wafers and the shed corrosion products were enclosed with fibrous tissue capsules that severely impeded both uranium solubilization and transport of UO_2 particles to local lymph nodes. For the four rats that survived longer than 1 y, 72 ± 4 % of the total amount of uranium absorbed from implant to death was absorbed during the first 354 d.

A wound uranium retention equation was obtained for each rat (Equations B.20a to B.20f in Table B.10) using its kinetic data for systemic absorption and excretion of solubilized uranium in the wound model. The estimated rates of transfer of uranium oxide particles to and dissolution of uranium in local lymph nodes with release of UO_2^{2+} to blood were taken into account in the modeling. The parameters of Equation B.20 in Table B.10, describe the average wound uranium retention for the six rats implanted with DU metal wafers.

TABLE 4.9—*Parameters of multiexponential wound retention equations for radioactive solids i.m. or s.c. implanted in rats and rabbits.*[a]

Study Conditions	Retention Equation Parameters[a]				Equation Numbers
	A_1 (%)	λ_1 (d^{-1})	A_2 (%)	λ_2 (d^{-1})	
DU metal wafers; i.m., rats[b]	0.50	8.6×10^{-3}	99.48	6.5×10^{-6}	B.20
Plutonium metal wire; s.c., rabbits[c]	0.50	8.9×10^{-3}	99.50	2.8×10^{-6}	B.16
Plutonium and americium in particles of local fallout (aluminum, iron, plastic); s.c., rats[d]	0.24	2.0×10^{-2}	99.76	3.3×10^{-8}	B.21
Plutonium metal wire; s.c., rats[c]	0.14	9.0×10^{-3}	99.86	1.6×10^{-6}	B.17
Plutonium and americium in particles of local fallout (constituents of soils, UO$_2$); s.c., rats[e]	—	—	100	3.5×10^{-7}	B.22

[a]Retention equations of the form, $R(t) = \sum_i A_i e^{-\lambda_i t}$, $R(0) = 100$ %.

[b]DU; uranium retention equation developed using wound model (Appendix B.3.4, Table B.10).

[c]Plutonium metal wire; plutonium retention equations estimated by simulation modeling or matching to individual DU rats (Appendix B.1.5).

[d]Minispheres of local nuclear weapons test fallout composed mainly of construction materials contaminated with plutonium and americium (Appendix B.4.2).

[e]Minispheres of local nuclear weapons test fallout composed mainly of UO$_2$ or soil constituents, plutonium and americium presumed to be incorporated (Appendix B.4.2).

TABLE 4.10—*Transfer rates of wound model for retention of actinides introduced into wounds as solid fragments of plutonium or DU metal or minispheres of local weapons test fallout.*

Implanted Material	DU Metal[a]	Plutonium Metal[b]	Fallout Particles[c]
Animal	Rat	Rabbit	Rat
Implant Mode	i.m.	s.c.	s.c.
Pathway	Wound Model Transfer Rates (d^{-1})		
Fragments to PABS	7.9×10^{-3}	9×10^{-3}	—[d]
PABS to TPA	0.72	1.4	2×10^{-2}
TPA to PABS	5×10^{-4}	7×10^{-4}	0
Fragments to soluble	0	0	—[d]
PABS to soluble	0	0	4.6×10^{-4}
PABS to lymph nodes	4×10^{-3}	5.4×10^{-3}	3×10^{-6}
Lymph nodes to blood	2.9×10^{-2} [c]	2.9×10^{-2}	2×10^{-2}
Soluble to blood	3.1[e]	0.9[e]	0.9[e]

[a]DU metal introduced into fragments compartment of wound model. Mean transfer rates for six rats obtained by modeling systemic uranium data for individual rats (Appendix B.3.4; Section 4.5.1).

[b]Plutonium metal wire introduced into fragments compartment of wound model. All transfer rates were fixed for simulation modeling (Appendix B.1.5; Section 4.5.2).

[c]Minspheres of local weapons test fallout composed mainly of aluminum alloy, carbon steel, or plastic (structural materials) introduced into PABS compartment of the wound model. All transfer rates of plutonium and americium constituents combined were fixed for simulation modeling (Appendix B.4.2; Section 4.5.3).

[d]Not applicable when fragments compartment is excluded.

[e]Fixed parameter value.

The results of fitting the wound model to the systemic data from a representative rat (96) is shown graphically in Figure 4.23 together with the transfer rates. The systemic data points were derived from the DU urine excretion data as explained previously. According to the fit, essentially all of the solubilized uranium reaches the blood *via* the lymph nodes, with little if any uranium coming as a result of dissolution from fragment or PABS. This result is considered to be an artifact of the fit, which is due to the absence of wound retention or lymph-node data. It is not reasonable that no uranium would come directly from the wound site. A second artifact noted in the fit result is the prediction that 99 % of the DU fragment would be transformed into particles (in PABS or TPA) by 300 d after implantation. Based on direct visualization of the DU wafers at necropsy, this was clearly not the case. However, notwithstanding these known or suspected artifacts, the model results could not be changed by fitting the data as they exist from the Hahn *et al.* (2002) study without fixing essentially all of the transfer rates. Because the internal kinetics among compartments within the wound site did not affect the net wound-site retention, this was not done. Therefore, the simulation of the average biokinetics of DU implanted in wafers in rats was based on the average uranium urinary excretion (Figure 4.24), and the default transfer rates taken directly from this simulation. It is clear that results from a future well-designed study with DU wafers implanted in animals would be very useful in rectifying the internal artifacts described here.

4.5.2 *Plutonium Metal Wire Implanted Subcutaneously in Rabbits and Rats*

Absorption of plutonium into the tissues of rabbits and rats was measured after s.c. implantation of little pieces of clean plutonium wire. The animals were observed for lifespan, and the time course of the changes in the status of the implants and implant sites were monitored (Appendices B.1.5 and B.6.3; Lisco and Kisieleski, 1953). Excreta were collected periodically during the first 300 d, and selected soft tissues and bones taken at death were radioanalyzed to measure plutonium absorption. The plutonium absorption and excretion data are reproduced in Table B.6; plutonium absorption, which was considered to be equal to the plutonium clearance from the wound site, was not well correlated with the amount of plutonium implanted or the time elapsed between implant and death. Excretion of plutonium by the rats was not detectable until 70 d after the implant; it peaked at ~100 d and declined toward much lower levels thereafter. The very low level of plutonium excretion

Transfer rates for wound-site retention of DU i.m. implanted as wafers into rat legs.[a]

Pathway	Transfer Rate (d^{-1})
Fragment to soluble	4×10^{-12}
Fragment to PABS	0.014
Soluble to systemic	3.1[b]
PABS to TPA	0.014
TPA to PABS	0.0[b]
PABS to soluble	4×10^{-12}
PABS to lymph nodes	0.91×10^{-5}
Lymph nodes to blood	0.11

[a]Material injected into fragment compartment.
[b]Parameter value fixed.

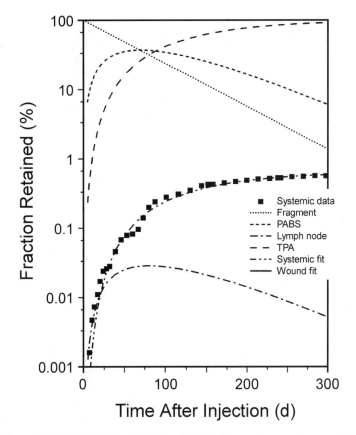

Fig. 4.23. Model fit of retention of DU in a representative rat (96; see Table B.9 and Figure B.7) implanted with DU wafers.

Transfer rates for wound-site retention of DU i.m. implanted as wafers into rat legs.[a]

Pathway	Transfer Rate (d^{-1})[b]
Fragment to soluble	0.0
Fragment to PABS	0.0079
Soluble to systemic	3.1
PABS to TPA	0.72
TPA to PABS	0.0005
PABS to soluble	0.0
PABS to lymph nodes	0.0039
Lymph nodes to blood	0.029

[a]Material injected into fragment compartment.
[b]Parameter value fixed.

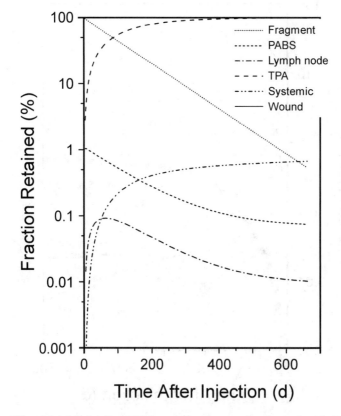

Fig. 4.24. Model fit of DU retention in rats implanted with DU wafers (based on mean transfer rates of the six experimental rats).

by the rabbits, close to the limit of detection at all times is not unexpected, because rabbits excrete little soluble injected plutonium (Finkle *et al.*, 1947).

Periodic radiographic examinations of the implant sites during life and visual inspection of the implant sites and surrounding tissues at autopsy showed that the plutonium wire rapidly corroded and disintegrated into smaller fragments and particles of hydrous plutonium oxides. Within ~300 d the plutonium fragments and particles at the implant site were completely embedded in or encapsulated by mineralizing fibrous tissue.

It is likely that some of the newly formed plutonium oxide particles were small enough to be phagocytized, and that solubilization of plutonium occurred at the slightly reduced pH of lysosomes within macrophages at the wound site and/or in local lymph nodes. Small phagocytized particles can also be expected to have been transported from the wound site to the major draining lymph nodes. Unfortunately, macrophage transport of plutonium oxide particles cannot be demonstrated by this study, because lymph nodes were not analyzed or inspected either visually or histologically.

Transport of plutonium oxide particles to lymph nodes by macrophages would have occurred within the same time frame as solubilization of phagocytized particles at the wound site. Once the plutonium fragments and particles at the implant site were embedded in or enclosed by a fibrous capsule, most likely by the end of the first year, release of plutonium solubilized at the wound site and macrophage transport of particulate plutonium to lymph nodes would be expected to occur at rates so slow as to be indistinguishable from zero.

The data for wound plutonium retention in the animals s.c. implanted with bits of plutonium wire were insufficient for analysis using the wound model. However, the wound plutonium retention patterns of these animals were similar to those of individual rats i.m. implanted with DU metal wafers. The wound model transfer rates obtained from modeling the systemic uranium data from the most suitable DU rat(s) were used as starting parameter values to simulate wound plutonium retention curves for the rabbits (Equation B.16). The uranium retention equation for DU Rat 86 (Table B.10) was considered to be a reasonable surrogate for wound plutonium retention in the rats implanted with plutonium wire (Equation B.17).

The wound plutonium retention equation developed for the rabbits is probably more reliable than the surrogate plutonium retention equation adopted for the rats. More rabbits were studied over a longer span of post-implant time, and because rabbits excrete so little systemic plutonium, the plutonium contents of their tissues at death is a good approximation of total plutonium absorption (wound retention) (Appendix B.1.5).

4.5.3 Minispheres of Nuclear Weapons Test Fallout Contaminated with Plutonium and Americium Implanted Subcutaneously in Rats

Minispheres (1 mm average diameter) of fused structural materials, nuclear weapons debris (UO_2), or soil constituents containing radionuclides were collected from a former nuclear weapons test site. Particles composed mainly of aluminum, polystyrene, or carbon steel were considered to have originated from structural materials, those composed mainly of UO_2, from weapons debris, and those composed mainly of limestone or clay, from soil constituents. The plutonium content of the particles ranged from 8.2 kBq for particles composed mainly of high impact polystyrene to 390 kBq for particles composed mainly of clay. The chemical and physical histories of the particles and their behavior *in vivo* suggest that the actinides were probably incorporated into the matrices of the particles composed mainly of UO_2 or soil constituents, while they were part of a surface coating on the particles composed mainly of structural materials.

Particles of each composition category were s.c. implanted in rats, one particle per rat, by surgical insertion beneath the skin of the ventral surface of a hind paw. At autopsy at 30 or 180 d, liver, both femora, regional lymph nodes, the implanted paw, the remainders of both legs, and the residual carcass were analyzed radiochemically for plutonium and americium (Appendix B.4.2; Harrison et al., 1990; 1993).

The fractions of the contained actinides translocated from the implanted particles to all of the body parts except the wounded foot were summed to estimate total plutonium and americium absorption for each of the six categories of implanted fallout particles. On average, the fractions of plutonium and americium translocated in 180 d from the particles composed mainly of structural materials were ~40 times greater than from those composed mainly of UO_2 or soil constituents.

At 180 d, the local lymph nodes contained 1 to 6 % of the actinide translocated from the particles. The liver, bones, carcass, and lymph nodes contained from 20 % (clay particles) to 95 % (limestone particles) of the translocated actinides. The remainder of the actinides that had been translocated from the implant site in the paw was apparently bound firmly by tissue constituents in the leg proximal to the paw. Histological sections and autoradiographs, prepared from a few rats killed ~1 y after implantation of minispheres composed mainly of aluminum, polystyrene, or carbon steel, showed that all of the particles were completely enclosed by fibrous capsules. The particles were intact except for minor corrosion of the surfaces of the metallic particles. The autoradiographs showed single alpha tracks associated with hair follicles, sebaceous glands, and blood vessels and aggregations of alpha tracks emanating from macrophages located within and around the fibrous tissue of the capsules. The combined evidence from radioanalysis of the tissues and the autoradiographs of the implant sites and surrounding tissues supports the view that the actinides were slowly leached from the solid particles in soluble form.

The data were insufficient for individual analysis of the translocation of plutonium or americium from the implant sites of the six categories of fallout minispheres using the wound model. However, the patterns of translocation of plutonium and americium from the fallout particles composed mainly of structural materials (Table B.11) were similar to the translocation patterns of uranium in some individual rats i.m. implanted with DU metal fragments (Table B.9). The absorption patterns of the two actinides associated with those three categories of fallout particles were sufficiently similar to one another at each of the two post-implant sampling times that they could be combined into a single data set. The wound model transfer rates obtained from modeling uranium absorption for the most closely matching rats implanted with DU were used as starting parameter values to simulate the average wound retention of plutonium and americium contained in fallout particles of those three composition categories (Equation B.21). Log-linear regression analysis of the combined data for translocation of plutonium and americium from the more refractory minispheres composed mainly of UO_2 or soil constituents yielded an exponential wound actinide retention equation with a single term (Equation B.22).

4.5.4 *Summary for Solid Radioactive Materials*

Equations describing wound site retention (Table 4.9) and systemic absorption are presented for several actinides implanted in animals in solid forms. The solid forms were DU metal wafers implanted in rats, bits of plutonium metal wire s.c. implanted in rats and rabbits, and minispheres of local nuclear weapons test fallout containing plutonium isotopes and [241]Am s.c. implanted in rats.

Those four equations are recommended as useful analytical tools for assessing wounding events involving contamination with those specific materials, as well as large fragments of chemically similar solids.

The equations describing wound retention of uranium in rats implanted with DU metal wafers (Equation B.20), plutonium in rabbits implanted with plutonium metal wires (Equation B.16), and plutonium and americium associated with fallout particles composed mainly of structural materials (Equation B.21) were calculated from measurements of systemic actinide absorption using the wound model (Appendix 4.4.7.4). In the case of the metal fragments, the modeling took account of the early chemical phases of corrosion, shedding of oxide particles, and slow dissolution of the oxidation products, most particles being too large to be phagocytized. Account was also taken of the biological processes of transport of some phagocytized oxide particles to local lymph nodes and eventual isolation or entrapment of the residual metal fragments and shed particles within fibrous capsules.

The equation describing wound retention of plutonium and americium associated with the fallout minispheres, composed mainly of UO_2 or soil constituents (Equation B.22), was obtained empirically from the actinide absorption data.

Even though the animal species and implant sites and chemical composition, surface areas, and reactivity *in vivo* of the implanted solids differed, the local tissue responses appeared to be similar and proceeded on much the same time schedule. By the end of the first year, the implanted solids and their associated particulate corrosion products were encapsulated by fibrous tissue.

In all cases, <1 % of the implanted actinide was translocated to the tissues at a moderate initial rate (half-time ~60 d on average). Actinide absorption after the first implant year slowed dramatically (half-time ~800 y on average), presumably because absorption to blood was impeded by the fibrous capsules surrounding the solid source materials.

The combined results for both animal species and both implant modes (Table 4.9) indicated that actinide retention at an implant site of solids composed of or containing actinides is in the order: plutonium and americium in weapons test fallout particles composed mainly of weapons debris (UO_2) or soil constituents (limestone, clay) > plutonium and americium in fallout particles composed mainly of construction materials (aluminum, carbon steel, plastic) > plutonium metal wire (in rabbits) > DU metal wafers. Actinide absorption is in the reverse order.

The somewhat greater absorption of uranium and plutonium from those implanted metals can be attributed mainly to their oxidation in extracellular water at physiological pH, yielding UO_2 and PuO_2 particles, some of which were apparently small enough to be phagocytized and dissolved, albeit slowly, within macrophage lysosomes at the implant site or in local lymph nodes. The substantially greater absorption of uranium from implanted DU metal is attributable to its advantageous chemistry *in vivo* (*i.e.*, to further slow oxidation of UO_2 to soluble UO_2^{2+}), which can be stably complexed and removed by the abundant HCO_3^- in tissue fluid. Nevertheless, the total amount of uranium transported from the wound site was still very small.

Absorption of plutonium and the americium from the implanted fallout minispheres, composed mainly of UO_2 or soil constituents, was much slower than that of the same actinides implanted in or associated with the other solid forms, and these particles may be considered as a special class of contaminated solid. The major constituents of these radionuclide-retentive particles and their likely formation in the fireball of surface or tower-burst nuclear explosions suggest that they were refractory glasses. The surfaces of such particles would be resistant to attack under the mild chemical conditions *in vivo*, and their amorphous internal structure would be unfavorable to the leaching of highly charged actinide cations.

The more efficient leaching of the actinides from the implanted fallout minispheres composed mainly of structural materials (compared with those composed mainly of UO_2 or soil constituents) supports the view that cooling vaporized fission products and actinides collected as surface coatings on these particles (Appendix B.4.2). Mild corrosion of the surfaces of the particles composed mainly of aluminum alloy or carbon steel would have somewhat increased the surface area, creating more favorable conditions for actinide leaching.

The several wound retention equations predict that, if those solids were allowed to remain undisturbed for 10 y, the fractional amounts of actinide translocated from a wound site would be 3 % of the implanted DU metal, 1.4 % of the implanted plutonium metal, 0.25 % of the plutonium and americium associated with the implanted fallout particles composed mainly of structural materials, and 0.13 % of the plutonium and americium contained in the implanted fallout particles composed mainly of UO_2 or soil constituents.

4.5.5 *Application of the Wound Model to Animal Data for Retention of Radionuclides in Implanted Solids*

The wound model was used to obtain sets of intercompartmental transfer rates that described wound retention and systemic absorption of actinides implanted as solid fragments (1 mm diameter) in simulated wounds in animals. Those transfer rates (Table 4.10) are recommended for use as analytical tools in investigations of accidental woundings with fragments of uranium or DU metal, plutonium metal, or minispheres of structural materials such as aluminum or steel contaminated with radionuclides.

4.5.5.1 *Depleted Uranium Metal Wafers Implanted Intramuscularly in Rats.* The study of DU metal wafers implanted in rats (Appendix B.3.4) provided six independent sets of uranium absorption data, each sufficient for analysis with the wound model.

The implanted DU metal wafers rapidly corroded and shed particles of hydrous uranium oxide corrosion products at the implant site. At death, the major draining lymph nodes contained microscopically visible black particles of oxide transported from the implant site by macrophages (Appendix B.3.4.2).

There is evidence for the dissolution of a small fraction of implanted uranium metal. However, uranium oxides are insoluble in water, and it is reasonable to conclude that, regardless of their anatomical location (at the wound site or in the lymph nodes) macrophage lysosomes were the principal, if not the only, sites of uranium oxide dissolution.

The DU metal wafers were introduced into the fragments compartment of the wound model. Disintegration of the DU metal was accounted for by allowing transfer to the PABS compartment, and direct dissolution of the DU at the surfaces of the metal wafers was allowed by transfer from the fragments to the soluble compartment. Material in the PABS compartment was allowed to transfer to the TPA compartment to account for encapsulation by fibrous tissue, to the lymph-nodes compartment to account for the presence of black uranium oxide particles in the lymph nodes at death, or to the soluble compartment to allow for dissolution of uranium at the wound site. In all, the six wound model compartments listed in Table 4.10 were sufficient to describe uranium retention at the wound site, systemic uranium absorption, and transient accumulation of uranium in lymph nodes. The wound model parameters for retention of uranium implanted in the form of DU metal wafers are collected for the six individual rats in Appendix B.3.4, and the mean parameters for the group are given in Table 4.10. The mean absorption values for the rats and the wound model simulation curves are shown in Figure 4.23.

Two wound parameters were fixed as in the case of rats injected with $^{235}UO_2$ particles (Appendix 4.4.3.2). The transfer rate, soluble to blood, was fixed at 3.1 d^{-1}, and the rate of dissolution of uranium particles in lymph nodes, lymph nodes to blood, was set to 0.029 d^{-1}. For modeling the data from four of the rats implanted with DU metal, the transfer rate, PABS to lymph nodes, was fixed at 0.0054 d^{-1}, the average rate of transfer of PuO_2 particles s.c. implanted in dogs (Table 4.8). However, better fits to the systemic uranium data of Rats 90 and 100 were obtained when the latter transfer rate was fixed at 0.001 d^{-1}, the rate used for modeling the implanted $^{235}UO_2$ particles.

Model solutions that included a lymph-node compartment with input from PABS (presumably phagocytized uranium oxide particles) and outflow to blood (presumably of soluble $UO_2{}^{2+}$), rejected direct dissolution of the DU metal wafers or of uranium oxide particles at the wound site. That is, the transfer rates generated by the model calculations, fragments to soluble and PABS to soluble, were too small (<10^{-8} d^{-1}) to be distinguishable from zero. This model structure implies that dissolution of uranium occurred only within lymph-node macrophages. Neither the study of $^{235}UO_2$ particles i.m. injected in rats which provided only wound retention data (Appendix B.3.1 and 4.4.5.2) nor this study in which only systemic uranium data were available, allowed a model solution that discriminated between dissolution of UO_2 at the wound site or in lymph nodes.

On average, the half-time of the modeled transfer pathway representing disintegration of the pieces of implanted solid metal into smaller shards and corrosion products, fragments to PABS, was ~90 d. The average half-time of 1 d, obtained for the transfer rate, PABS to TPA, supports the view that the transitions from solid metal to smaller metal shards and particles of corrosion products, phagocytosis of the smaller particles, and development of the fibrous tissue capsule were taking place simultaneously.

Systemic absorption of uranium, measured by urinary uranium excretion, nearly ceased by 350 d after the DU metal wafers were implanted in four of the six rats. Absorption of uranium in the other two rats (Rats 90 and 100) continued, but at slower than previous rates. The wound model solutions for the latter two rats showed non-zero transfer rates from TPA back to PABS and the smallest relative transfer rates, (PABS to TPA) (TPA to PABS)$^{-1}$, suggesting that isolation of the DU metal, shards and corrosion product particles by the fibrous capsule was more effective in some rats than others.

4.5.5.2 *Plutonium Metal Wire Implanted Subcutaneously in Rabbits.* The data for plutonium absorption in seven rabbits s.c. implanted with bits of plutonium metal wire (Table B.6) were insufficient for analysis with the wound model. Similarly to implanted DU metal, the plutonium metal fragments rapidly corroded and shed hydrous-oxide particles at the wound site. At the same post-implant times plutonium absorption in the rabbits was similar to the absorption of uranium from DU metal implanted in rats, in particular to that of Rat 102. The model structure adopted for simulation is the same as that used to model uranium absorption in rats implanted with DU metal (Section 4.5.1). The plutonium metal was introduced into the fragments compartment of the wound model. The intercompartmental transfer rates obtained from modeling uranium absorption in Rat 102 were used as starting parameter values for the simulation. Macrophage transport of plutonium oxide particles from the wound site to local lymph nodes was accommodated by introducing a rate of transfer, PABS to lymph nodes, of 0.0054 d^{-1}, and dissolution of plutonium oxide particles within macrophages was accommodated by introducing a rate of transfer, lymph nodes to blood, of 0.029 d^{-1} (Sections 4.4.5.2 and 4.5.1). The rate of transfer of dissolved plutonium, soluble to blood, 0.9 d^{-1}, was adopted from analysis of the data for particulates of PuO_2 s.c. implanted in dogs (Section 4.4.5.1).

The transfer rates shown in Table 4.10 are those that provided the best visual fit to all of the systemic plutonium data for the rabbits. Not surprisingly, those transfer rates are similar to the mean rates obtained from modeling the systemic uranium data from the six rats implanted with DU metal.

In the plutonium case, the transfer rates, fragments to PABS and TPA to PABS, are somewhat faster than those for the DU case, suggesting that the plutonium corrosion products might be more readily available for absorption. However, the rate of plutonium oxide particle entrapment, PABS to TPA, is nearly twice that for the uranium oxide particles, implying that the plutonium particles are sequestered more rapidly. Considering that the rates of encapsulation by fibrous connective tissue appear to have been about the same in both cases, the rate-limiting step is likely to be chemical. The great stability and insolubility of Pu^{4+} hydroxides and oxides are, by themselves, substantial impediments to plutonium dissolution and absorption. It should be noted that chemical transitions to highly insoluble forms, accumulation in macrophages at the wound site, and development of a fibrous tissue physical barrier all contributed to the transfer pathway designated PABS to TPA, and the wound model does not discriminate among them.

4.5.5.3 *Minispheres of Nuclear Weapons Test Fallout Contaminated with Plutonium and Americium Implanted Subcutaneously in Rats.* Simulation modeling was used to provide a set of wound model transfer rates suitable to describe plutonium and americium absorption from fallout particles composed mainly of structural materials (aluminum alloy, carbon steel, high-impact polystyrene) s.c. implanted in rats (Appendices B.4.2 and 4.5.3). The patterns of absorption of plutonium and americium from the fallout particles with these compositions were similar (Table B.11), and the six small data sets were combined. Six small sets of corresponding lymph-node plutonium and americium data were also available, and these were also combined (Table B.11).

The fallout minispheres were introduced into the PABS compartment of the wound model, because tissue sections of the implant sites of other rats implanted with fallout particles of these same compositions showed that during the first implant year the particles had remained essentially intact and surface corrosion was minor. A rate of 0.9 d^{-1} was adopted for transfer of dissolved actinide (soluble to blood). At the same post-implant times absorption of plutonium and americium was similar to the absorption of uranium in some of the rats i.m. implanted with DU metal. The appropriate intercompartmental transfer rates obtained for Rat 86 were used as starting parameter values for the simulation. The four transfer rates, PABS to TPA, PABS to lymph nodes, PABS to soluble, and lymph nodes to blood, were adjusted until the simulated absorption curves included (0, 0) and the mean absorbed actinide fractions at 30 and 180 d, and a reasonable fit was obtained to the mean lymph-node actinide contents at 30 and 180 d. These transfer rates are shown in Table 4.10.

Inclusion of the lymph-node data allowed the model to partition the outflow from the PABS compartment between the soluble and lymph-node compartments as well as to entrapment in the TPA compartment. The ratio of the transfer rates, (PABS to soluble) (PABS to lymph nodes)$^{-1}$, 150 to 1, is in reasonable agreement with the measured ratio of actinide absorption to lymph-node content of ~100 to 1.

If the transfer rate, PABS to TPA, represents mainly the rate of development of the fibrous connective tissue capsule and the rates of particle encapsulation are not dependent on their specific composition, then the appropriate transfer rates, PABS to soluble and

PABS to lymph nodes, for the more refractory particles composed mainly of UO_2 or fused solid constituents would be expected to be <10 % of those shown in Table 4.10 for the less retentive particles of structural materials.

4.6 Default Biokinetic Parameters for Radionuclides in Wounds

One of the purposes for developing a biokinetic model for radionuclides in wounds was to provide a unified, descriptive formalism useful for predicting the retention of a given radionuclide within a wound site, as well as the absorption rates to blood, and hence excretion in urine. Although the present wound model is one of several different models that have been presented and published (*e.g.*, Falk *et al.*, 2006; Piechowski, 1995), this model has been conceived using a mechanistic framework of chemical and biological principles, and has been shown to satisfy the above goal. To facilitate the use of the model for radiation protection (*i.e.*, in prospective dose assessment), two sets of default parameters have been determined based on the data, analyses and discussions presented in this Section and in Appendices A, B and C. Table 4.11 gives the default coefficients of two- or three-component exponential equations that describe the retention of the various categories of radionuclides in wounds. This mathematical representation of wound-site retention is simple and accurate for cases in which significant transfer of radionuclide to the wound-draining lymph nodes does not occur. Where such lymph-node transfer occurs, the absorption rate to blood will be overestimated as will the urinary excretion rate. For the four categories of initially soluble radionuclides, significant transfer to lymph nodes is rarely the case. However, when the physiochemical form of the radionuclide involves a particulate or solid phase, then lymph-node drainage is expected and can be significant.

The second set of default parameters is the transfer rates for the wound model for each of the seven categories defined in this Report (Table 4.12). In general, the use of the wound model for describing the biokinetics of radionuclides deposited in wounds is more accurate in that it is a materials-balance approach that accounts for the time-dependent presence of the radionuclide not only in the wound site, but also in the lymph nodes and blood. Coupling the wound model with the appropriate element-specific systemic model will also provide the time-dependent radionuclide content of the systemic organs, and excreta. The tradeoff is that the simple representation by a single equation is lost, and simulation modeling software or analytical solution of the models is most often required.

TABLE 4.11—Default parameters for equations describing the retention of various categories of radionuclides in wounds.[a]

Category	Wound Retention Equation Parameters					
	A_1 (%)	λ_1 (d^{-1})	A_2 (%)	λ_2 (d^{-1})	A_3 (%)	λ_3 (d^{-1})
Weak[b]	55	55	40	6.0	5.0	0.1
Moderate[b]	55	55	35	0.5	10	0.02
Strong[b]	50	1.0	30	0.03	20	0.001
Avid[b]	19	37	81	0.001	—	—
Colloid[c]	15	3.0	8	0.055	77	7×10^{-4}
Particle[c]	5	0.05	95	4×10^{-4}	—	—
Fragment[c]	0.5	0.009	99.5	6.5×10^{-6}	—	—

[a]Wound retention equations of the form, $R(t) = \sum A_i e_i^{-t}$, where $R(t)$ is percent of injected amount retained at the wound site and t is days after injection.

[b]Radionuclides initially in solution.

[c]Radionuclides initially sparingly soluble or insoluble in water.

TABLE 4.12—*Default transfer rates for the wound model for the various categories of radionuclides in wounds.*

Transfer	Transfer Rate (d^{-1})						
	Radionuclides Initially in Solution				Colloids[a] (injection to CIS)	Particles[a] (injection to PABS)	Fragments[a] (injection to fragment)
	Weak	Moderate	Strong	Avid			
Soluble to blood	45	45	0.67	7.0	0.5	100	—
Soluble to CIS	20	30	0.6	30	2.5	—	—
CIS to soluble	2.8	0.4	2.4×10^{-2}	0.03	2.5×10^{-2}	—	—
CIS to PABS	0.25	6.5×10^{-2}	1.0×10^{-2}	10	5×10^{-2}	—	—
CIS to lymph nodes	2×10^{-5}	2×10^{-5}	2×10^{-5}	2×10^{-5}	2×10^{-3}	—	—
PABS to soluble	8×10^{-2}	2×10^{-2}	1.2×10^{-3}	0.005	1.5×10^{-3}	2×10^{-4}	0.0
PABS to lymph nodes	2×10^{-5}	2×10^{-5}	2×10^{-5}	2×10^{-5}	4×10^{-4}	3.6×10^{-3}	0.004
PABS to TPA	—	—	—	—	—	4×10^{-2}	0.7
TPA to PABS	—	—	—	—	—	3.6×10^{-3}	5×10^{-4}
Lymph nodes to blood	—	—	—	—	3×10^{-2}	6×10^{-4}	3×10^{-2}
Fragment to soluble	—	—	—	—	—	—	0.0
Fragment to PABS	—	—	—	—	—	—	8×10^{-3}

[a]Sparingly soluble or insoluble in water; colloids and particles based on plutonium data, fragments on uranium metal data.

It should be noted that the default parameters are most useful for prospective assessments in which knowledge of the form and composition of the contaminating radionuclide is not available. For retrospective dose assessments involving radionuclide-contaminated wounds, if material-specific information of the contaminant is known, it should be given preference over the default values. This is particularly true in cases involving colloids, particles and fragments, in which the size, mass, chemical form, specific activity, etc., can affect the biokinetics. Longer-term monitoring data could also be used to develop case-specific retention parameters. In addition, it must be remembered that medical intervention is likely to affect the applicability of the wound model to any actual case (Bailey *et al.*, 2003).

It should also be noted that the wound model was developed based on data from deep puncture wounds, typically i.m. If a particular wound in question is other than a deep puncture wound, then the caveats described in Section 4.3 need to be considered.

5. Exposure Assessment and Dosimetry of Radionuclide-Contaminated Wounds

In order to assess the dosimetric and medical consequences of a contaminated wound, it is necessary both to identify the radionuclide(s) present, and, if at all possible, quantify the radioactive material present. Any radiological measurements performed fall under the heading of "bioassay," that is, determining the amount of radioactive material present in the body, or being excreted from it. Typically both direct measurements (*i.e.*, radiation detection at the wound site with an external detector), and indirect measurements (*i.e.*, quantification of radioactive material in excreta samples), are performed to determine the appropriateness and later the effectiveness of medical interventions.

5.1 Wound Assessment

Direct measurements are normally made at the wound site to quantify the radioactive material present, and thereby to provide guidance for medical management of the injury. Subsequent to the initial measurements, follow-up measurements are used to indicate the effectiveness of decontamination or surgical excision. In addition, measurements may be made at anatomical sites distant from the wound location to determine if radioactive material has migrated from the wound site to regional lymph nodes (Graham and Kirkham, 1983), or to organs that are known deposition sites for the radionuclides involved, such as the thyroid for radioiodines and the skeleton and liver for transuranics. In some cases, such as a wound contaminated with a highly soluble radionuclide (*e.g.*, ^{137}Cs) rapid transport of contamination from the wound site may mean that rapid treatment of the systemic burden is more important than assessment and treatment of the wound itself.

5.1.1   *Wound Monitors*

The choice of detector is driven by the radiations emitted by the contaminant. Those that emit photons are easily detectable, even those emitting only low-energy gamma or x rays (*e.g.*, ^{239}Pu, ^{241}Am) because there is typically little attenuation by overlying soft tissue for most wounds. Radionuclides that emit energetic beta particles without accompanying photons (*e.g.*, ^{32}P, ^{90}Y) can be detected directly if near the surface of the skin or from the bremsstrahlung created as the betas interact with tissue. Most radionuclides that emit alpha particles also emit photons that can be detected with the appropriate instruments, but low-energy beta-emitting radionuclides (*e.g.*, ^{3}H) that are embedded in a wound are difficult to detect. Usually some contamination remains on the surface of the skin at or near the wound site and external measurements with a survey meter or contamination survey instrument gives the first quantitative estimate of the potential radiological consequences of the wound. Detectors intended for measurement of radioactive material in a wound are normally calibrated with a point source of the radionuclide of interest, covered by an appropriate thickness of tissue-equivalent absorber. A discussion of detectors commonly used for wound monitoring and their calibration is included in Appendix E to this Report.

A common problem encountered in calibration for radionuclides that emit only particulate and/or low-energy photon radiations is quantifying the effects of self-absorption in the embedded material. For all but the smallest metallic or oxide particles, all alpha emissions and most beta emissions occur only from the surface of the particle, whereas photons that are being detected externally may be emitted from the entire volume. Consequently, it is important to quantify the effects of self-absorption in actual samples of the embedded material, if such can be obtained. Self-absorption of emitted radiations in the fragment or particle will also affect the dose received by surrounding tissue.

5.1.2   *Survey Meters*

Usually the first and sometimes the only direct measurements of radioactive material in a contaminated wound will be made with a survey meter. These instruments are commonly used to detect surface contamination, and usually consist of a Geiger-Mueller tube (in any of several configurations) coupled to a rate meter. Detectors typically have thin windows that permit the detection of beta, and sometimes even alpha particles, as well as photons.

Typical detection efficiency for beta particles with a "pancake" detector is ~10 %, and a rule of thumb is that contamination is detected if the observed counting rate is equal to three times the background rate. Since a typical background is ~0.5 counts per second (cps), a survey meter can detect surface contamination of ~15 Bq if the detected radiation is emitted in each decay. However, because a detector will typically not be calibrated for wound measurements, survey-meter results are usually made to indicate only whether or not a wound is in fact contaminated, and if so, to provide a qualitative estimate of the amount of contamination present. Many facilities require all wounds incurred in a radioactive materials area to be assayed with a dedicated wound monitor, even if initial survey-meter results are negative.

5.1.3 *Sequential Measurements*

Most frequently, sequential measurements are used to determine the success of surgical intervention in removing the radioactive material from the wound site. However, sequential measurements may also be used to determine the retention of radioactive material at the wound site without intervention. For these measurements to be meaningful, constant geometry and calibration of the detector must be maintained. However, several processes can affect both the geometry and the calibration:

- an embedded particle or fragment may slowly dissolve, thereby changing both its own shape and the distribution of radioactive material at the wound site and elsewhere in the body;
- it may change location in the wound, working its way closer to the surface due to muscle flexion; and
- biological processes such as inflammation, localized edema, and encapsulation may also change the absorption of emitted radiations by overlying soft tissue.

If sequential measurements are to be used to determine the loss of radioactive material from the wound site, care must be taken to ensure that the geometry and calibration of subsequent measurements reproduce those of the original measurement as closely as possible. Otherwise loss of efficiency may be interpreted as loss of material.

5.2 Local Dosimetry Models

A radionuclide-contaminated wound presents two problems in dose assessment. The first, and typically the more important for radiation protection considerations, is the estimation of the committed organ dose and/or the effective dose to the individual from radioactive material absorbed into the systemic circulation from the wound site. The second is the assessment of radiation dose to the tissues immediately adjacent to the wound site. Although few specific dosimetry models for wound sites have been developed, a number of dosimetry models commonly used in health physics can be applied to contaminated wounds.

5.2.1 *Skin (Shallow) Dosimetry Models*

Many contaminated wounds occur as chemical burns or abrasions in which much of the skin may remain intact. In this case, dosimetry models for external contamination of intact skin are appropriate for use. NCRP Report No. 106, *Limit for Exposure to "Hot Particles" on the Skin* (NCRP, 1989) and Report No. 130, *Biological Effects and Exposure Limits for "Hot Particles"* (NCRP, 1999) described a number of skin dosimetry models that may be applied to contaminated wound scenarios. These detailed discussions will not be repeated here, but briefly, dose estimates are obtained from point kernels that describe the absorbed dose distribution about a point, isotropic source in an infinite, homogeneous medium (water is usually used to simulate soft tissue). The tables developed by Berger (1971) are still considered valid for use in dose calculations, and form the basis of the VARSKIN® program (Oak Ridge National Laboratory, Oak Ridge, Tennessee), described below. Doses can also be estimated by Monte-Carlo methods in which millions of individual particles (betas and photons) are tracked from their points of origin through various interactions in a uniform medium (again, usually water) and the energy deposited as a function of distance from the source is tabulated. The International Commission on Radiation Units and Measurements (ICRU) reviewed Monte-Carlo calculations in beta-particle dosimetry in ICRU Report 56, *Dosimetry of External Beta Rays for Radiation Protection* (ICRU, 1996), and concluded that results have sufficient accuracy for use in radiation protection. Kocher and Eckerman (1987) and Chaptinel *et al.* (1988) have published tables of skin dose coefficients for numerous radionuclides, for both surface contamination and penetration of the radionuclide into the epidermis. Some of their values are included in Tables 5.1 and 5.2.

TABLE 5.1—*Shallow dose coefficients for selected radionuclides on skin surface.*

Radionuclide	NCRP (1991)	IAEA (1996b)	Chaptinel *et al.* (1988)
	$(\text{mSv h}^{-1} \text{ cm}^2 \text{ MBq}^{-1})$		
^{14}C	305	320	320
^{22}Na	1,870		1,700
^{32}P	2,397	1,900	1,900
^{35}S	332	350	350
^{36}Cl	2,178		1,800
^{45}Ca	884		850
^{54}Mn		62	62
^{57}Co	78[a]		120
^{59}Fe	1,283	960	
^{60}Co	1,146	780	780
^{63}Ni		6.5×10^{-4}	6.5×10^{-4}
^{67}Ga	324[a]		340
^{90}Sr	4,272[b]	1,600	3,600[b]
^{99m}Tc	243[a]	250	250
^{111}In	376[a]		380
^{123}I	365[a]		370
^{125}I	417	21	21
^{131}I	1,694	1,600	1,600
^{137}Cs	1,941[c]	1,600	1,600[c]
^{147}Pm	612		500
^{192}Ir	1,592		1,900
^{201}Tl	343		280
^{204}Tl	1,803		1,600

[a]For application of this value see NCRP Report No. 111 (NCRP, 1991).
[b]Assumes ^{90}Y in secular equilibrium.
[c]Assumes ^{137m}Ba in secular equilibrium.

TABLE 5.2—*Local dose rates in a contaminated wound (Piechowski and Chaptinel, 2004).*

Radionuclide	Equivalent Dose Rate[a] (mSv h^{-1} kBq^{-1})
^{3}H	6.3×10^{-3}
^{14}C	5.4×10^{-2}
^{32}P	7.7×10^{-1}
^{51}Cr	4.8×10^{-3}
^{54}Mn	1.6×10^{-2}
^{57}Co	1.4×10^{-2}
^{58}Co	5.0×10^{-2}
^{60}Co	1.5×10^{-1}
^{90}Sr-^{90}Y	1.2
^{95}Zr-^{95}Nb	2.0×10^{-1}
^{99m}Tc	1.5×10^{-2}
^{106}Ru-^{106}Nb	1.6
^{110m}Ag	1.2×10^{-1}
^{125}I	1.6×10^{-2}
^{131}I	2.1×10^{-1}
^{137}Cs-^{137m}Ba	2.8×10^{-1}
^{144}Ce-^{144m,144}Pr	9.1×10^{-2}
^{201}Tl	3.7×10^{-2}
^{235}U	8.4×10^{1}
^{238}U	9.2×10^{1}
^{238}Pu	1.2×10^{2}
^{239}Pu	1.1×10^{2}
^{241}Pu	5.7×10^{-3}
^{241}Am	1.2×10^{2}

[a]To a 10 mm diameter sphere of tissue-equivalent medium surrounding a point source.

5.2.1.1 *The VARSKIN® Program.* The U.S. Nuclear Regulatory Commission (NRC) has approved the use of the VARSKIN® code (Durham, 1991; 1992; 2006; Durham *et al.*, 1991; Traub *et al.*, 1987) by licensees to calculate skin doses for regulatory and reporting purposes. The dose of interest for regulatory purposes is averaged over an area of 10 cm^2, at the "shallow" or "skin" dose depth of 70 μm (*i.e.*, 7 mg cm^{-2}). For contaminated wounds in which the skin is largely intact, these dose calculations may be directly applicable. For embedded contamination, Berger's point kernels may be integrated over the depth of interest.

5.2.1.2 *Shallow Dose Coefficients.* Dose assessment for a contaminated wound includes the shallow dose received by the skin, evaluated at the assumed depth of the basal-cell layer (*i.e.*, 70 μm). Shallow, or skin dose coefficients for selected radionuclides have been published by NCRP in Report No. 111 (NCRP, 1991), by IAEA (1996b), by Chaptinel *et al.* (1988), and by numerous other authors. Selected values are given in Table 5.1.

As an example, calculate the shallow dose rate from skin contaminated with ^{60}Co over an area of 10 cm^2, if a direct measurement with a pancake detector [efficiency (*i.e.*, cps Bq^{-1} ^{60}Co) of 10 %] yields 10,000 net cps:

surface activity = 10,000 cps / (0.1 × 10 cm^2) = 10 kBq cm^{-2},
shallow dose rate = 10 kBq cm^{-2} × 1,146 mSv h^{-1} cm^2 MBq^{-1}
 × 10^{-3} MBq kBq^{-1} = 11.5 mSv h^{-1}.

The regulatory limit of NRC for shallow dose is 500 mSv y^{-1} to the skin of any extremity; thus, in the above example, no regulatory limit would be exceeded if contamination were removed within 40 h.

5.2.2 *Dosimetry of Penetrating Wounds*

A key issue in estimating the local dose to tissues surrounding a contaminated wound is the definition of the volume of tissue for which the dose is to be calculated. In the case of short-range radiations such as alpha particles and low-energy beta particles (sometimes referred to as nonpenetrating radiations), the energy emitted is absorbed within a short distance from the source. Consequently, the larger the volume of tissue for which the dose is calculated, the lower the absorbed dose will be, since the energy absorbed remains constant while the mass of tissue increases. If the activity in the wound is known, as well as the configuration of the source (particle, fragment, etc.) and its exact location, dose calculations may be limited to the volume of tissue actually irradiated, as the ranges of the various radiations in tissue are known. However, for radionuclides that emit penetrating radiations only, or some combination of penetrating and nonpenetrating radiations, or if the identity and configuration of the embedded radionuclides are unknown, the volume of tissue irradiated may be a matter of conjecture. This Report recommends that in the absence of sufficient information to determine the exact volume of irradiated tissue, a default value of 1 cm³ be used. Several specific instances are described below.

5.2.2.1 *Line Sources.* A puncture wound with a narrow, sharp, contaminated object, such as a needle stick, may be treated as a line source of radioactive material deposited in tissue. To a first approximation, the concentration of radioactive material along the length of the wound may be assumed to be constant. In this case, the absorbed dose rate, $\dot{D}$ (Gy Bq^{-1} h^{-1}) at a distance d (centimeters) perpendicular to the line of the wound is given by:

$$\dot{D}(h) = 5.76 \times 10^{-7} \frac{S}{h\,d} \bar{\varepsilon}\, \frac{\mu_{en}(\bar{\varepsilon})}{\rho} F(\theta, \mu d), \qquad (5.1)$$

where S is the activity of the line source (becquerel) of length h (centimeters), $\bar{\varepsilon}$ is the mean energy (million electron volts) per transformation of the photon emission, μ_{en}/ρ is the mass energy absorption coefficient (cm² g^{-1}) for photons of energy $\bar{\varepsilon}$ in soft tissue, μ is the linear attenuation coefficient (cm^{-1}) in soft tissue, and $F(\theta, \mu d)$ is the sievert integral (or secant integral) which is frequently tabulated in books addressing radiation shielding (Shultis and Faw, 1996).

For an alpha- or beta-emitting radionuclide, the absorbed dose rate could be calculated as follows: the volume of tissue irradiated will be a cylinder of length h, equal to the length of the wound, with a radius equal to the range of the particulate radiation in soft tissue, plus two hemispherical end caps whose radii are also equal to that range. To get an average dose rate, determine the average energy of the particulate emissions, and then determine their range in soft tissue (or water). The absorbed dose rate $\dot{D}$ (Gy s^{-1}) would then be approximately:

$$\dot{D} = 1.6 \times 10^{-10} \frac{A\,\bar{\varepsilon}}{\pi\, r^2\, h + 1.33\, \pi\, r^3}, \qquad (5.2)$$

where A is the total activity (becquerel) in the wound, $\bar{\varepsilon}$ is the mean energy (million electron volts) per transformation of the particulate radiation, r is the range (centimeters) of that radiation in tissue, and h is the length (centimeters) of the contaminated wound. It should be noted that the above equation is exact for alpha particles and monoenergetic electrons that have a defined range. However, since the energies of the beta particles emitted in beta decay have a range from zero to a maximum value (characteristic of the radionuclide), the dose rate is nonuniform with distance from the source. In this case, r should be set to the range of the maximum energy betas. The dose rate will then apply to consideration of the entire volume irradiated, but not for any subdivision of that volume.

5.2.2.2 *Volume Sources.* Because injection of radioactive material in the form of a liquid is frequently encountered in nuclear medicine practice, dose models derived for that practice are available and may be used for wound analysis. To estimate the dose to a spherical volume of tissue uniformly containing a radioactive solution, the computer program MIRDOSE (Stabin, 1996) included a module that contains the results of Monte-Carlo calculations of the so-called S-factors (energy absorbed per nuclear transformation) used in the dosimetry schema of the Medical Internal Radiation Dose Committee of the Society of Nuclear Medicine (Loevinger *et al.*, 1991). The program allowed the user to specify the radionuclide of interest and then to calculate the self-dose to unit-density spheres of various volumes from 0.01 to 6,000 cm^3. A volume of 1 cm^3 is appropriate to use in the absence of other data.

Piechowski and Chaptinel (2004) have published values for the mean dose rate from an embedded source of different radionuclides in a uniform, tissue-equivalent medium. The source is in the middle of a target sphere of 10 mm diameter of soft tissue. This is representative of a critical volume in a wounded finger or palm. As the soft tissues are not immobile, the mean dose rate around the source is rather representative of the actual dose rate they receive. Values of the dose rate from various radionuclides are shown in Table 5.2 as taken from Table 1 of Piechowski and Chaptinel (2004).

5.3 Systemic Dosimetry

5.3.1 *Indirect Bioassay Measurements*

Indirect bioassay measurements subsequent to a contaminated wound incident are normally of two types; measurements of material surgically removed from the wound site, and measurements of radioactive material excreted in urine. The former are used, together with initial direct measurements of the wound site, to determine the effectiveness of the surgical intervention, and frequently the material undergoes extensive radiochemical analysis to identify all radionuclides present. Other material subsequently removed from the wound site, such as eschar or scab, is similarly analyzed. Urinalysis is used to determine if radioactive material has been absorbed into the systemic circulation from the wound site, and also to monitor the effectiveness of systemic decorporation therapy, if administered. The radioanalytical methods used are the same as those used for routine exposure monitoring, and are described in NCRP Report No. 58, *A Handbook of Radioactivity Measurements Procedures* (NCRP, 1985).

5.3.2 *Bioassay Data Interpretation*

Results of both direct and indirect bioassay measurements for contaminated wounds have been difficult to interpret, because of the lack of a standard model for wounds such as those published for inhalation and ingestion intakes. It should be noted that reference values such as the annual reference level of intake (NCRP, 1993) and the annual limits on intake (ICRP, 1979; 1991a) cannot be used directly for contaminated wounds, because the published values are derived from inhalation or ingestion models. In addition, reference levels such as the annual reference level of intake and the annual limits on intake are intended for application to routine occupational exposures, and by definition, a contaminated wound is not a routine exposure.

5.3.3 *Intake Retention Fractions*

Once a retention model for a contaminated wound has been established, as shown in Section 4 of this Report, it can be used to derive intake retention fractions for use with subsequent direct bioassay measurements. The intake retention fraction $[m(t)]$ is defined as that fraction of the initial activity taken into the body that either remains in the body (or in a specific organ) at a given time, t, after intake. The intake retention fraction is specific to the radionuclide involved, and is a function of the biokinetic models used to describe the intake of radioactive material, the transfer of radioactive material to the systemic circulation, and the subsequent deposition, retention and excretion of systemic radioactive material. Tables of intake retention fractions for intakes by inhalation and ingestion have been published by NRC (Lessard *et al.*, 1987), IAEA (2004), and ICRP (1997).

For direct measurements at a wound site, an intake retention fraction can be calculated if the retention function for radioactive material in the wound is known. Examples for uranium calculated from the wound model are provided in Appendix D, and tables of intake retention (and excretion) fractions for other radionuclides should be forthcoming. As an example, consider an incident in which a worker is pipetting a solution of natural uranium as UO_2Cl_2, and incurs a laceration when the pipette breaks, but does not report the injury until the next day. A direct measurement at the wound site gives a result of 26 Bq or ~1 mg of natural uranium. The intake is calculated as follows:

$$\text{intake} = \frac{1 \text{ mg}}{0.0676} = 14.8 \text{ mg}, \tag{5.3}$$

where 0.0676 is the intake retention factor at 1 d at the wound site for weakly-retained uranium (Table D.2).

5.3.4 *Excretion Fractions*

For excreta measurements, the excretion fraction is defined as the fraction of the intake that appears in a day's urine or fecal excretion. This excretion fraction is obtained from the time derivative of the systemic retention function, multiplied by the fraction of excretion that occurs *via* either urine or feces, and integrated over the time period of excreta collection (usually 24 h). As is the case with intake retention fractions, most published values of excretion fractions cannot be applied directly to the excretion of activity from a contaminated wound, because they already contain the biokinetic model for the specific intake route of inhalation or ingestion.

Excretion fractions that relate radioactive material in excreta directly to the intake *via* a contaminated wound may be developed from the wound model presented in this Report, by convoluting the wound retention function of the specific radionuclide with its systemic retention and excretion functions. Excretion fractions for uranium based on the wound model are provided in Appendix D, and excretion fractions for other radionuclides based on the wound model should be forthcoming. In the interim, a "worst case" analysis for potential internal dose can be performed by assuming all activity measured at the wound site will become systemic. Tables of systemic excretion fractions (*i.e.*, excretion per unit uptake to blood) have been published by IAEA (2004), ICRP (1997), and Piechowski *et al.* (1992).

Consider the above case of a laceration contaminated with natural uranium. After the direct measurement, a 24 h urine sample is then collected and found to contain 0.8 mg of uranium above background. What was the intake and effective dose?

$$\text{Intake} = \frac{0.8 \text{ mg}}{0.0516} = 15.5 \text{ mg}, \qquad (5.4)$$

where 0.0516 is the excretion fraction for day two from Table D.2.

5.3.5 *Multiple Intake Routes*

Frequently, an accident situation involves the release of radionuclides that may produce, in addition to contaminated wounds, intakes by inhalation, and oral contamination leading to intakes by ingestion, as well as contamination of intact or damaged skin. Inhalation intakes may be initially assessed by collection and analysis of nasal swabs or nose blows, and the oral cavity should also be swabbed. Analysis of collected material may be used to identify the radionuclide(s) involved, and possibly also their chemical and physical forms. Only limited guidance on the interpretation of nasal swabs has been published (Heid and Jech, 1969; Smith, 2003) and assessment of internal dose will rely on subsequent bioassay measurements. However, the interpretation of the measurement results will be complicated by the additional source term from the contaminated wound(s), and an intake/retention model specific to the individual circumstances will have to be developed.

5.3.6 *Systemic Dose Coefficients*

Dose coefficients relate a dose parameter to a unit intake of a given radionuclide by inhalation or ingestion, and usually have units of Sv Bq^{-1}. Depending on the particular reference, the dose parameter may be committed dose equivalent or committed equivalent dose to a single organ (H_T), or committed effective dose equivalent or committed effective dose (E). The respective dose coefficients have the symbols h_T and e, and are specific for the route of intake and solubility characteristics of the radioactive material. Tables of dose coefficients have been published by Eckerman *et al.* (1988), IAEA (1996a), and ICRP (1979; 1989; 1993; 1994b; 1995a; 1995b; 1997). However, none of these publications contains dose coefficients for unit activity intake *via* a contaminated wound, because of the previous lack of a consensus model for the uptake of radioactive materials from wounds.

Approximate dose coefficients for systemic uptake of selected radionuclides have been published in NCRP Report No. 111, *Developing Radiation Emergency Plans for Academic, Medical or Industrial Facilities* (NCRP, 1991). These factors were obtained by dividing the organ-specific dose coefficients for ingestion by the gastrointestinal absorption factor. This latter factor represents the fraction of the ingested material that becomes systemic, if the physical half-life of the radionuclide(s) in question is long compared to the assumed 42 h transit time of the gastrointestinal tract. However, this methodology ignores any possible contributions of gut doses to the effective dose.

Other tables of dose coefficients for systemic activity have been published by IAEA (2004) and Piechowski *et al.* (1992). These factors may be used with direct measurements of the activity at a wound site, with the assumption that all the radioactive material will become systemic. The activity measured at the wound site (becquerel) is multiplied by the systemic dose conversion factor (Sv Bq^{-1}) to obtain either committed dose to a given target organ or effective dose. Although such a calculation produces only a crude upper bound for the internal dose resulting from a contaminated wound, it can serve as a quick indication of whether or not decorporation therapies should be initiated. Table 5.3 shows dose coefficients for systemic activity, based on the ICRP Publication 68 biokinetic models (ICRP, 1994b), and was provided by Eckerman.[3]

5.3.7 Systemic Dose Coefficients for Uranium Derived from the Wound Model

Appendix D provides systemic dose coefficients for uranium based on the wound model. As an example, consider the above case of a wound intake of 15 µg of uranium, as determined by initial direct and urine monitoring. What are the maximum potential organ equivalent and effective doses? From Table D.1, the maximum organ dose is to bone surfaces, and the dose coefficient is 3.5×10^{-5} Sv Bq^{-1}. The committed organ dose to bone surfaces is then:

$$15 \text{ mg} \times 26 \text{ Bq mg}^{-1} \times 3.5 \times 10^{-5} \text{ Sv Bq}^{-1} = 14 \text{ mSv} \tag{5.5}$$

---

[3]Eckerman, K.F. (2006). Personal communication (Oak Ridge National Laboratory, Oak Ridge, Tennessee).

TABLE 5.3—*Systemic dose coefficients for selected radionuclides.*[a]

Nuclide	h_T (Sv Bq^{-1})[b]	Target Organ	e (Sv Bq^{-1})[c]
^{3}H	1.83E–11	All same	1.83E–11
^{14}C	5.78E–10	All same	5.78E–10
^{22}Na	6.44E–09	Bone surface	3.13E–09
^{32}P	1.04E–08	Bone surface	2.26E–09
^{35}S	3.25E–10	LLI wall[d]	1.24E–10
^{36}Cl	2.12E–09	UB wall[d]	8.89E–10
^{45}Ca	2.06E–08	Bone surface	1.64E–09
^{51}Cr	1.57E–10	LLI wall	5.64E–11
^{54}Mn	9.77E–09	Liver	3.00E–09
^{57}Co	1.55E–09	Liver	6.38E–10
^{58}Co	3.16E–09	Liver	1.54E–09
^{59}Fe	2.95E–08	Liver	8.47E–09
^{60}Co	4.27E–08	Liver	1.95E–08
^{67}Ga	1.21E–09	Bone surface	1.17E–10
^{85}Sr	2.71E–09	Red marrow	1.11E–09
^{89}Sr	1.99E–08	Bone surface	3.15E–09
^{90}Sr	1.36E–06	Bone surface	8.80E–08
^{95}Zr	2.19E–07	Bone surface	1.02E–08
^{99m}Tc	1.30E–10	Thyroid	1.93E–11
^{106}Ru	4.11E–08	LLI wall	3.01E–08
^{110m}Ag	1.47E–07	Liver	2.18E–08
^{111}In	1.01E–09	Kidneys	2.54E–10
^{124}Sb	2.61E–08	Bone surface	3.68E–09
^{125}Sb	9.04E–08	Bone surface	5.40E–09
^{123}I	4.24E–09	Thyroid	2.24E–10
^{125}I	3.10E–07	Thyroid	1.56E–08

TABLE 5.3—*(continued).*[a]

Nuclide	h_T (Sv Bq^{-1})[b]	Target Organ	e (Sv Bq^{-1})[c]
^{129}I	2.13E–06	Thyroid	1.07E–07
^{131}I	4.38E–07	Thyroid	2.20E–08
^{134}Cs	2.26E–08	LLI wall	1.94E–08
^{137}Cs	1.67E–08	LLI wall	1.36E–08
^{144}Ce	1.91E–06	Liver	1.66E–07
^{147}Pm	8.72E–07	Bone surface	2.88E–08
^{192}Ir	3.67E–08	Liver	6.72E–09
^{201}Tl	2.87E–10	LLI wall	8.87E–11
^{204}Tl	6.73E–09	LLI wall	1.25E–09
^{203}Hg	1.41E–08	Kidneys	1.70E–09
^{226}Ra	6.23E–05	Bone surface	1.37E–06
^{228}Ra	1.12E–04	Bone surface	3.48E–06
^{228}Th	4.90E–03	Bone surface	1.22E–04
^{232}Th	2.36E–02	Bone surface	4.55E–04
^{234}U	3.93E–05	Bone surface	2.29E–06
^{235}U	3.70E–05	Bone surface	2.13E–06
^{238}U	3.56E–05	Bone surface	2.06E–06
^{238}Pu	1.48E–02	Bone surface	4.47E–04
^{239}Pu	1.65E–02	Bone surface	4.93E–04
^{240}Pu	1.65E–02	Bone surface	4.93E–04
^{241}Am	1.81E–02	Bone surface	3.99E–04
^{242}Cm	3.72E–04	Bone surface	1.37E–05
^{244}Cm	9.86E–03	Bone surface	2.36E–04
^{252}Cf	5.85E–03	Bone surface	1.53E–04

[a]Eckerman, K.F. (2006). Personal communication (Oak Ridge National Laboratory, Oak Ridge, Tennessee).
[b]h_T = committed equivalent dose to a single organ per unit intake.
[c]e = committed effective dose per unit intake.
[d]LLI = lower large intestine; UB = urinary bladder.

and the effective dose is:

$$15 \text{ mg} \times 26 \text{ Bq mg}^{-1} \times 2.03 \times 10^{-6} \text{ Sv Bq}^{-1} = 0.8 \text{ mSv}, \qquad (5.6)$$

where 2.03×10^{-6} Sv Bq^{-1} is the effective dose coefficient from Table D.1.

Because of the magnitude of these doses, medical intervention is not indicated for radiological considerations. However, because the primary hazard from intakes of natural uranium is chemical toxicity to the kidney, competent medical advice should be sought; in fact, in this case the intake exceeds tolerable daily intake levels (Bleise *et al.*, 2003).

5.3.8 *Lymph-Node Dosimetry*

The mass of "fixed lymphatic tissue" is given by ICRP (1975) as 700 g in males and 580 g in females, and includes the mass of the lymphocytes normally present in the nodes. The total number of lymph nodes in the body has been estimated to be in the range of ~500 to 700 (ICRP, 1975), and most have a length of <2.5 cm along their longest axis (Marieb, 1992). ICRP (1994a) has provided dosimetry models for only the thoracic and extra-thoracic lymph nodes as part of the human respiratory tract model. However, it is generally considered that the lymph nodes are not at radiogenic risk. The dose to lymph nodes predicted by the wound model would be calculated by determining the total number of decays in the lymph-node compartment, and multiplying by the sum of the energy emitted per decay in the form of particles, and the fraction of the photon energy emitted per decay that is absorbed in a 1 cm radius sphere, all divided by a mass of 700 g. Similarly, the wound model could be used to calculate the dose to specific lymph nodes, such as the axillary nodes draining a wound site in the arm or hand, by assuming all decays in the lymph-node compartment occur in those nodes, and dividing the total absorbed energy by the mass of those nodes, if that can be determined.

6. Medical Management of Radionuclide-Contaminated Wounds

6.1 Evaluation and Treatment of Radionuclide-Contaminated Wounds

Most published reports of medical management of radionuclide-contaminated wounds are concerned with transuranic materials, especially plutonium. Therefore plutonium-contaminated wounds serve as an archetype, and the principles used in this Report in evaluating and treating radioactive material wounds tend to be those used for plutonium wounds. Nontransuranic radionuclide-contaminated wounds may be handled with these same basic principles, and with the use of either the same or other medical and surgical measures as appropriate. However, nontransuranic radionuclide-contaminated wounds may be less likely to be surgically debrided because of the lower toxicity of the contamination. An excellent summary of the etiology and care of radionuclide-contaminated wounds is given by Ilyin (2001). Guidebooks for the assessment and treatment of contaminated wounds have been published by IAEA (1978; 1996b), NCRP (1980), and by the Commission of the European Communities jointly with DOE (Gerber and Thomas, 1992). Other useful references include: *Medical Management of Radiation Accidents* (Gusev *et al.*, 2001), *Decorporation of Radionuclides from the Human Body* (Henge-Napoli *et al.*, 2000), *Treatment of Accidental Intakes of Plutonium and Americium: Guidance Notes* (Menetrier *et al*, 2005), and *Decorporation of Radionuclides* (Stradling and Taylor, 2005).

A common question is what level of activity in a wound should indicate medical intervention. As is the case for all medical treatment, the ultimate responsibility for treating patients rests with the treating physician. However, medical decision making can and should be informed by dosimetric considerations. No definitive guidance is available; the truism "every case is different" always applies. Nevertheless, the health physicist can compute "saved dose" by standard techniques (Toohey, 2002; 2003b) and advise the treating physician. For a relatively innocuous intervention (*e.g.*, administration of DTPA) (see below), saved doses on the order of

1 to 10 times the annual limit may indicate therapy should be undertaken; for more drastic intervention (*e.g.*, surgical excision), saved doses exceeding 10 times the annual limit may be more appropriate. Local doses can be computed from the data in Table 5.2 and a direct measurement of activity in the wound. Maximum effective doses can be computed from the data in Table 5.3 and the measured activity, assuming all will become systemic. More realistic effective doses will be computable when systemic dose coefficients for activity in a wound have been developed.

6.2 General Principles in the Initial Evaluation and Care of a Wound Incident

The following is provided as guidance for care and not as prescriptive recommendations. Emergency life- or limb-threatening conditions must always receive primary consideration. It is the responsibility of first medical responders and responding physicians and nurses to preserve life and provide such emergency treatment as might be necessary to stabilize the patient. Such life- and limb-saving medical procedures always take precedence and must not be delayed by considerations related to contamination or reporting requirements. Initially, if indicated, remove the victim(s) from further contamination or other exposures and begin initial medical treatment. In those situations where the wounded individual(s) may be further contaminated, exposed to external ionizing radiation, or chemicals, it is prudent to move the person(s) to a clean area, as soon as possible.

In wound first aid and medical assessment, it is first necessary to achieve hemostasis and take whatever medical and surgical measures that may be indicated to preserve physiologic and anatomic function. Depending on the availability of equipment and supplies, and the training and experience of the responders, the medical evaluation and treatment may range from simple first aid to more advanced medical care prior to transportation to a medical facility capable of a more sophisticated level of medical care.

After the patient is medically stable, health-physics assessment is begun in order to identify the presence of radioactive contaminants and as possible, achieve an initial quantitative dosimetry estimate. Decontamination of an open wound takes priority over other actions because of the direct access of contamination to the bloodstream, so usually the wound is irrigated and visible fragments removed before a quantitative assessment of wound contamination is made (Section 6.4). After wound irrigation, decontamination of body orifices and then intact skin is performed, and, depending on the location of the wound, assessment of remaining activity may be performed simultaneously. Often this quantitative estimate of wound activity is achieved by wound counting using either a specialized wound probe or simply an appropriate type of radiation detector (Appendix E). Later measurements of a photon emitter may use an intrinsic germanium detector. For a wound containing plutonium/americium mixtures, this detector has the added advantage of superior resolution over older NaI(Tl) systems, and so the depth of remaining contamination in the wound may often be estimated by observing the relative attenuation of the various L-shell x-ray lines (Section 5 and Appendix E).

In those cases where radioactive material may be or is present in a wound, an assessment of type, amount and form of radioactive material by an experienced health physicist is essential to determining the best approach to medical treatment. Since many wounds are found on the hands, consultation with a hand surgeon may be advisable. In many cases, surgical debridement of the wound may be achieved, either by sharp excision, or by use of a 3 to 4 mm skin biopsy instrument. Historically, within the DOE complex where most plutonium wounds have occurred, reviews of medical records indicate that prompt patient evaluation and subsequent surgical excision of contaminated tissue were undertaken.

6.3 Consideration of Chelation or Other Systemic Medical Therapy

For some radionuclides that become deposited in a wound, such as radioisotopes of the lanthanides and actinides (e.g., plutonium, americium), systemic chelating agents such as the calcium- or zinc-DTPA can be used in those cases where there is a risk of systemic absorption of the radionuclide from the wound. Chelating agents bind metals into complexes that are stable in biological fluids, thus preventing tissue uptake and allowing urinary excretion. It is desirable to give such agents as soon as the risk is identified, since their effectiveness is greatest when given as soon after the exposure as possible. A more detailed description of DTPA administration is given at the end of this Section. Guidance for the use of other decorporation or blocking agents for intakes of other radionuclides is provided in NCRP Report No. 65 (NCRP, 1980).

6.4 Wound Decontamination with Irrigation and Removal of Visible Foreign Materials

Once the patient is stable, the next priority with a radionuclide-contaminated wound is removal of contamination in the open wound. Open wounds may allow rapid incorporation of radionuclides into the body, so they should be copiously irrigated with physiologic saline solution for several minutes. If contamination persists, surgical debridement may be necessary (Conklin *et al.*, 1983). Studies at Hanford (Norwood and Fuqua, 1969) indicate that scrubbing action employed in cleansing the wound may be more important than the cleansing agent. However, scrubbing should not be so vigorous as to cause increased trauma to the wound or to cause skin hyperemia in surrounding intact skin. Often microscopic fissures from vigorous scrubbing may allow more rapid transdermal absorption than if the skin were maintained intact.

Depending on the radionuclide present in the wound, the use of local chelating agents as irrigating solutions or injected locally around the wound site may be considered. Wounds contaminated with transuranics (plutonium and americium) may be irrigated with DTPA, which will bind and solubilize the contaminant, enhancing physical removal. The solubilized material will also be more likely to be absorbed into the bloodstream, but will be rapidly excreted in the urine. An effective irrigating solution consists of 1 g calcium-DTPA and 10 mL of 2 % lidocaine in 100 mL of 5 % glucose solution or isotonic saline (NCRP, 1980).

In decontaminating skin surrounding the wound, care should be taken not to contaminate the wound. Decontamination of intact skin usually requires only gently scrubbing with soap and warm water. Use of hot water is contraindicated because of the subsequent vasodilation. If more aggressive decontamination is necessary, a mixture of half corn meal and half laundry detergent has been shown to be effective. Hair can usually be decontaminated with soap and water. If this is inadequate, the hair should be clipped rather than shaved, to avoid disruption of the skin barrier.

Persons participating in decontamination should wear standard surgical gowns, gloves, aprons, and shoe and head covers. Health-physics monitoring may indicate the need for additional protective gear, but this has been rare in practice. If indicated, surgical exploration and excision of contaminated tissue/foreign material may be necessary, occasionally assisted by a health physicist using a wound probe. However, excision of tissue from a wound solely to remove radioactive contamination should be performed only upon the advice of a physician expert in radiological emergencies. Nevertheless, rapid excision of tissue bearing radioactive material is frequently the treatment of choice, and a review of >500 wound cases indicates that this has been done in most cases. However, it is important to consider the maintenance of functional capability and so consultation with a surgical subspecialist is often necessary. There is no contraindication to the use of standard local or systemic anesthetic agents in managing these types of wounds.

A wound containing radioactive material is usually treated by primary closure once adequate decontamination has taken place. For wounds that have had delayed care and where infection is likely, secondary closure may be advisable. If drains are used, any dressing must be monitored for activity. Wound eschar should also be collected and monitored for activity. If a radiation accident victim has received external exposure high enough to induce the acute radiation syndrome, surgical treatment of wounds must be completed within the first 48 h since exposure before immunosuppression occurs (Bushberg and Miller, 2004).

6.5 Wound Dressing and Follow-Up

Additional health physics and medical consideration should include:

- Contamination control and establishment of a radiological control area as required, to avoid further contamination of personnel, equipment or facilities. Experienced staff should establish appropriate control lines and controlled area boundaries, so the area can be properly surveyed, decontaminated and returned to normal use.
- In the response to a radiation accident it is necessary to ensure rescuer protection with avoidance of unnecessary contamination and/or external radiation exposure. Rescuers responding to an accident involving radioactive material should use appropriate personnel protective clothing and gear, if that is possible. This, however, should be a secondary priority to responding to and stabilizing injured victims.
- Communication with any wounded victim(s) requires a calm, measured approach that provides a careful explanation of the victim(s)' status and how the situation will probably be handled. Psychological support should also be offered to the victim and his or her family members (Berger and Sadoff, 2002).
- Reporting requirements regarding radiation accidents should also be considered along with the initial emergency medical management. It is required that appropriate authorities and/or supervisors be notified immediately of the status of the accident situation. In all instances, this

will be a secondary consideration when manpower is necessarily focused on medical emergencies.

- Continued physical and psychological follow-up care of the victim should be arranged, along with preservation of relevant data for scientific use.

6.6 Response Personnel

Prior planning and anticipation of credible accident scenarios, including radiological attack, are essential. NCRP Report No. 138 (NCRP, 2001b) provides planning guidance for radiological terrorist attacks that is adaptable to other credible scenarios. The existence of an appropriately trained emergency team is mandatory to ensure a rapid and appropriate response to a radiation accident. Policies and procedures must be well considered and practiced on a regular schedule. Equipment and supplies should be readily available and routinely checked and calibrated. Provision should be made for the administration of decorporation or blocking agents in a field situation by emergency medical technicians under the direction of the supervising physician.

6.7 Obtaining Emergency Information and Expert Advice

Oak Ridge Institute for Science and Education operates REAC/TS, an emergency response asset of DOE. Expert advice and information on managing radiation accidents is available at any time by calling (865) 576-1005. In addition, REAC/TS provides training courses that prepare hospital and emergency personnel to manage the medical response to radiation accidents. Information about these courses can be obtained by writing to REAC/TS, Oak Ridge Institute for Science and Education, P.O. Box 117, Oak Ridge, Tennessee 37831, USA; by calling (865) 576-3131; or on the web at http://orise.orau.gov/reacts (ORISE, 2007). Another source of medical advice is the Medical Radiological Assistance Team at AFRRI in Bethesda, Maryland [http://www.afrri.usuhs.mil (AFRRI, 2007)].

Each state in the United States maintains a radiation protection division in either the public health or environmental protection department that can provide guidance in setting up radiation protection programs. These professionals may also help with the assessment of radiation accidents and in dealing with ionizing radiation issues in industry, health care settings, and research and development projects. In most states, the state radiation protection agency is involved with licensing, auditing, inspecting or accrediting groups that use ionizing equipment and materials. A list of state contacts is maintained on the Conference of Radiation Control Program Directors website at http://www.crcpd.org/Map/map.asp (CRCPD, 2007).

6.8 Use of DTPA in the Management of Actinide-Contaminated Wounds

DTPA is a synthetic polyamino polycarboxylic acid that forms stable complexes (metal chelates) with a large number of metal ions. The drug effectively exchanges one metal (calcium or zinc) for another metal of greater binding power and carries it to the kidneys where it is excreted into the urine. The plasma half-life of DTPA is 20 to 60 min in adult humans. Almost the entire administered dose is excreted in 12 h. DTPA undergoes only little metabolic change in the body. Following i.v. administration, DTPA is rapidly distributed throughout the extracellular fluid space. A small fraction is bound to plasma proteins with a half-life >20 h, and ternary compounds of DTPA, plutonium and plasma proteins may be formed. The urinary excretion half-life of plutonium-DTPA is ~5 d in adult humans, so that after one injection of DTPA the excretion of plutonium is enhanced for approximately two to three weeks when compared to plutonium excretion without DTPA (Schofield et al., 1974).

DTPA is available as the calcium and zinc salts. Calcium-DTPA is somewhat more effective than zinc-DTPA for initial chelation of transuranics. Therefore, calcium-DTPA is the form of choice for initial patient management unless contraindicated. Approximately 24 h after exposure, zinc-DTPA is as effective as calcium-DTPA. This comparable efficacy, coupled with its lesser toxicity for long-term therapy, makes zinc-DTPA the preferred agent for protracted therapy. Calcium- and zinc-DTPA effectively chelate several transuranic ions (e.g., plutonium, americium, berkelium, curium and californium). Their most common clinical use has been for treatment of internal contamination with plutonium and americium. The efficacy of calcium- and/or zinc-DTPA treatment is good for internal contamination with the soluble plutonium salts, such as the nitrate or chloride, but is not very effective for insoluble compounds, such as the high-fired oxide. The same efficacy is noted in animal experiments when a soluble (monomeric) form of plutonium is administered that gradually converts to less-soluble forms as it is distributed and deposited in various tissues in the body. Thus, effective chelation is highly dependent not only on the actual metal, but also on the chemical and physical characteristics of the compound at the time of DTPA administration. Because the efficiency of DTPA chelation decreases with time, it should be given promptly after exposure. The effectiveness of the treatment diminishes the longer the interval between exposure and treatment.

Calcium- and zinc-DTPA were approved by the U.S. Food and Drug Administration (FDA) on August 11, 2004 for treatment of intakes of certain radionuclides. These drugs are available by prescription and should only be given under the supervision of a physician. Detailed information is available at the FDA website [http://www.fda.gov (FDA, 2007)] and the Centers for Disease Control and Prevention (CDC) website [http://www.cdc.gov (CDC, 2007)] or by calling the CDC at (800) 311-3435.

6.8.1 *Dosage and Administration*

An adult dose of calcium-DTPA is 0.5 to 1 g and doses should not be fractionated. The route of administration may be either slow i.v. push of the drug over a period of 3 to 4 min or i.v. infusion (1 g in 100 to 250 mL D_5W, Ringer's Lactate, or normal saline). Each i.v. administration should not last >2 h.

Calcium-DTPA may be administered undiluted by i.m. injection when i.v. administration is not practical, although significant pain at the injection site has resulted when this route is used. The addition of 1 to 2 % procaine or lidocaine to the undiluted calcium-DTPA prior to i.m. injection has proven to be helpful in reducing injection site pain.

DTPA may be given by inhalation in a nebulizer (1:1 dilution with water or normal saline). The effect will be slower and the absorbed dosage is less predictable by this method than by i.v. or i.m. injection. Smith (1974) reported that the residence time in the body of calcium-DTPA administered by nebulizer is a factor of two greater than when i.v. administered, and Stather *et al.* (1976) reported that calcium-DTPA administered by nebulizer soon after exposure was more effective in removing soluble forms of plutonium deposited in the lung than was the i.v. administered agent. The only contraindication to nebulizer administration is preexisting lung pathology (NCRP, 1980).

Regardless of administration route, the chelating efficacy is greatest immediately or within 1 h of exposure when the radionuclide is circulating in or available to tissue fluids and plasma. However, post-exposure intervals longer than 1 h do not preclude the administration and effective action of calcium-DTPA.

6.8.2 *Combined Calcium- and Zinc-DTPA Therapy Guidelines*

It should be noted that the statements above are general guidelines for DTPA therapy and that treatment must be specifically
tailored for each individual patient. Calcium- and zinc-DTPA may
be thought of as two components of transuranic decorporation therapy. If there is any contraindication to the use of calcium-DTPA,
the same dose of zinc-DTPA may be substituted. A generic protocol
follows:

1. On assurance that a credible incident has occurred and that
   the exposed person(s) at risk has, in all likelihood, received
   internal transuranic contamination:

   a. Obtain baseline blood samples for complete blood count
      with differential, blood urea nitrogen, and serum creati-
      nine, and urine samples for urinalysis and urine radio-
      bioassay, and as medically indicated thereafter.

   b. Administer 1 g calcium-DTPA by the most appropriate
      route (do not wait for the results of radioanalysis of the
      first urine sample).

   c. Begin collection of 24 h urine and fecal samples for bioas-
      say. Chest, liver, skull and/or wound counting should also
      be performed as appropriate. At very early times after a
      large, acute exposure, blood assays may prove helpful if
      the initial urinalysis is positive for transuranic contami-
      nation.

   d. If long-term use of calcium-DTPA is contemplated, one
      should consider the use of supplemental zinc therapy
      (one 220 mg zinc sulfate tablet daily delivers 50 mg zinc
      systemically).

   e. Repeat doses of 1 g calcium- or zinc-DTPA may be admin-
      istered daily for up to 5 d in the first week if the radiobio-
      assay data or history indicate the need for additional
      chelation. Note that the majority of patients in the past
      have received only one dose of DTPA. However, one
      patient who in an industrial accident received the high-
      est intake of ^{241}Am ever reported, received daily injec-
      tions of zinc-DTPA for 11 months, followed by thrice-
      weekly injections for the next 11 months; injections con-
      tinued at reduced frequency thereafter (Breitenstein,
      1983).

   f. Although no significant side effects of DTPA at the rec-
      ommended dosage level are known and there are no

known contraindications to its use, urinalysis and complete blood counts should be done at the time of the initial treatment and as medically indicated thereafter. The patient's pulse and blood pressure also should be monitored during each drug infusion. Bioassay results and any side effects should be noted and recorded on the standard treatment form.

g. Additional tests may be ordered at the discretion of the treating physician and with the consent of the patient.

2. Before, during and after chelation therapy, pertinent measurements for excretion and retention of radioactive material should be made to determine the efficacy of treatment. By the fifth day, evaluate bioassay data for intake/uptake estimation and decide whether further chelation is necessary. If continued chelation therapy is needed, a zinc-DTPA treatment regimen should be implemented.

a. Begin the therapy regimen by administration of zinc-DTPA on a two-dose per week basis, 1 g zinc-DTPA per dose, until such time as the urine excretion rate of the transuranic is not increased by zinc-DTPA administration.

b. Subsequently it may be indicated to wait four to six months, then reestablish a baseline urinary excretion-rate value and give a 1 g zinc-DTPA dose by an appropriate route. Obtain bioassay measurements to determine whether the zinc-DTPA increased excretion of the contaminant.

c. If medically indicated, begin a second course of zinc-DTPA treatment on a two-dose per week basis as in 2.a above.

d. If medically indicated, more frequent administration of zinc-DTPA may be performed (Carbaugh et al., 1989).

3. Total length of chelation treatment after an accident is dictated by the nature and magnitude of the accident and by the medical judgment of the attending physician.

4. When the patient is released from treatment, he/she should be followed at the routine intervals established by the occupational practice of the facility where the individual is employed. A urinalysis including radiobioassay is recommended at these examinations.

5. It is recommended that at the time of an employment termination, the treating physician should forward a copy of the

medical history to a physician of the patient's choice. This should be done to ensure continuity of patient care and to assist if he/she should again become contaminated and require therapy elsewhere.

6. Patients who have received extensive chronic incorporation of transuranics require unusual therapy and will be treated largely according to the discretion of the physician. In the past, treatment has not exceeded three 1 g doses during any 24 h period. Doses should be administered by the route considered most appropriate for the particular patient (Breitenstein, 1983).

7. Summary

This Report presents a comprehensive review and in some cases, reanalysis of animal data relating to the biokinetic behavior of radionuclides in wounds. The data have been used to derive the parameters of a comprehensive compartmental model for contaminated wounds, while the structure of the model itself is grounded in the biochemical and physiological response of the body to a wound. Information is also presented on the etiology of radionuclide-contaminated wounds, and the biological processes of wound healing, including foreign-body responses and carcinogenesis. Human data from occupational, military and medical exposures are provided to relate the animal data to human experience. Dose coefficients for local doses are presented, as is a summary of wound monitoring methodology. The development of systemic dose coefficients based on the wound model for all commonly encountered radionuclides is beyond the scope of this Report, but should be undertaken in the future. Finally, current procedures for the medical management of contaminated wounds are discussed.

7.1 Human Experience

The literature contains reports of >2,100 cases of contaminated wounds incurred by radiological workers, mostly in nuclear weapons complexes (Section 3.1). However, because the vast majority of these wounds received prompt medical treatment, including excision and/or decorporation therapy, they do not provide data that can be used to develop parameters of the wound model specifically for humans.

Another set of human data comes from military personnel wounded with DU shrapnel during the first Gulf War (Section 3.2). In many cases, embedded DU shrapnel was not surgically removable without risk of substantial damage to healthy tissue or loss of function, and so was left in place. Medical follow-up of wounded personnel has provided data on the urinary excretion of DU from embedded shrapnel, but has not revealed any clinically significant health effects.

A brief description of wound healing and pathobiology is provided in Section 3, with more detail in Appendix F.

7.2 The Wound Model

The wound model developed in this Report (Figure 4.1) comprises seven compartments, of which five describe radionuclide behavior at the wound site, and two can receive radionuclides transported from the wound site. The seven compartments are:

- fragment
- soluble
- colloid and intermediate state
- particles, aggregates and bound state
- trapped particles and aggregates
- blood
- lymph nodes

The compartments that come into play for any given wound depend on the physico-chemical properties of the radionuclide in the wound (Figures 4.2 to 4.5).

The animal data show that radionuclides i.m. injected in initially soluble form could be divided into four categories, based on their retention at the wound site, namely weak, moderate, strong and avid (Table 4.1; Section 4.2.2.2). On average, weakly-retained radionuclides have 2.8 % of the injected amount present at the wound site at 1 d post-injection, and 1.2 % present at 16 d. Moderately-retained radionuclides have 31 % of the injected amount present at the wound site at 1 d, and 3.9 % present at 64 d. Strongly-retained radionuclides have 66 % of the injected amount present at the wound site at 1 d, and 19 % present at 64 d. Avidly-retained radionuclides have 86 % of the injected amount present at the wound site at 1 d, and 62 % present at 64 d.

The parameters (partition coefficients and rate constants) of the default wound retention equations for the four retention types and for colloids, particles and fragments are given in Table 4.11, and the default transfer rates between the various pairs of model compartments for the four retention types and for colloids, particles and fragments are given in Table 4.12.

7.3 Management of Contaminated Wounds

The management of radionuclide-contaminated wounds is relatively straightforward. Although medical considerations always take priority in the treatment of any serious injury, the vast majority of contaminated wounds are not life-threatening, and the victim remains medically stable. Consequently, radiological assessment is usually performed promptly, first with portable instrumentation, and then, especially if initial results are positive, with more sophisticated monitoring equipment. Data on both the amount of radioactive material and its local distribution at the wound site can normally be obtained, and serve to inform medical decision making for wound excision and decorporation therapy. Details on wound monitoring are provided in Appendix E.

Tables of dose coefficients are provided in Section 5 for the shallow dose rate to the skin at the wound site and the local dose rate within the wound site for the radionuclides commonly encountered in the workplace (Tables 5.1 and 5.2). In addition, dose coefficients for other organs and tissues are shown in Table 5.3, based on the assumption that all activity at the wound site will become systemic.

The wound model presented in this Report will be used to derive dose coefficients that will take into account the retention of the radionuclide at the wound site. The input to the blood compartment of the wound model is the input to the transfer compartment of the systemic biokinetic model recommended by ICRP for the radionuclide. As a result, systemic dose coefficients will be generated in terms of unit activity injected at the wound site, without the assumption that all of it will become systemic. A detailed example of the generation of such parameters for the case of wounds contaminated with uranium is provided in Appendix D. NCRP believes this next step in the application of the wound model will produce better decision making for the management of contaminated wounds, although the worse-case assumption still has a place in the rapid assessment of a serious wound, or in a mass casualty situation as could occur as a result of a serious industrial accident or the use of an explosive radiological dispersal device.

Guidance for the medical treatment of patients with contaminated wounds is provided in Section 6. Recommended steps to be taken for the radiological protection of response personnel and detailed procedures for wound decontamination, dressing and follow-up, and the use of DTPA as a decorporation agent for transuranics are included.

7.4 Animal Data

Appendices A and B of this Report present a comprehensive review and discussion of data obtained over the past 60 y from experimental animals wounded with radioactive substances. Animal models include the rat, rabbit, dog, miniature swine, and monkey, and data for a total of 54 radionuclides are included. Wounding mechanisms include i.m. and s.c. injection or implantation, laceration, and direct application to intact, abraded, and thermally or chemically-burned skin. The physico-chemical forms of the administered radionuclides include solutions, colloidal suspensions, insoluble particles, and fragments such as wires and metal disks. Parameters including injected mass, volume, radionuclide concentration, solution pH, and the solubility of the nuclide at physiologic pH all affect the biokinetic behavior of the contaminant.

The animal experiments provide data on the retention of the contaminant at the wound site and its translocation to other deposition sites, both by the transfer compartment (blood and other bodily fluids such as lymph) and by phagocytosis and migration of macrophages to regional lymph nodes (Appendix C). The analysis of the retention and translocation of the contaminant as functions of the parameters mentioned above is used first to generate partitioning and rate constants for generic wound retention equations and then to develop recommended transfer coefficients among the various compartments of the wound model.

Appendix A

Dissolved Radionuclides in Experimental Wounds: Sources and Data

A.1 Puncture Wounds: Intramuscular Injection

This Appendix summarizes the studies of retention of radionuclides at an experimental puncture wound site. These investigations, nearly all done in rats, provide a systematic database for quantifying and classifying retention of soluble radionuclides deposited in deep wounds.

A.1.1 *Radionuclide Biokinetics Studies at the University of California Radiation Laboratory*

Early in 1942, Dr. Joseph G. Hamilton and a team of nuclear chemists, analytical chemists, and biologists working at the Crocker Laboratory, University of California Radiation Laboratory (UCRL) (now the Lawrence Berkeley National Laboratory), began the systematic preparation, separation and quantitative description of the biokinetics in rats of the products and heavy byproducts of nuclear fission (Hamilton, 1943; 1947a; 1947b; Lanz *et al.*, 1946; Scott *et al.*, 1947; 1948a; 1948b; 1949; Van Middlesworth, 1947). Those studies were later expanded to include the biokinetics of the entire lanthanide series and many previously unstudied or poorly understood transition group metals and heavy elements (Crowley *et al.*, 1949; Durbin, 1960; 1962; Durbin *et al.* 1956; 1957; 1958; Hamilton, 1948a; 1948b; 1948c; 1948d; 1948e; 1949a; 1949b; 1949c; 1949d; 1950a; 1950b; 1950c; 1951a; 1951b; 1951c; Kawin *et al.*, 1950; Lanz *et al.*, 1950; Scott and Hamilton, 1950; Scott *et al.*, 1951). The results of those studies were used to develop the earliest protection standards for many internally-deposited radionuclides (ICRP, 1959; NBS, 1953).

The radionuclides were administered to rats by i.m. injection in most of the UCRL biokinetic studies, but because the purpose of the program was to describe the distribution and excretion of radionuclides absorbed into the blood, the published data for each radionuclide were expressed as percent of the absorbed fraction of the injected activity. The fraction of the injected radionuclide retained at the wound site was often not included in the published reports. However, the original project work records were available in the Lawrence Berkeley National Laboratory archives.

The archived publications, progress reports, and work records of the UCRL group for the years 1942 to 1960 were searched, and the data were assembled for the studies in which uncomplexed radionuclides were administered by i.m. injection. A summary was prepared for each study, which included the chemical form of the radionuclide, the amount of radioactive material injected, the volume and pH of the injected solution, and the fraction of injected radionuclide retained at the wound site at the post-injection times investigated. The experimental conditions of the suitable UCRL studies are presented in Table A.1. The retention data (unabsorbed fraction remaining at the i.m. site) are presented in Table A.2.

Radionuclides were diluted in isotonic saline (0.14 mol L^{-1} NaCl) at pH 2 to 7, and injected volumes ranged from 0.1 to 1 mL. Groups of three 2 to 4 month old male or female rats were injected in the thigh muscles of the left leg. The muscle tissue was expected to act as a filter that would permit entry into the blood only of ions that are soluble at physiological pH or are complexed by circulating bioligands. The intact injected leg and the separated bones and muscle of the uninjected leg were radioanalyzed. Sample preparation and radioanalysis procedures were reported in many of the publications. The mean recovered radioactive material (i.e., the sum of the retained fraction in the left leg plus the sum of the activity in the bones and muscle of the right leg) each expressed as percent of the amount of radioactive material injected [percent injected dosage (% ID)] for each three-rat group was normalized to 100 % of the injected dosage, and the retained fraction was calculated as follows:

$$\text{retained fraction} = \text{fraction in the left leg} \tag{A.1}$$
$$- \text{fraction in the bones and muscle of the right leg}.$$

Although practical and efficient, that method of assessing radionuclide retention in the injected leg slightly overestimates retention,

TABLE A.1—*Intramuscular injections in rats of radionuclides in solution: Experimental conditions.*[a]

Radionuclide	Amount injected		Solution			References
	(Bq)[b]	(μg)[c]	(mL)[d]	(mol L^{-1})[e]	(pH)[f]	
Anions and complex oxo- and chloro-metal ions						
$^{131}I^-$	7.4×10^4	1.6×10^{-5}	2.5×10^{-2}	4.9×10^{-9}	3	Ilyin and Ivannikov (1979)
$^{71}GeO_3^{2-}$	1.8×10^5	3.0×10^{-5}		1.4×10^{-9}	7	Hamilton (1948b)
$^{71}GeO_3^{2-}$	1.8×10^5	1.0×10^3		4.7×10^{-2}	7	Hamilton (1948b)
$^{48}VO_3^-$	2.2×10^5	3.5×10^{-5}		2.4×10^{-9}	6	Scott et al. (1951)
$^{74}AsCl_5^{2-}$	2.8×10^5	7.4×10^{-5}	5×10^{-1}	2.0×10^{-9}	6	Lanz et al. (1950)
$^{124}SbO_3^-$	3.7×10^4	5.7×10^{-5}		1.5×10^{-9}	6	Hamilton (1948a)
$^{75}SeO_4^{2-}$	3.3×10^5	6.6×10^{-4}		2.9×10^{-8}	6	Hamilton (1948b; 1948c)
$^{127m, 129m}TeO_4^{2-}$	2.6×10^4	5.1×10^{-5}	4×10^{-1}	5.1×10^{-10}	6	Scott et al. (1947)
$^{181}WO_4^{2-}$	5.6×10^4	2.9×10^{-4}	2×10^{-1}	1.1×10^{-8}	7	Durbin et al. (1957)
$^{95,96}TcCl_6^{2-}$	3.7×10^6	2.4×10^{-3}		8.3×10^{-8}	6	Durbin et al. (1957)
$^{106}RuCl_5^{2-}$	1.1×10^6	8.8×10^{-3}		2.8×10^{-7}	3	Scott et al. (1947)
$^{185}OsO_5^{2-}$	7.4×10^5	2.8×10^{-3}	7×10^{-1}	2.1×10^{-8}	6	Durbin et al. (1957)
$^{185}RhCl_6^{3-}$	1.7×10^5	5.4×10^{-6}	2×10^{-1}	2.6×10^{-10}	6	Durbin et al. (1957)
$^{191,193}PtCl_4^{2-}$	3.0×10^5	4.2×10^{-5}	1×10^{-1}	1.5×10^{-9}	6	Durbin et al. (1957)

TABLE A.1—(continued)

Radionuclide	Amount injected		Solution			References
	$(Bq)^b$	$(\mu g)^c$	$(mL)^d$	$(mol\ L^{-1})^e$	$(pH)^f$	
Monovalent cations						
^{86}RbCl	1.8×10^4	6.3×10^{-6}		2.4×10^{-10}	4	Hamilton (1948b)
^{134,137}CsCl	5.6×10^4	1.8×10^{-2}		4.3×10^{-7}	3	Scott et al. (1947)
^{137}CsCl^g	7.4×10^4	2.3×10^{-2}	2.5×10^{-2}	6.6×10^{-6}	3	Ilyin and Ivannikov (1979)
^{105,106,111}AgCl	3.7×10^4	3.8×10^{-5}		1.2×10^{-9}	6	Scott and Hamilton (1950)
^{105,106,111}AgCl	3.7×10^4	1.0×10^3		3.2×10^{-2}	6	Scott and Hamilton (1950)
^{237}NpO$_2$NO$_3$	2.6 to 3.9×10^3	1.0 to 1.5×10^2	1×10^{-1}	4.3 to 6.4×10^{-3}	2	Morin et al. (1973a) Nenot et al. (1972a)
Divalent cations						
^{7}BeCl$_2$	7.4×10^5	5.7×10^{-5}	1×10^0	8.1×10^{-9}	3	Crowley et al. (1949)
^{45}CaCl$_2$	1.8×10^5 b	2.6×10^{-4}	2×10^{-1}	2.9×10^{-8}	6	Hamilton (1948c)
^{90}SrCl$_2$	1.8×10^5 b	3.2×10^{-2}	2×10^{-1}	1.8×10^{-6}	7	Hamilton (1948c)
^{133}BaCl$_2$	1.1×10^5 b	1.2×10^{-2}	2×10^{-1}	4.6×10^{-7}	5	Scott et al. (1947)
^{223}RaCl$_2$	5.6×10^4	2.9×10^{-5}	1×10^{-1}	4.4×10^{-10}	4	Durbin et al. (1958)
^{64}CuCl$_2$	1.5×10^5	1.0×10^{-6}		5.3×10^{-11}	7	Hamilton[h]
^{64}CuCl$_2$	1.5×10^5	1.0×10^3		5.3×10^{-2}	7	Hamilton[h]
^{230}UO$_2$Cl$_2$	3.7×10^3	4.1×10^{-6}		5.3×10^{-11}		Hamilton (1948c)
^{233}UO$_2$Cl$_2$	1.3×10^4	3.7×10^1		5.3×10^{-4}	5	Hamilton (1948a)

^{239}PuO$_2$Cl$_2$	3.7×10^4	1.6×10^1	1×10^0	6.7×10^{-5}	2	Kawin et al. (1950) Scott et al. (1948a) Van Middlesworth (1947)
^{239}PuO$_2$(NO$_3$)$_2$	4.6×10^4	2.0×10^1	1×10^{-1}	8.4×10^{-4}	2	Kisieleski and Woodruff (1947)
Trivalent cations						
^{46}ScCl$_3$	7.4×10^4 b	6.0×10^{-5}	2×10^{-1}	8.7×10^{-9}	6	Hamilton (1950b; 1950c; 1951c)
^{88}YCl$_3$	7.4×10^5	1.4×10^{-3}		5.3×10^{-8}	3	Hamilton (1948c) Scott et al. (1947)
^{140}LaCl$_3$	1.8×10^5	9.1×10^{-6}		2.2×10^{-10}	3	Hamilton (1943) Scott et al. (1947)
^{140}LaCl$_3$	1.8×10^5	1.0×10^3		2.4×10^{-2}	3	Hamilton (1948c)
^{67}GaCl$_3$	2.2×10^5	1.0×10^{-5}		5.0×10^{-10}		Hamilton (1949a)
^{114m}InCl$_3$	1.8×10^4	2.0×10^{-5}		4.5×10^{-10}	6	Durbin et al. (1957) Hamilton (1948a)
^{51}CrCl$_3$	3.7×10^4 b	1.1×10^{-5}		7.3×10^{-10}	5	Hamilton (1950b)
^{95}NbCl$_3$	3.1×10^5	2.2×10^{-5}	3×10^{-1}	7.7×10^{-10}	3	Scott et al. (1947) Durbin et al. (1957)
Trivalent lanthanides						
^{144}CeCl$_3$	3.7×10^4	3.2×10^{-4}		7.3×10^{-9}	3	Scott et al. (1947)
^{143}PrCl$_3$	9.2×10^3	3.7×10^{-6}		8.7×10^{-11}	3	Scott et al. (1947)
^{143}PrCl$_3$	9.2×10^3	1.0×10^3		2.4×10^{-2}	3	Hamilton (1949b)
^{147}NdCl$_3$	1.8×10^6	5.9×10^{-4}		1.5×10^{-8}	3	Hamilton (1949a)

TABLE A.1—(*continued*)

Radionuclide	Amount injected		Solution			References
	$(Bq)^b$	$(\mu g)^c$	$(mL)^d$	$(mol\ L^{-1})^e$	$(pH)^f$	
$^{147}NdCl_3$	1.8×10^6	1.0×10^3		2.5×10^{-2}		Hamilton (1949a)
$^{147}PmCl_3$	9.2×10^5	2.5×10^{-2}		5.7×10^{-7}	3	Hamilton (1947a; 1948f; 1949e)
$^{154,155}EuCl_3$	8.1×10^4	6.0×10^{-1}		1.3×10^{-5}		Hamilton (1948d; 1948e; 1949b)
$^{160}TbCl_3$	2.8×10^5	6.0×10^{-1}	5×10^{-1}	7.6×10^{-6}	4	Hamilton (1950b; 1951a)
$^{166}HoCl_3$	5.2×10^5	5×10^1		1.0×10^{-3}		Hamilton (1949d)
$^{170}TmCl_3$	2.8×10^5	2.5×10^0	2×10^{-1}	7.5×10^{-5}	5	Hamilton (1950c; 1951c)
$^{175}YbCl_3$	5.2×10^5	3.3×10^1		6.3×10^{-4}		Hamilton (1949d)
$^{177}LuCl_3$	2.7×10^5	6×10^0		1.1×10^{-4}		Hamilton (1949d)
Trivalent actinides						
$^{227}AcCl_3$	4.6×10^4 b	1.7×10^{-2}		2.5×10^{-7}		Hamilton (1948b; 1948c)
$^{239}PuCl_3$	3.7×10^4	1.6×10^1	1×10^0	6.7×10^{-5}	3	Scott et al. (1948a)
$^{241}AmCl_3$	3.7×10^4	3×10^{-1}	1×10^0	1.2×10^{-6}	5	Scott et al. (1948b)
$^{241}Am(NO_3)_3$ [i]	2×10^2 to 3.8×10^2	1.6×10^{-3} to 3×10^{-3}	1×10^{-2}	6.6×10^{-7} to 1.9×10^{-6}	1	Gray et al. (1994) Harrison et al. (1978b) Stradling et al. (1993; 1995b)
$^{241}Am(NO_3)_3$ [i]	3.2×10^4 to 1.8×10^5	2.5×10^{-1} to 1.5×10^0	1×10^{-1}	1×10^{-5} to 6×10^{-5}	2	Lafuma et al. (1971) Morin et al. (1973b) Nenot et al. (1972a)

^{242}CmCl$_3$	3.7×10^4	3×10^{-4}	1×10^0	1.2×10^{-9}	5	Scott et al. (1949)
^{244}Cm(NO$_3$)$_3$ [i]	3.7×10^2	1.2×10^{-4}	1×10^{-2}	5×10^{-8}	1	Harrison et al. (1978b)
^{242}Cm(NO$_3$)$_3$	3.7×10^4	3×10^{-4}	1×10^{-1}	1.2×10^{-8}	2	Morin et al. (1973b) Nenot et al. (1972b)
^{242}Cm(NO$_3$)$_3$	1.8×10^5	1.5×10^{-3}	1×10^{-1}	6.0×10^{-8}	2	Nenot et al. (1972a)

Tetravalent and pentavalent cations and actinides

^{95}ZrCl$_4$	2.6×10^5	3.3×10^{-4}	5×10^{-1}	5×10^{-9}	2.5	Scott et al. (1947)
^{113}SnCl$_4$	7.4×10^4	1.9×10^{-4}		5.7×10^{-9}		Hamilton, (1948a; 1949a)
^{210}Po(NO$_3$)$_4$	7.4×10^4	4.4×10^{-4}	1×10^{-1}	2.1×10^{-8}	2	Ilyin et al. (1977)
^{233}PaCl$_5$	3.7×10^5	4.7×10^{-4}		6.7×10^{-9}	2.6	Lanz et al. (1946)
^{234}ThCl$_4$	3.7×10^5	4.2×10^{-4}		6×10^{-9}	2.6	Lanz et al. (1946)
^{228}Th(NO$_3$)$_4$	6×10^2	2×10^{-5}	1×10^{-2}	8.8×10^{-9}	1	Stradling et al. (1995a)
^{238}Pu(NO$_3$)$_4$	2.6×10^1	4×10^{-5}	1×10^{-1}	1.7×10^{-8}	1	Harrison et al. (1977b)
^{238}Pu(NO$_3$)$_4$	7.3×10^3	1.1×10^{-2}	1×10^{-1}	4.6×10^{-6}	1	Harrison et al. (1977b)
^{238}Pu(NO$_3$)$_4$	3.7×10^4 to 1.5×10^5	5×10^{-2} to 2.3×10^{-1}	1×10^{-1}	2.1×10^{-6} to 9.7×10^{-6}	2	Lafuma et al. (1971) Morin et al. (1972; 1973b) Nenot et al. (1972a; 1972b);
^{239}Pu(NO$_3$)$_4$ [i,j]	2.5×10^1	1.1×10^{-2}	1×10^{-1}	4.6×10^{-6}	1	Harrison et al. (1978a) Nenot and Stather (1979)

TABLE A.1—(continued)

Radionuclide	Amount injected			Solution		References
	$(Bq)^{b}$	$(\mu g)^{c}$	$(mL)^{d}$	$(mol\ L^{-1})^{e}$	$(pH)^{f}$	
$^{239}Pu(NO_3)_4{}^{i,j}$	2.3×10^{2} to 1.1×10^{3}	1×10^{-1} to 4.8×10^{-1}	1×10^{-1}	4.2×10^{-5} to 2×10^{-4}	1	Gray et al. (1994) Harrison and David (1977; 1978) Harrison et al. (1977a; 1977b; 1978a; 1978b) Nenot and Stather (1979)
$^{239}Pu(NO_3)_4{}^{i,j}$	3.7×10^{3} to 7.4×10^{3}	1.6×10^{0} to 3.2×10^{0}	5×10^{-3} to 1×10^{-1}	6.7×10^{-5} to 2.7×10^{-3}	1	Harrison et al. (1978a) Nenot and Stather (1979) Taylor (1967) Taylor and Sowby (1962)
$^{239}Pu(NO_3)_4{}^{i,j}$	2×10^{4}	8.8×10^{0}	1×10^{-1}	3.4×10^{-3}	<0	Volf (1974a; 1974b; 1975)

[a]Radionuclide injected into the thigh muscle of rats, except see footnotes g, i, and j.

[b]Activity of radionuclide injected (becquerel); reported values, except six designated radionuclides, for which injected dosage was calculated from the counting rate of the dosing standards and the detection system efficiency.

[c]Mass of element injected (micrograms); calculated from the injected activity using Equation A.3. for carrier-free radionuclides, or total mass when radionuclide was added to carrier solution.

[d]When injected volume was not reported, a default value of 0.3 mL was assumed.

[e]Molar concentration (mol L^{-1}) of radionuclides in solutions injected was calculated from the injected mass and volume using Equation A.5.

[f]When solution of pH was not reported, a default value of pH 4 was assumed.

[g]Cesium-137 injected in "skin-muscle wound" (Ilyin and Ivannikov, 1979).

[h]Hamilton, J.G. (1948). Personal communication (University of California Radiation Laboratory, Berkeley, California).

[i]Includes hamsters i.m. injected in thigh muscle.

[j]Includes rats i.m. injected in muscle of foreleg.

TABLE A.2—*Intramuscular injections in rats of radionuclides in solution: Retention at the wound site.*[a]

Radionuclide	Mass (μg)	Fraction Retained in the Wound (percent injected amount) at Time t (days post-injection) Time (d)[b]												Retention Class[c,d]
		0.042	0.167	1	4	6–8	14–16	28–32	60–64	90	120	180	256	
Anions and complex oxo- and chloro-metal ions														
$^{131}I^-$	1.6×10^{-5}	8.0	2.5	1.0										W
$^{71}GeO_3^{2-}$	3.0×10^{-5}		12	3.4	0.44									W
$^{71}GeO_3^{2-}$	1.0×10^{3}			10										m
$^{48}VO_3^-$	3.5×10^{-5}			27	22		8.4		4.8					M
$^{74}AsCl_5^{2-}$	7.4×10^{-5}			1.0										W
$^{124}SbO_3^-$	5.7×10^{-5}			0.36	0.14		0.08							W
$^{75}SeO_4^{2-}$	6.6×10^{-4}			2.4	1.4		0.26							W
$^{127m,129m}TeO_4^{2-}$	5.1×10^{-5}			55	22		9.0	7.3						M
$^{181}WO_4^{2-}$	2.9×10^{-4}		46	0.5										W
$^{95,96}TcCl_6^{2-}$	2.4×10^{-3}			2.2		0.46								W
$^{106}RuCl_5^{2-}$	8.8×10^{-3}				28	1.3	17		20					S
$^{185}OsO_5^{2-}$	2.8×10^{-3}			25	7.5									M
$^{185}RhCl_6^{3-}$	5.4×10^{-6}			11		7.3	7.1							M
$^{191,193}PtCl_4^{2-}$	4.2×10^{-5}				9.4	7.3		4.4						M
Monovalent cations														
$^{86}RbCl$	6.3×10^{-6}				0.85									W

TABLE A.2—(continued)

Radionuclide	Mass (μg)	Fraction Retained in the Wound (percent injected amount) at Time t (days post-injection) Time (d)[b]												Retention Class[c,d]
		0.042	0.167	1	4	6–8	14–16	28–32	60–64	90	120	180	256	
^{134,137}CsCl[e]	2×10^{-2}	20	11	5.6	6.4		2.6							W
^{105,106,} ^{111}AgNO$_3$	3.8×10^{-5}			26	12		9.0	3.0						M
^{105,106,} ^{111}AgNO$_3$	1.0×10^{-3}					46								s
^{237}NpO$_2$NO$_3$	1.0 to 1.5×10^2			75	57	54	53	36						s
Divalent cations														
^{7}BeCl$_2$	5.7×10^{-5}			60	46	24	30	24	18					S
^{45}CaCl$_2$	2.6×10^{-4}				2.6									W
^{90}SrCl$_2$	3.2×10^{-2}				5.1									W
^{133}BaCl$_2$	1.2×10^{-2}			4.0	2.0	2.0								W
^{223}RaCl$_2$	2.9×10^{-5}			41		14	9.3		$(0.23)^f$					M
^{64}CuCl$_2$	1.0×10^{-6}			4.9										W
^{64}CuCl$_2$	1.0×10^{3}			37										m
^{230}UO$_2$Cl$_2$	4.1×10^{-6}			5.3	5.0		1.2	2.1						W
^{233}UO$_2$Cl$_2$	3.7×10^{1}			4.0	3.1		1.5		1.0				0.3	w
^{239}PuO$_2$Cl$_2$	1.6×10^{1}				69	48	30		35				13	s
^{239}PuO$_2$(NO$_3$)$_2$	2.0×10^{1}					51	46	37	40	31			22	s

Trivalent cations

									A
46ScCl₃	6.0×10^{-5}	88							A
88YCl₃	1.4×10^{-3}	71	75		26	28	8.2		S
140LaCl₃	9.1×10^{-6}	66	35						S
140LaCl₃	1.0×10^{3}	98	30	36					a
67GaCl₃	1.0×10^{-5}	32	36						S
114mInCl₃	2.0×10^{-5}	48	31		18	19	11		S
51CrCl₃	1.1×10^{-5}	50			41				S
95NbCl₃	2.2×10^{-5}	61	44		41		18		S

Trivalent lanthanides

144CeCl₃	3.2×10^{-4}	62	40		27		10		S
143PrCl₃	5.7×10^{-6}	72	55		37	32	30		S
143PrCl₃	1×10^{3}	91	86						a
147NdCl₃	5.9×10^{-4}	73	57		36	35			S
147NdCl₃	1×10^{3}	97	98		96		97		a
147PmCl₃	2.5×10^{-2}	54	51		39	32	16	4.3	S
154, 155EuCl₃	6×10^{-1}	73	72		65	56	40	21	S
160TbCl₃	6×10^{-1}	62	50		32	32		11	S
166HoCl₃	5×10^{1}	96	96						a
170TmCl₃	2.5×10^{0}	68	51		38	37		14	S

TABLE A.2—(continued)

Radionuclide	Mass (µg)	Fraction Retained in the Wound (percent injected amount) at Time t (days post-injection)												Retention Class[c,d]
		Time (d)[b]												
		0.042	0.167	1	4	6–8	14–16	28–32	60–64	90	120	180	256	
^{175}YbCl$_3$	3.3×10^1			95	96									a
^{177}LuCl$_3$	3×10^1			89										a
Trivalent actinides														
^{227}AcCl$_3$	1.7×10^{-2}			68	42			31	18				4.2	S
^{239}PuCl$_3$	1.6×10^1				79		74		40				22	s
^{241}AmCl$_3$	3×10^{-1}			42	16		8.2		6.6				1.6	m
^{241}Am(NO$_3$)$_3$ [g]	1.6×10^{-3} $- 3 \times 10^{-3}$			80		62		40		33			22	S
^{241}Am(NO$_3$)$_3$ [g]	2.5×10^{-1} $- 1.5 \times 10^0$			90		42		43		16	15			S
^{242}CmCl$_3$	3×10^{-4}			15	7.5		6.6		2.4				4.5	m
^{244}Cm(NO$_3$)$_3$	1.2×10^{-4}			82		61		35		30		22		S
^{242}Cm(NO$_3$)$_3$	3×10^{-4}			82				44		19	22			S
^{242}Cm(NO$_3$)$_3$	1.5×10^{-3}			82		57		46		31				S
Tetravalent and pentavalent cations and actinides														
^{95}ZrCl$_4$	3.3×10^{-4}			80	86		80	78	66					A
^{113}SnCl$_4$	1.9×10^{-4}			90	84	79								A

Radionuclide	Mass (g)							Retention class[c]
$^{210}Po(NO_3)_4$	4.4×10^{-4}	74	50	52	26			S
$^{233}PaCl_5$	4.7×10^{-4}		85	82	73	59		A
$^{234}ThCl_4$	4.2×10^{-4}		91	86	83	78	61	A
$^{228}Th(NO_3)_4$	2×10^{-5}		65	37	35			A
$^{238}Pu(NO_3)_4$	4×10^{-5}					16		S
$^{238}Pu(NO_3)_4$	1.1×10^{-2}		33	33		8.8		S
$^{238}Pu(NO_3)_4$[h]	5×10^{-2} – 2.3×10^{-1}	79	36	21	15	11		S
$^{239}Pu(NO_3)_4$	1.1×10^{-2}		34	32	15			S
$^{239}Pu(NO_3)_4$[g]	1×10^{-1} – 4.8×10^{-1}	76	56	40	22	12		S
$^{239}Pu(NO_3)_4$[g]	1.6×10^{0} – 3.2×10^{0}		64	48	31			S
$^{239}Pu(NO_3)_4$	8.8×10^{0}	88[a]	69	64				a

[a] Radionuclide identity and mass provide links to the appropriate references cited in Table A.1.

[b] Time intervals are indicated to accommodate data generated in differing experimental designs.

[c] Assigned wound retention class: W = weak, M = moderate, S = strong, A = avid.

[d] Retention classifications shown in lower case have been assigned to radionuclides or masses of radionuclide plus stable carrier, for which the experimental conditions made them unsuitable for use in defining the retention classes (e.g., element mass >5 μg). Assignments were made based on wound retention behavior similar to that of the assigned class.

[e] Pooled data for $^{137}Cs^+$ (Ilyin and Ivannikov, 1979; Scott et al., 1947).

[f] Retention of $^{223}Ra^{2+}$ shown in parentheses in "60 to 64 d" column was measured at 48 d.

[g] Pooled data from all studies of these actinides in rats and hamsters, in which the i.m.-injected mass was within the indicated range (sources cited in Table A.1).

[h] Pooled data from all studies of $^{238}Pu(NO_3)_4$ in rats, in which the i.m.-injected mass was within the range indicated (sources cited in Table A.1).

because it fails to account for the small fractions of absorbed radionuclide contained in the skin and tissues of the paw of the injected leg.

A.1.1.1 *Injected Radioactive Material.* With few exceptions, the quantities of radioactive material injected in the UCRL studies ranged from 18 to 740 kBq. Radionuclide dosage, originally expressed in microcuries, was available from project records for 52 of the 58 suitable UCRL studies. The original work sheets for the other six studies contained the counting rates of the dosing standards, which could be converted to becquerel using the 21.5 % beta counting efficiency determined for the geometric configuration of the sample mounting, sample holder, and the large diameter thin window Geiger-Mueller tubes in routine use at that time.

A.1.1.2 *Injected Radionuclide Mass.* Most of the radionuclides studied at UCRL were short-lived, carrier-free, beta-emitting isotopes produced on the 60 inch cyclotron at the Crocker Laboratory or were separated from mixed fission products or natural decay chains (Garrison and Hamilton, 1951; Lanz *et al.*, 1946; Scott *et al.*, 1947). Radioisotopes of the heavy lanthanides were prepared by neutron capture, and the mass of the irradiated samples was used to calculate the mass injected (Durbin *et al.*, 1956). The injected masses of all other radionuclides in the studies at UCRL and elsewhere were calculated from their activity and half-lives (Kocher, 1981; Schirmer and Waechter, 1968).

The number of atoms (N) in a radioactive sample is:

$$N = \frac{A\ T_{1/2}}{\ln(2)}\,, \tag{A.2}$$

where A is the activity (becquerel) and $T_{1/2}$ is the half-life of the radionuclide in seconds. The sample mass m (micrograms) is:

$$m = 10^6 \frac{A_r}{N_A} N\,, \tag{A.3}$$

where A_r is the isotopic weight (g mol^{-1}) and N_A is the Avogadro constant (6.022×10^{23} mol^{-1}). Combining Equations A.2 and A.3 and all of the constant terms:

$$m = 2.4 \times 10^{-18}\ A\ A_r\ T_{1/2}\,, \tag{A.4}$$

where $T_{1/2}$ is the physical half-life (Kocher, 1981).

A.1.1.3 *Injected Solution Volume.* Injected volumes were recorded for 23 of the suitable UCRL studies (Table A.1). They ranged from 0.1 to 0.7 mL, but were as large as 1 mL for six early studies of the transuranics and ^{7}Be. Excluding those unusual studies, the mean injected volume was 0.29 ± 0.017 mL. A default value of 0.3 mL was adopted when the actual amount was not recorded.

A.1.1.4 *Radionuclide Concentrations in Injected Solutions.* The data in Table A.1 can be used to calculate the molar concentrations of the study radionuclides (mol L^{-1}) in the injected solutions:

$$\text{molar concentration} = 10^{-6} \frac{m}{A_r V}, \qquad (A.5)$$

where m is the injected mass (micrograms), A_r is the isotopic weight (g mol^{-1}), and V is the injected volume (liters).

A.1.1.5 *Solution pH.* It was important to distinguish between cations in solution and those that may have been present in the injection media as colloidal hydrolysis products. In the absence of a complexing agent, the aqueous solubility of a cation is given by:

$$K_{sp} = (M^{n+})(OH^-)^n, \qquad (A.6)$$

where K_{sp} is the solubility product and (M^{n+}) and (OH^-) are the respective concentrations (mol L^{-1}) of the cation and the hydroxide ions. The simplified expression for the ionization of pure water is:

$$K_w = (H^+)(OH^-) = 10^{-14}, \qquad (A.7)$$

where $(H^+) = (OH^-) = 10^{-7}$, and the solution pH defines both (H^+) and (OH^-). There was no record of the pH of the injection solutions used in 13 of the suitable UCRL studies. A pH of four was assumed for those radionuclide solutions with incomplete records.

A.1.1.6 *Radionuclide Solubility in the Injected Solutions.* Several transition and heavy metals were injected in highly oxidized states as complex oxo- or chloro-anions, which are not subject to hydrolysis. The hydroxides of the monovalent alkali metals and Ag$^+$ and NpO$_2^+$ and the divalent alkaline earth elements are soluble at physiological pH, and K_{sp} ranges from 10^{-9} (NpO^{2+}) to 10^{-4} (Ba^{2+}). The range of K_{sp} for divalent Be^{2+}, Cu^{2+}, UO$_2^{2+}$, and PuO$_2^{2+}$ is 10^{-22} to 10^{-18}, and for trivalent cations, including the lanthanides and actinides, the range of K_{sp} is from 10^{-31} (Ga^{3+}) to 10^{-20} (Ac^{3+}). Hydrolysis of these divalent and trivalent cations and formation of microcolloids become important at physiological pH. The tetra- and pentavalent cations, a group that includes important chemical forms of thorium, neptunium and plutonium form insoluble hydroxides at low pH. The range of K_{sp} is 10^{-54} (Np^{4+}, Pu^{4+}) to 10^{-37} (Po^{4+}) (Baes and Mesmer, 1976; Figgins, 1961; Latimer, 1952; Martell and Smith, 1976; Rai et al., 1998a; 1998b; Shannon, 1976; Sillen and Martell, 1964; 1971; Smith and Martell, 1989).

The molar concentration and pH data in Table A.1 were used to calculate the ion product (M^{n+}) $(OH^-)^n$, for each radionuclide solution injected. The ion products of the injection solutions used in the studies included in Tables A.1 and A.2 did not exceed their respective K_{sp} and were usually many orders of magnitude less. Those injected solutions were unlikely to have contained insoluble hydrolysis products. The nature of the $^{113}Sn^{4+}$ solution is uncertain, because the pH was not recorded. The ion product would have exceeded K_{sp} at pH 5, resulting in hydrolysis of the $^{113}Sn^{4+}$, but hydrolysis would have been avoided at pH $\leq$ 3.

A.1.2 Studies in Other Laboratories

The experimental conditions and wound retention data for the studies described below are included in Tables A.1 and A.2, respectively.

Hexavalent $^{239}PuO_2(NO_3)_2$ was injected in rats, and retention at the injection site was measured radiochemically from 10 to 406 d (Kisieleski and Woodruff, 1947).

Several soluble actinides in dilute HNO_3 viz $^{238}Pu^{4+}$, $^{241}Am^{3+}$, $^{242}Cm^{3+}$, and $^{237}NpO_2^+$, were injected in rats, and retention at the wound site was measured radiochemically from 1 to 90 d (Lafuma et al., 1971; Morin et al., 1972; 1973a; Nenot et al., 1972a; 1972b).

Polonium as $^{210}Po(NO_3)_4$ was i.m. injected in rats in solution, and ^{210}Po retention at the wound site was determined radiochemically from 1 to 16 d (Ilyin, 2001; Ilyin and Ivannikov, 1979; Ilyin et al., 1977).

The influence on retention at an i.m. wound site of the mass and activity of deposited $^{238}Pu^{4+}$ or $^{239}Pu^{4+}$ was investigated in i.m. injected rats and hamsters. Retention at the wound site and accumulation in the regional lymph nodes were determined radiochemically from 1 to 180 d (Harrison and David, 1977; 1978; Harrison et al., 1977a; 1977b; 1978a; 1978b).

Several studies assessed the efficacy of chelation therapy for reducing actinide retention at an i.m. wound site in rats and for diverting chelated actinide to excretion. The untreated controls in these studies provide wound retention data for $^{238}Pu^{4+}$, $^{239}Pu^{4+}$, $^{228}Th^{4+}$, and $^{241}Am^{3+}$ (Gray *et al.*, 1994; Stradling *et al.*, 1993; 1995a; 1995b; Taylor, 1967; Taylor and Sowby, 1962).

Early clearance of two rapidly absorbed radionuclides was investigated in rats. $Na^{131}I$ was injected in the thigh muscle, and $^{137}CsCl$ was s.c. injected in a hind paw. Radionuclide retention at the wound site was measured by external photon counting (Ilyin, 2001; Ilyin and Ivannikov, 1979).

In a study of tumor induction by alpha radiation, 50 mice were s.c. injected with 1.2 µg of ^{239}Pu in an "ionic" form (Brues *et al.*, 1965; Lindenbaum and Westfall, 1965). The chemical form of $^{239}Pu^{4+}$ was not defined, but it was likely to have been $^{239}Pu(NO_3)_4$ in dilute HNO_3. Slow transport away from the injection site was indicated by the delayed appearance of bone tumors (Finkel and Biskis, 1962). At 1.5 to 2 y (midpoint 640 d), 3 % of the injected $^{239}Pu^{4+}$ remained at the wound site (Brues *et al.*, 1966). This is the only known measurement of retention in a puncture wound in a rodent of ≤ 5 µg of $^{239}Pu^{4+}$ in solution at a post-injection time longer than 90 d.

A.1.3 *Data Used in Model Development*

Statistical measures of variability of radionuclide retention at a wound site were not published. In 40 UCRL studies, the standard deviations of radionuclide retention in the injected leg were on the order of ±10 % of the mean values for groups of three rats. Because the purpose of this Report is to provide general descriptions of the behavior of many radionuclides that might contaminate wounds and to identify trends, only mean values, rounded to two significant figures, of the retention at the wound site are given in Tables A.2 to A.6.

Not all of the experimental data shown in Table A.2 were included in the development of the kinetic model described in Section 4 for retention of radionuclides in a puncture wound. The kinetic modeling used only data from studies in which:

- the radionuclide was in solution when injected;
- the mass of soluble radionuclide deposited was ≤ 5 µg;
- the fraction of radionuclide retained at the injection site was measured by radiochemical analysis or by well standardized external photon counting of the isolated limb; and
- the volume of solution injected was <1 mL (except for ^7Be for which no other data are available).

TABLE A.3—*Retention at a puncture wound site of weakly held monovalent and divalent cations and anions or anionic metal complexes for i.m. injection in rats of <5 µg of radionuclide in isotonic saline.*[a]

Radionuclide	Fraction Retained in Wound (percent of injected amount) at Time t (days post-injection)					
	0.042	0.167	1	4	8	16
$^{131}I^-$	8.0	2.5	1.0			
$^{71}GeO_3^{2-}$		12	3.4	0.44		
$^{74}AsCl_5^{2-}$			1.0			
$^{124}SbO_3^{2-}$			0.36	0.14		0.08
$^{75}SeO_4^{2-}$			2.4	1.4		0.26
$^{181}WO_4^{2-}$		46	0.5			
$^{95,96}TcCl_6^{2-}$			2.2	1.3	0.46	
$^{86}Rb^+$				0.85		
$^{137}Cs^{+ b}$	20	11	5.6	6.4		2.6
$^{45}Ca^{2+}$				2.6		
$^{90}Sr^{2+}$				5.1		
$^{140}Ba^{2+}$			4.0	2.0	2.0	
$^{64}Cu^{2+}$			4.9			
$^{230}UO_2^{2+}$			5.3	5.0		1.8
Mean	14	20	2.8	2.5	1.2	1.2
±SD	8.5	23	2.0	2.2	1.1	1.2
Number of radionuclides	2	4	11	10	2	4

[a]Data from Table A.2.
[b]Pooled data of Ilyin and Ivannikov (1979) and Scott et al. (1947).

TABLE A.4—*Retention at a puncture wound site of moderately held monovalent and divalent cations and anionic metal complexes for i.m. injection in rats of <5 µg of radionuclide in acidic isotonic saline.*[a]

Radionuclide	Fraction Retained in Wound (percent of injected amount) at Time t (days post-injection)						
	1	4	7 – 8	15 – 16	32	48	64
$^{48}VO_3^-$	27	22		8.4			4.8
$^{127m,129m}TeO_3^{2-}$	55	22		9.0	7.3		
$^{185}OsO_5^{2-}$	25						
$^{105}RhCl_6^{3-}$	11	7.5					
$^{191,193}PtCl_4^{2-}$		9.4	7.3	7.1	4.4		
$^{110}Ag^+$	26	12		9.0	3.0		3.0
$^{223}Ra^{2+}$	41		14.5	9.3		0.23	
Mean	31	15	10.5	8.6	4.9		3.9
±SD	15	7.0	4.7	0.9	2.2		1.3
Number of radionuclides	6	5	2	5	3		2

[a]Collected data from Table A.2.

The grouped data used to define four distinct wound retention classes of soluble radionuclides are shown in Table A.3 (weakly retained), Table A.4 (moderately retained), Table A.5 (strongly retained), and Table A.6 (avidly retained). With few exceptions, the entries in those four tables are the results of one study with each radionuclide. In five cases ($^{137}Cs^+$, $^{241}Am^{3+}$, $^{242,244}Cm^{3+}$, $^{238}Pu^{4+}$, and $^{239}Pu^{4+}$), the results from several studies were combined, because their retention at the i.m. wound site was not systematically affected by the deposited masses within the ranges indicated. The criteria used to assign a radionuclide to one of these four classes are discussed in Section 4.2.2.2.

TABLE A.5—*Retention at a puncture wound site of strongly held multivalent cations and one anionic metal complex for i.m. injection in rats of <5 µg of radionuclide in isotonic saline.*[a]

Radionuclide	Fraction Retained in Wound (percent of injected amount) at Time t (days post-injection)									
	1	4	6–8	14–16	28–32	64	90	120	180	256
$^7Be^{2+}$	60	46	24	30	24	18				
$^{51}Cr^{3+}$	50			41						
$^{67}Ga^{3+}$	32	26								
$^{88}Y^{3+}$	71	35		26	28	8.2				
$^{95}Nb^{3+}$	61	44		41		18				
$^{106}RuCl_5^{2-}$		28		17		20				
$^{114m}In^{3+}$	48	31		18	19	11				
$^{140}La^{3+}$	66	30	36							
$^{143}Ce^{3+}$	62	40		27		10				
$^{143}Pr^{3+}$	72	55		37	32	30				
$^{147}Nd^{3+}$	73	57		38	35					
$^{147}Pm^{3+}$	54	51		39	32	16				4.3

	1	2	3	4	5	6	7	8	9	10
154,155Eu³⁺	73	72		65	56	40				21
160Tb³⁺	62	50			32					11
120Tm³⁺	68	51		38	37					14
227Ac³⁺	68	42			31	18				4.2
241Am³⁺,b,c	85		55		41		23	15	22	
142,244Cm³⁺,b,c	82	57	55		40		26	22	22	
210Po⁴⁺	74	50	52	26						
238Pu⁴⁺,b	79		50	26	26		14	11		
239Pu⁴⁺ 0.04–11 ng			34		32		15			
239Pu⁴⁺,b,c 0.10–3.2 µg	76		58	64	41		24		12.5	
Mean	66	45	46	36	34	19	20	16	19	11
±SD	13	12	12	14	8.8	10	5.5	5.6	5.5	7.1
Number of radionuclides	20	17	8	15	15	10	5	3	3	5

[a]Collected data from Table A.2.
[b]Mean of pooled data from all i.m.-injection studies (sources cited in Table A.1).
[c]Studies include i.m. injections in hamsters.

TABLE A.6—*Retention at a puncture wound site of avidly held trivalent, tetravalent and pentavalent cations for i.m. injection in rats of ≤5 µg of radionuclide in acidic isotonic saline.*[a]

Radionuclide[b]	Fraction Retained in Wound (percent of injected amount) at Time t (days post-injection)					
	1	4	8	16 – 17	32	64
$^{46}Sc^{3+}$	88	75				
$^{95}Zr^{4+}$	80	86		80	78.5	66.5
$^{113}Sn^{4+}$	90	84	79			
$^{233}Pa^{5+}$		85		82	73	59
$^{228,234}Th^{4+\,c}$		91	75	83	78	61
Mean	86	84	77	82	77	62
±SD	5.3	5.8	2.8	1.6	2.9	3.8
Number of radionuclides	3	5	2	3	3	3

[a]Collected data from Table A.2. Note that except for ^{228}Th, these radionuclides are short-lived beta-gamma emitters.
[b]See Table A.1 for references.
[c]Data for ^{228}Th and ^{234}Th combined.

A.1.4 Supporting Studies of Intramuscularly Injected Radionuclide Solutions

The studies described in the following paragraphs were unsuitable for inclusion in the basic data set for various reasons. However, they support the conclusions drawn from the basic data sets.

A.1.4.1 $^{239}Pu(NO_3)_4$ *in a Dilute Acid.* Male and female rats were injected in the thigh muscle with 14 to 17 kBq (6 to 7.2 µg) of $^{239}Pu(NO_3)_4$ in 0.1 mL of 0.1 mol L^{-1} HNO$_3$ to investigate cancer induction in the body and at the i.m.-injection site (Bazhin *et al.*, 1984). Retention of the ^{239}Pu at the wound site, measured from 1 h to 512 d, was reported only as the ranges of five of the six parameters of a three-component exponential equation [*i.e.*, $R(t) =$

$$\sum_i A_i\, e^{-\lambda_i t}$$, as follows: A_1 (10 to 21 %), A_2 (61.2 to 63.7 %), A_3 (8.9 to

10.1 %), λ_2 (1.8 to 1.9×10^{-2} d^{-1}), λ_3 (2 to 3×0^{-3} d^{-1}), and λ_1 was not defined]. The text implies that the first component, A_1, would be exhausted in 1 d. If A_1 were reduced to 1 % of its initial value in 1 d, the rate constant, λ_1, would have been 4.6 d^{-1}. Retention at the i.m. wound site can be reasonably estimated by assigning $\lambda_1 = 4.6$ d^{-1}, using the mid-ranges of the other rate constants, and normalizing total retention to 100 % at $t = 0$:

$$R(t) = 18e^{-4.6t} + 71e^{-0.018t} + 11e^{-0.0025t}. \tag{A.8}$$

In this study of i.m.-injected ^{239}Pu^{4+} (~6.6 µg in solution at pH 1), the calculated wound retention, 81 % at 1 d and 31 % at 64 d, meets the criteria for a strongly-retained radionuclide, and the wound retention curve defined by Equation A.8 lies closer to the composite curve for small masses of strongly-retained i.m.-injected radionuclides than that for the avidly-retained radionuclides (Sections 4.2.2.2.3, 4.2.2.2.4, and Figure 4.13).

A.1.4.2 ^{239}Pu(NO$_3$)$_4$ in Strong Acid. Rats were i.m. injected with 18 to 22 kBq (8 to 9.7 µg) of ^{239}Pu(NO$_3$)$_4$ in 0.005 to 0.01 mL of 3 mol L^{-1} HNO$_3$ (Volf, 1974a; 1974b; 1975). The experimental conditions and retention data for ^{239}Pu at the i.m. wound site are included in Tables A.1 and A.2, respectively. The strong acid suppressed hydrolysis of the ^{239}Pu^{4+} in the injection medium, but prompt hydrolysis in situ and local tissue damage caused by the injected acid were to be expected. Log-linear regression analysis of the data yielded a three-component exponential retention curve for ^{239}Pu^{4+} from 1 to 30 d, where t is days:

$$R(t) = 8e^{-1.2t} + 21e^{-0.18t} + 72e^{-0.004t}. \tag{A.9}$$

Wound retention of 8.8 µg of Pu^{4+} in this study is close to, but slightly less than the retention curve for much smaller masses of avidly-retained radionuclides (Section 4.2.2.2.4 and Figure 4.13). Even though injected in strong acid, this larger mass of ^{239}Pu^{4+} was avidly retained.

A.1.4.3 Short-Term Russian Studies. Ilyin (2001) and Ilyin and Ivannikov (1979) reviewed the literature dealing with animal studies of the retention of radionuclides deposited in various kinds of wounds, including their own studies, which emphasized the early stages of contamination, after i.m. injection of $^{144}CeCl_3$ or $^{241}AmCl_3$ in rats. Retention of those radionuclides at the injection site was estimated by summing the amounts of radionuclide recovered in the radioanalyzed tissues. Retention of $^{144}Ce^{3+}$ was estimated to be 91 % at 1 d. Retention of $^{241}Am^{3+}$ was estimated to be 81, 72 and 51 % and 1, 4 and 64 d, respectively.

Retention of $^{140}LaCl_3$ at an i.m.-injection site in rats, estimated by a method similar to that described above, was 91 and 76 % at days one and four, respectively (Moskalev, 1961a). The results of the three Russian studies agree reasonably well with the retention of small masses of the same radionuclides determined by radioanalysis of the dissected i.m. wound site (Table A.2).

A.1.4.4 $^{85}SrCl_2$ *in Rhesus Monkeys.* Rhesus monkeys (*Maccaca mula*) were used to investigate clearance of 370 to 3,700 kBq of $^{85}SrCl_2$ from a puncture wound (0.1 mL of a saline solution injected into the thigh muscle). The activity at the wound site and in the same site on the opposite leg was monitored by external photon counting for 2 h. The $^{85}Sr^{2+}$ at the injection site, corrected for the ^{85}Sr content of the uninjected leg (to allow for detection in the injected leg of activity not associated with the wound site), was cleared at one fast rate (half-time ~10 min), and absorption, demonstrated by uptake to blood and accumulation in bone, was essentially complete in 1 h (Ducuosso *et al.*, 1974).

A.1.4.5 *Radiolabeled Soluble Inorganic Salts.* A study was conducted to determine whether the retention of some aerosolized cations in the lung could be correlated with their chemical properties (ultrafilterability from serum) and/or with their retention at an i.m. wound site. Ten radiolabeled cations encompassing a broad range of lung clearance behavior were i.m. injected in rats in 0.5 mL of 0.006 mol L^{-1} solutions, pH range about two to four (Morrow *et al.*, 1968). The masses of the metal ions deposited at the injection site ranged from 15 to 61 µg. Retention of the metal ions in the injected leg was determined for as long as 100 d by external counting of the gamma-emitting radiolabels. The data for filterability from serum and for retention at the i.m. site, expressed as retention half-time(s), are shown in Table A.7. The trend of retention at an i.m. site for this set of cation salts was, $1^+ < 2^+ \ll 3^+$, in agreement with their chemical properties and their ultrafilterability from serum, and it supports the detailed data for much smaller masses (≤5 µg) of those same radionuclides administered by i.m. injection as shown in Tables A.3 to A.6. The wound retention of 15 to 61 µg

TABLE A.7—Comparison of retention at an i.m.-injection site in rats and ultrafilterability from serum of selected soluble radiolabeled cations (data of Morrow et al., 1968).

Radiolabeled Compound	Injected Mass (μg)[a]	Retention Half-Time(s) at i.m.-Injection Site[b] (d)	Ultrafilterable from Serum[c] (%)	Retention Classification[d]
$^{134}CsCl$	41	0.003	93	w
$^{85}SrCl_2$	26	0.02/>19	84	w
$^{133}BaCl_2$	40	0.7/>70	23	m
$^{58}CoCl_2$	17	0.02/>9	11	w
$^{51}CrCl_3$	15	>150	9	a
^{203}Hg (acetate)$_2$	61	1/30	4.1	m
$^{54}MnCl_2$	16	1/10	2	m
$^{59}FeCl_3$	18	0.1/>100	2	a
$^{141}CeCl_3$	42	~300	1.7	a
$^{65}Zn(NO_3)_2$	20	1/140	1.5	s

[a]Prepared by mixing radiolabel with stable carrier cation in solution. Injected mass was calculated by assuming 0.05 mL of 6×10^{-3} mol L^{-1} solution.

[b]When two half-time values are shown (a/b), retention was bi-phasic.

[c]Concentration of cations dispersed in bovine serum at ~6 × 10^{-3} mol L^{-1}; centrifugal ultrafiltration through cellophane membrane (4.5 nm pore diameter).

[d]Retention classifications shown in lower case have been assigned to radionuclides or masses of radionuclide plus stable carrier, for which the experimental conditions made them unsuitable for use in defining the retention classes (e.g., element mass >5 μg). Assignments were made based on wound retention behavior similar to that of the assigned class.

quantities of these cations i.m. injected in solution can be classified as follows:

- weak: $CsCl_2$, $SrCl_2$, $CoCl_2$
- moderate: $MnCl_2$, $BaCl_2$, Hg acetate
- strong to avid: $Zn(NO_3)_2$, $FeCl_3$, $CrCl_3$, $CeCl_3$

A.1.4.6 *Mixed Fission Products Injected Intramuscularly in Rats and Monkeys.* Mixed fission products [FP (87 d old)] were chemically separated from a large mass of uranyl nitrate irradiated with cyclotron produced fast neutrons. Rats were i.m. injected with the FP in a NaCl solution at pH 2.5 (Scott *et al.*, 1947). In a second study, FP (spallation products) were produced in uranium metal irradiated with cyclotron deuterons (chemical separation method not published), and rats and monkeys were i.m. injected when the FP were 32 d old (Hamilton, 1952). Fractional losses of some FP probably occurred during the chemical separations of the FP from the uranium matrices; all of the iodine and some of the ruthenium were volatilized during dry ashing of the biological samples at 500 °C. Dosing standards were prepared to correct the measured activity in the biological samples for radioactive decay and the limitations of the homemade Geiger-Mueller tubes. Those detectors were ill suited for detection of photons, decay by electron capture, isomeric transitions, or beta particles with average energies <50 keV. Self-absorption curves were prepared to correct for the poor penetration by low energy beta particles of the considerable masses of the ashed tissue and excreta samples.

In general, the wound retention of the 32 and 87 d old FP, shown in Table A.8, is >1 SD greater than the mean for moderately-retained radionuclides (Table A.4), but within 1 SD less than the mean for strongly-retained radionuclides (Table A.5).

The 87 d old FP mixture was also administered orally to rats that were killed at 4 or 16 d after administration; 7.5 to 11 % of the orally administered radioactive material was absorbed from the gastrointestinal (GI) tract. Skeleton and urine accounted for 90 % of the absorbed fraction of the radioactive material, soft tissues accounted for 10 %, and liver for only 0.3 %. The authors concluded that the radionuclides absorbed from the GI tract were almost entirely isotopes of strontium and barium, and that their absorption was independent of the presence of the isotopes of the less well absorbed components of the FP mixture (Scott *et al.*, 1947). Quantitative analytical chemical methods were used to separate the constituent radioelements of the 87 d old FP mixture and determine their proportional contributions to its total activity. The

TABLE A.8—*Measured and predicted retention of mixed fission products at an i.m.-injection site in rats and monkeys and proportional contributions of readily and poorly absorbed radioelements to the total activity of those fission product mixtures at the times biological samples were measured.*[a,b]

Parameter	Fraction Retained in Wound (percent of injected amount) at Time t (days post-injection)						
	Rats[a]			Rats[b]		Monkeys[b]	
	4	16	64	1	4	1	4
Age of FP when samples were measured, t(d)[c]	110	120	165	47	50	47	50
Injected leg							
Measured	30.5	24.8	14.1	44.2	34.6	32.0	27.3
Predicted[d]	35.1	28.6	15.5	45.7	31.4	—	—
Proportion of FP activity at time t (d) after fission (%)[e,f]							
Readily absorbed FP (strontium, barium, cesium, tellurium)	22.5	21.2	18.6	32		32	
Poorly absorbed FP	77.5	78.8	81.5	68		68	

[a]Fission products (0.14 mol L[-1] NaCl, pH 2.5) were 87 d old when injected (Scott et al., 1947).

[b]Fission products (0.14 mol L[-1] NaCl, pH 2.5) were 32 d old when injected (Hamilton, 1952).

[c]Method of estimating fission product age at times biological samples were measured is described in the text.

[d]Predicted wound retention was calculated by using Equation A.10.

[e]Proportional contributions to the detectable beta activity of readily and poorly absorbed radioelements in 110, 120 and 165 d old fission product mixtures were reported by Scott et al. (1947). The poorly absorbed fraction includes small amounts of [234]Th and [234]Pa.

[f]The data of Petrov et al. (1963) were used to estimate the abundances at 50 d after fission of readily and poorly absorbed radioelements as described in the text.

results of that original assay were used to calculate the relative abundances of the principal constituents at the later times when biological samples were measured. At ~110 d after fission, when samples from the rats killed at 4 d after FP administration were measured, 22 % of the administered FP radioactive material was associated with isotopes of readily absorbed strontium, barium, cesium and tellurium, and the remaining 78 % was associated with isotopes of the poorly absorbed lanthanides yttrium, zirconium, and the beta-emitting ^{238}U daughters, ^{234}Th and ^{234}Pa.

If absorption of the individual FP radionuclides from a deep puncture wound is similarly independent, it should be possible to predict the gross wound retention of mixed FP from the composition of the mixture at the time wound retention is measured and the mean retentions of the radionuclide (radioelement) categories shown in Tables A.3 to A.6.

Laboratory records indicated that at least 14 d were needed to process the biological samples from each timed study group. The FP ages at the times biological samples were radioanalyzed can be estimated by summing the post-injection interval when each group of rats was killed, the sample processing time (14 d), and the age of the FP mixture when it was administered. The proportional contributions of readily and poorly absorbed radionuclides to the total FP activity were reported by Scott et al. (1947) for the times when samples from rats killed at 4, 16 or 64 d after i.m. injection of the 87 d old FP mixture were measured (i.e., at FP ages of 110, 220 and 165 d, respectively).

The data given by Petrov et al. (1963) were used to estimate the proportional contributions of readily and poorly absorbed radionuclides to the total activity of an FP mixture at the times of radioanalysis (FP age ~50 d) of the samples from the rats and monkeys killed at 1 and 4 d after i.m. injection of 32 d old FP (Hamilton, 1952). Petrov et al. (1963) tabulated the abundances of the 30 d old products of thermal neutron fission of ^{235}U. They also compared the abundances of the major products of thermal and fast neutron fission and of high energy neutron spallation, and concluded that they did not differ greatly. The proportional distribution of the activity of the 50 d old FP were based on those reported for 30 d old FP corrected for radioactive decay to 50 d. Some radionuclides were omitted from that reconstruction of the FP abundances in a 50 d old mixture; those with half-lives <7 d, those that contributed <0.02 % of the total activity, those with decay characteristics such that their detection was unlikely using the instruments available to Hamilton (1952) and Scott et al. (1947), and the iodine and ruthenium isotopes that would have been lost in the sample processing.

In all cases, it was assumed that the time elapsed between the FP injection and radioanalysis of the biological samples was sufficient to reestablish radioactive equilibria of parent-daughter pairs that may have been separated biologically (e.g., [140]Ba from [140]La).

The fractions of the total FP activity present at the times when biological samples were measured that were contributed by radionuclides expected to be weakly or moderately retained in a puncture wound (strontium, barium, cesium, tellurium) and the fractions contributed by strongly and avidly-retained radionuclides are shown in Table A.8. The composition of the 87 d old FP mixture used by Scott et al. (1947) after 110 to 120 d decay agrees well with that of 100 d old FP [data of Petrov et al. (1963), edited as described above], in which strontium, barium, cesium and tellurium isotopes contribute 22 % of the total activity.

Wound retention of a FP mixture, $R_{FP}(t)$, at any time after deposition, can be predicted by Equation A.10:

$$R_{FP}(t) = R_w(t) fr_w(T) + R_S(t) fr_S(T) , \qquad (A.10)$$

where t is time in days after FP deposition in the wound, $R_W(t)$ and $R_S(t)$ are, respectively, the wound retentions of weak and strong category radionuclides at t days after deposition, T is the age in days of the unseparated FP mixture at the time the wound content is measured, and $fr_W(T)$ and $fr_S(T)$ are, respectively, the fractions of the activity of the FP mixture at T days of age contributed by weakly and strongly-retained radionuclides. On average, the predicted wound retentions shown in Table A.8 agree within ±10 % of the reported values.

Although tellurium is moderately retained (Table A.4) and zirconium, [234]Th, and [234]Pa are avidly retained at an i.m. wound site in rats (Table A.6), the best predictions of wound site retention at times from 1 to 64 d after deposition were obtained by combining tellurium with the weakly-retained radionuclides and zirconium, thorium and protactinium with the strongly-retained radionuclides.

Retention of mixed FP injected into the thigh muscle of the monkeys was ~25 % less than that injected into the thigh muscle of mature rats. It may be suggested that somewhat greater absorption was the combined result of dilution in the greater volume of tissue fluid of the larger muscle mass of the monkeys and the higher rate of physical activity of the monkeys, both of which tend to enhance the rate of tissue fluid flow.

A.2 Subcutaneous Puncture Wounds

A.2.1 *Subcutaneous Injections in Rats*

Only a few uncomplexed radionuclides in solution have been s.c. injected. That kind of puncture wound deposits the radionuclide solution into the loose connective tissue layer (hypodermis) between the skin (pelt of a furbearing mammal) and the underlying muscle.

In a series of investigations of the efficacy of chelation treatment for removing deposited actinides and of comparative retention of actinides at differing wound sites, rats were s.c. injected in a limb with small volumes of weakly acidic solutions containing small masses of $^{228}Th^{4+}$, $^{241}Am^{3+}$, $^{238}Pu^{4+}$, or $^{239}Pu^{4+}$. The injected limb was dissected and the retained radionuclide was measured radiochemically (Gray *et al.*, 1994; Harrison *et al.*, 1978b; Stradling *et al.*, 1993; 1995a; 1995b). (Experimental conditions and retention of these radionuclides at an i.m. wound site are given in Tables A.1 and A.2, respectively.)

Metabolic studies of some s.c.-injected radionuclides were conducted by Kalistratova *et al.* (1968) and Moskalev (1961a; 1961b; 1961c; 1961d), but the locations of the s.c.-injection sites were not reported, nor did it appear that the injection sites (contaminated skin and underlying muscle) were dissected and radioanalyzed. In some of those studies, tissue distributions were reported for the same time intervals after the same radionuclide preparation was i.v. injected, and radionuclide retention at the s.c. site could be estimated:

$$R = 100[1 - (\text{tissues}_{s.c.})(\text{tissues}_{i.v.})^{-1}] , \qquad (A.11)$$

where $(\text{tissues}_{s.c.})$ and $(\text{tissues}_{i.v.})$ are the tissue radionuclide contents (% *ID*) or concentrations (% *ID* g^{-1}) after s.c. and i.v. injection, respectively. In other studies, fractional retention at the s.c. site was estimated as the difference between the amount injected and the total amount recovered in tissues and excreta, divided by the amount injected.

Information on the experimental conditions, retention of the radionuclides at the wound site to 16 d (length of longest study), and the sources of the s.c.-injection data are collected in Table A.9. The masses of the radionuclides s.c. injected were small (<5 µg), and solution pH was low (two to three in most cases); with the possible exception of $^{111}AgCl$, all of these cations were in solution when injected. The tri- and tetravalent cations would be expected to hydrolyze at the wound site.

A.2.2 $^{241}Am(NO_3)_3$ in the Foot Pad of a Dog

A solution of ^{241}Am(NO$_3$)$_3$ (33 kBq, 0.27 µg) was injected into the left carpal pad of a beagle dog. The injected volume and pH of the solution were not reported, but because of the small size of the footpad and its structure (dense fatty connective tissue covered with thick epidermis), the injected volume was likely to have been ≤0.1 mL. The ^{241}Am concentration would have been ~10^{-4} mol L^{-1}, and at pH ≤ 5, the ^{241}Am would have been in solution. Partial and whole-body counting with a large NaI(Tl) photon detector, standardized by body, liver and paw phantoms, were used to measure ^{241}Am retention in the injected paw, the liver region, nonliver tissue (mainly bone), and the whole body at intervals from a few minutes to 10 weeks after the injection (Lloyd et al., 1975).

Apparently no ^{241}Am was lost from the wound site by seepage, because the retention of ^{241}Am in the whole body was nearly 100 % during the first few days. Little ^{241}Am was excreted during the 74 d observation period. The data for ^{241}Am retention in the paw (% ID) to 74 d after injection, read from the published curve, can be described by a three-component exponential equation, where t is days after injection:

$$R(t) = 67e^{-1.8t} + 9e^{-0.083t} + 24e^{-0.009t}. \tag{A.12}$$

The much faster initial clearance to blood of ^{241}Am from this particular s.c.-injection site is the most important difference between the pattern of ^{241}Am retention at this s.c. site and that of the group of strongly-retained radionuclides (including ^{241}Am) at an i.m. wound site in rats (Section 4.2.2.2.3). Absorption of ~55 % of the injected ^{241}Am from the dog foot pad in 1 d compares favorably with that of ^{241}Am(NO$_3$)$_3$ s.c. injected in a small volume of dilute acid in a rat limb (76 % absorbed in 7 d, Table A.9).

A.2.3 Intradermal Injection of $^{239}Pu(NO_3)_4$ in Swine

Blond miniature swine were injected intradermally at permanently tattooed sites with ^{239}Pu(NO$_3$)$_4$ in 0.2 mol L^{-1} HNO$_3$. A total of 558 ^{239}Pu-injected sites (0.026 to 80 µg per site) and 57 HNO$_3$-injected sites were randomly distributed on the lateral shoulder to hip regions of 10 swine (~60 injected sites on each animal) (Cable et al., 1962).

TABLE A.9—*Experimental conditions and retention of some representative soluble radionuclides at a s.c. wound site in rats.*[a]

Radionuclide	Amount Injected		Solution			Fraction Retained at s.c. Site (percent of injected amount)			References
	Bq[b]	µg[c]	mL[d]	mol L^{-1}[e]	pH[f]	1 d	4 d	7 d	
^{137}CsCl	1.1×10^5	3.5×10^{-2}	5×10^{-1}	5.1×10^{-7}	3	~0			Moskalev (1961a)
^{137}CsCl	7.4×10^4	2.3×10^{-2}	2.5×10^{-2}	6.6×10^{-6}	3	3			Ilyin and Ivannikov (1979)
^{111}AgCl	3.7×10^4	1×10^{-5}	—[d]	1.8×10^{-10}	7.5	70[g]			Kalistratova *et al.* (1968)
^{140}BaCl$_2$	3.7×10^4	1.3×10^{-5}	—[d]	2.0×10^{-10}	3	5[g]			Moskalev (1961b)
^{140}LaCl$_3$	1.8×10^5	9.1×10^{-6}	—[d]	1.3×10^{-10}	3	94[g]	84[g]		Moskalev (1961c)
^{144}CeCl$_3$	3.7×10^4	3.2×10^{-4}	—[d]	4.4×10^{-9}	—	91[g]			Moskalev (1961d)
^{241}AmCl$_3$	7.4×10^4	5.8×10^{-1}	3×10^{-2}	8×10^{-5}	—	56[h]			Ilyin and Ivannikov (1979)
^{241}Am(NO$_3$)$_3$	$(2 - 3.5) \times 10^2$	$(1.6 - 2.8) \times 10^{-3}$	5×10^{-2}	1.8×10^{-7}	2			24[h]	Gray *et al.* (1994) Stradling *et al.* (1993; 1995b)
^{228}Th(NO$_3$)$_4$	6×10^2	2×10^{-4}	5×10^{-2}	1.8×10^{-8}	2			72[h]	Stradling *et al.* (1995a)

^{238}Pu(NO$_3$)$_4$	$(2-3.5) \times 10^2$	$(3-5) \times 10^{-4}$	5×10^{-2}	3.4×10^{-8}	2	22[h]	Gray et al. (1994) Stradling et al. (1993; 1995b)
^{239}Pu(NO$_3$)$_4$	$(2.2-4) \times 10^2$	1×10^{-1}	5×10^{-2}	8.4×10^{-6}	2	34[h]	Gray et al. (1994) Harrison et al. (1978a)

[a]Radionuclide injected between skin and muscle of rats.
[b]Amount of radionuclide injected (becquerel).
[c]Mass of element injected (micrograms); calculated from the injected activity using Equation A.3.
[d]Injected volume assumed to be 0.5 mL as in Moskalev (1961a).
[e]Molar concentration (mol L^{-1}) of radionuclides in solutions injected was calculated from the injected mass and volume by using Equation A.5.
[f]When solution pH was not reported, a default value of pH 4 was assumed.
[g]Retention estimated by comparing tissue levels with rats given same radionuclide by i.v. injection.
[h]Radioanalysis of dissected injection site or external monitoring of site.

The acid solution caused transient (12 to 36 h) reddening of the skin. At sites containing ≤0.64 µg of ^{239}Pu, skin lesions were few and minor. Sites containing >0.64 µg were edematous after 24 h. Sites containing ≥3.2 µg were ulcerated after 20 d, followed during the ensuing 20 to 40 d by scab formation and sloughing.

Average ^{239}Pu retention at the higher dosage sites (% *ID*) (3.2, 16, and 80 µg) was determined by external measurements to 565 d after injection, where t is days after injection:

$$R(t) = 88e^{-0.036t} + 12e^{-0.0037t}. \tag{A.13}$$

Loss of ^{239}Pu from the injected sites took place by absorption into the body, and at the higher dosage sites, also mechanically with sloughing of the scabs. Local lymph nodes contained from 2 to 13 % of the injected ^{239}Pu at 7 d. Equation A.13 is based only on data obtained from the sites injected with the three highest dosages, and mechanical loss (sloughing) dominates the first term. However, the rate constant of the second term, 0.0037 d^{-1}, which presumably describes subsequent loss of the small ^{239}Pu residue, is not very different from the last term of the Equation 4.4 that describes late loss of soluble avidly-retained elements i.m. injected in rats (Section 4.2.2.2.4).

A.3 Lacerations (Skin-Muscle Wounds)

Lacerations involve severance of blood and lymph vessels of the dermis, the s.c. connective tissue, and the underlying muscle. The local microcirculation is disrupted, and seeped and clotted blood and tissue fluid protein collect at the cut surfaces.

Some representative radionuclides have been applied to incisions made with scissors or sharp blades through the shaved skin and into the underlying muscle of rats (Ilyin and Ivannikov, 1979; Ilyin *et al.*, 1977; 2001; McClanahan and Kornberg, 1967; Oakley and Thompson, 1956) and of mice (Kusama *et al.*, 1986). Cuts, 1.5 to 2 cm long and 0.5 cm deep, were made on the lower back; smaller cuts were made on the lower backs of the rats. Radionuclide retention at the incision site was determined by external photon counting and/or by radiochemical analysis of the body and/or the dissected wound site. The experimental conditions of the studies and the data for radionuclide retention in the wounds are collected in Table A.10.

Retention of ^{85}Sr^{2+} was measured in rhesus monkeys after application to an incised wound or an i.m. injection (Appendix A.1.4.4;

TABLE A.10—*Experimental conditions and retention of soluble radionuclides in lacerated skin wounds in rats and mice.*

Radionuclide	Applied to Wound				Fraction Retained at Wound Site (percent of injected amount)			
	Bq	μg[a]	mL	pH	1 h	4 h	1 d	7 d
Na^{131}I [b]	7.4×10^4	1.6×10^{-5}	3×10^{-2}	—	12	10	7	
^{137}CsCl [b]	7.4×10^4	2×10^{-2}	3×10^{-2}	6 – 7	19	11	5	
^{89}SrCl$_2$ [b]	7.4×10^4	6.9×10^{-5}	3×10^{-2}	2	72	64	51	
^{60}CoCl$_2$ [c]	7.4×10^4	1.8×10^{-3}	1×10^1	—	70	—	—	
^{144}CeCl$_3$ [b]	7.4×10^4	6.2×10^{-4}	3×10^{-2}	3	—	—	98	
^{241}AmCl$_3$ [b]	7.4×10^4	5.8×10^{-1}	3×10^{-2}	3	—	—	94	
^{210}Po(NO$_3$)$_4$ [d]	7.8×10^5	4.7×10^{-3}	4×10^{-2}	1.5	99.7	98	90	
^{239}Pu(NO$_3$)$_4$	1.8×10^5 [e]	8×10^1	1×10^{-2}	2	—	—	—	82
	1.8×10^4 [f]	8×10^0	1×10^{-2}	1	—	—	99	
	1.8×10^4 [f]	8×10^0	1×10^{-2}	(10 mol L^{-1})	—	—	99.6	

[a] Calculated by using Equation A.4.
[b] Data of Ilyin and Ivannikov (1979). All radionuclides: 37 to 111 kBq in 0.01 to 0.05 mL at probable pH range of one to three; quoted in Ilyin (2001).
[c] Data of Kusama et al. (1986).
[d] Data quoted in Ilyin (2001), Ilyin and Ivannikov (1979), and Ilyin et al. (1977).
[e] Data of McClanahan and Kornberg (1967).
[f] Data of Oakley and Thompson (1956).

Ducousso *et al.*, 1974). The 2 × 2 cm lacerations were made on the upper lateral surface of one thigh. Retention of the $^{85}Sr^{2+}$ at the incision, measured for 2 h by serial external photon counting, was 65 % at 100 min; clearance was significantly slower than from an i.m. puncture wound, which was nearly complete in 1 h.

Absorption of soluble $^{131}I^-$ and $^{137}Cs^+$ from lacerated wounds in rats was as rapid and as efficient as from deep puncture wounds. Absorption of the less-soluble and more readily hydrolyzed and complexed multivalent cations ($^{144}Ce^{3+}$, $^{241}Am^{3+}$, $^{210}Po^{4+}$, and $^{239}Pu^{4+}$) applied to lacerations in rat skin was substantially less than from a puncture wound.

A.4 Application to the Skin

The keratinized upper layer of the skin (stratum corneum; Section 2.1) is ~13 % lipid and 74 % partially hydrated protein by weight, and total water content is 10 to 20 %. Although the intact stratum corneum is not impenetrable, it is an efficient barrier to water and dissolved polar solutes. In order to be absorbed through the skin into circulating fluids, a dissolved electrolyte must penetrate not only the stratum corneum but also five layers of cells before encountering the small blood and lymph capillaries of the dermis. Human skin is penetrated by epidermal appendages, hair follicles, and sweat gland ducts, which, depending on the anatomical location, occupy 0.1 to 1 % of the total skin surface. The skin of most furbearing animals lacks sweat glands, but it has densely packed hair follicles. Consequently, without verification using human skin, absorption measurement in furred laboratory animals is subject to uncertainties due to the differences in density and nature of the epidermal appendages, skin thickness, and lipid content. The skin of rodents has been found to be more permeable to many chemicals than human skin (Rice and Cohen, 1996).

The degree of absorption of a chemical through the intact skin (percutaneous absorption) depends on its chemical properties. Lipophilic substances permeate the skin more rapidly and to a greater degree than hydrophilic substances such as electrolytes in aqueous solution. Nonpolar (lipophilic) solvents and solutes diffuse rapidly through the intercellular lipid strands and the relatively dry protein. Polar substances in water diffuse slowly through the protein filaments of the outer surface of the stratum corneum and along the openings provided by the epidermal appendages. In general, percutaneous absorption of polar solutes in water is dependent on solute concentration and solubility at the pH of skin, exposure time, and the area exposed (Rice and Cohen, 1996).

A.4.1 *Penetration of Intact Skin*

Solutions of some representative radionuclides (1,110 kBq in 0.04 mL, pH 1 to 2) were applied to 1 to 6 cm^2 areas of shaved skin on the lower backs of rats. During the exposures (1 h to 5 d) the rats were restrained in special individual holders. Percutaneous absorption was determined by radioanalysis of blood and internal organs (Ilyin, 2001; Ilyin and Ivannikov, 1979; Ilyin *et al.*, 1982). The data for absorption of those radionuclides from shaved rat skin at 1 d are arranged in Table A.11 in the order of decreasing absorption, which is also the order of their increasing tendency to hydrolyze and/or to bind to protein. Earlier studies had been conducted of percutaneous absorption of ^{90}SrCl$_2$ (Budko, 1961) and ^{144}CeCl$_3$ (Rogacheva, 1961), in which comparable amounts of radionuclides were applied to similar areas of the shaved skin of singly caged rats, and absorption was also measured by radioanalysis of the skeleton and internal organs. Those results are in good agreement with the findings of Ilyin and coworkers; ^{90}Sr^{2+} absorption at 2 to 4 d was ~1 % of the amount applied, and that of ^{144}Ce^{3+} at 4 d was 0.13 %.

The early biological investigations with ^{239}Pu^{4+} conducted at the Hanford Laboratory (reviewed by Vaughan, 1973) included four measurements of absorption through the shaved skin of rats. In those studies, 0.005 to 0.1 mL of ^{239}Pu(NO$_3$)$_4$ solutions containing 3.2 or 18.3 kBq (1 or 8 µg) at pH 1 were applied to 0.5, 1, or 3 cm^2 areas of the shaved skin on the lower backs of the rats, and exposures were 1 to 5 d. Absorption of the ^{239}Pu^{4+} into the body was measured by radiochemical analysis of the skinned carcass (GI tract removed) (Oakley and Thompson, 1956; Weeks and Oakley, 1954; 1955). Absorption reported was 0.33 ± 0.3 % at 1 d and 0.05 to 0.29 ± 0.23 % at 45 d. Those absorbed fractions are ~20 times greater than were later observed by the Russian investigators in the experiments described above, and they are also greater than the absorbed fractions reported for similarly sparingly soluble and readily hydrolyzable ^{144}Ce^{3+}, ^{241}Am^{3+}, and ^{210}Po^{4+} (Table A.11). Absorption of ^{239}Pu^{4+} may have been overestimated in the Hanford studies; small, but in this case, substantial and nonreproducible amounts of ^{239}Pu^{4+} on the highly contaminated skin may have been mechanically transferred to the carcass during removal of the skin. Because the Russian studies of radionuclide absorption from rat skin were designed to avoid such technical difficulties, and because ^{239}Pu^{4+} studies were part of a systematically investigated series of radionuclides, only the data of Ilyin *et al.* (1982) for ^{239}Pu^{4+} are included in Table A.11.

TABLE A.11—*Absorption into the body at 1 d of some representative radionuclides applied to the intact or thermally-burned skin of rats (Ilyin, 2001; Ilyin and Ivannikov, 1979; Ilyin et al., 1982).*

Radionuclide	Fraction of Applied Radionuclide Absorbed (%)			
	Intact Skin	Burned Skin		
		Grade I	Grade II	Grade III
$^{131}I^-$	2.5	2.2	3.0	1.6
$^{137}Cs^+$	2.1	1.8	2.0	0.8
$^{204}Tl^+$	—	—	~1.0	—
$^{89}Sr^{2+}$	2.4	2.1	2.5	1.8
$^{140}Ba^{2+}$	—	—	~1.0	—
$^{60}Co^{2+}$	—	—	~1.0	—
$^{144}Ce^{3+}$ [a]	0.15	0.26	—	—
$^{241}Am^{3+}$	0.014	0.06	0.07	0.03
$^{210}Po^{4+}$	0.013	0.013	0.025	0.0015
$^{239}Pu^{4+}$	0.017	—	—	—

[a]Grigoryan (1966).

The fractional absorption at 1 d of $^{239}Pu(NO_3)_4$ in 0.1 mol L^{-1} HNO$_3$ (0.017 %) was not significantly different from that of a prepared $^{239}Pu^{4+}$ hydroxide polymer also applied in 0.1 mol L^{-1} HNO$_3$ (0.012 %) (Ilyin, 2001; Ilyin *et al.*, 1982). Those results imply that the dilute acidity of the applied solutions was effectively neutralized on the skin, allowing hydrolysis and protein binding of the $^{239}Pu^{4+}$ applied in solution.

Uranium compounds, ranging in aqueous solubility from soluble uranyl nitrate, $UO_2(NO_3)_2 \cdot 6H_2O$, to insoluble UO_2, were applied to the shaved skin of rats, mice, guinea pigs, and rabbits to determine acute toxicity (Orcutt, 1949). Absorption through the skin was not measured directly, but if it is assumed that equal amounts of UO_2^{2+} entering the circulation are equally toxic, absorption of the several uranium compounds can be estimated from their acute toxicity. Toxicity of $UO_2(NO_3)_2$ was studied in rabbits, guinea pigs, rats, and mice by applying a 70 % diethyl ether/30 % ethanol solution to the shaved skin. The dosage range (g U kg^{-1}) was broad enough to define the median lethal dose in each species. The exposed skin areas varied, because the larger dosages were spread over larger areas of skin. Total fractional absorption in 3 to 5 d can be estimated by comparing the species-specific acute toxicities (median lethal dose) of $UO_2(NO_3)_2$ applied to the skin with those after a single parenteral injection (Durbin and Wrenn, 1975). On that basis, absorption from the skin was as follows: rabbit, 0.17 %; guinea pig, 0.014 %; rat, 0.2 %; and mouse, 0.092 %. The $UO_2(NO_3)_2$ dried as crystals on the skin, and the ether-alcohol solution caused coagulation necrosis of the superficial skin layers, which may have altered absorption.

The toxicities of other uranium compounds were investigated only in the rabbits, the species most sensitive to UO_2^{2+} poisoning. Soluble uranium compounds were applied to the skin in aqueous solution, and the less-soluble diuranates and oxides were mixed with lanolin and spread on the skin. None of those uranium preparations caused a skin response. Their absorption can be estimated as before by comparing their toxic dosages with that of an equal weight of uranium as $UO_2(NO_3)_2$. UO_2F_2 was about as toxic as $UO_2(NO_3)_2$, and its absorption is probably similar. The toxicities of UCl_4, UO_3, and the diuranates were about one-half as great as those of the soluble uranium compounds, and their absorption was probably no more than one-half as great. Insoluble UF_4, UO_2, and U_3O_8 were essentially nontoxic when applied to the skin, from which it may be inferred that little, if any, of the uranium in those compounds was absorbed and subsequently oxidized to toxic UO_2^{2+}. The absorption of uranium from the skin, as assessed from these toxicity studies, particularly in the case of $UO_2(NO_3)_2$, may be an underestimate, because of the loss of the $UO_2(NO_3)_2$ crystals from the skin, and because the comparison of equal toxicity was made between an acute intraperitoneal injection (blood uranium very high for a brief interval) and the more protracted absorption from the skin (blood uranium relatively low, but sustained for many hours).

To summarize, the intact skin is an effective barrier to the absorption of the most soluble radionuclides investigated (Table A.11). Absorption of $^{131}I^-$, $^{137}Cs^+$, $^{89}Sr^{2+}$ from the shaved skin of rats was, on average, 2.5 % of the amounts applied during a 24 h exposure. Absorption of the less-soluble and readily hydrolyzed multivalent cations, $^{144}Ce^{3+}$, $^{241}Am^{3+}$, $^{210}Po^{4+}$, and $^{239}Pu^{4+}$ was severely inhibited. At 1 d, 0.013 to 0.15 % of the applied amounts of those radionuclides were absorbed.

A.4.2 *Abraded Skin*

Abrasion of the skin creates new open channels through the epidermal barrier. Some representative radionuclides were applied to small areas of shaved skin of rats (1 cm^2) or mice (0.8 cm^2) that had been mechanically damaged with a metal rasp or fine sandpaper (Ilyin, 2001; Ilyin and Ivannikov, 1979; Ilyin *et al.*, 1977; Kusama *et al.*, 1986). Radionuclide retention on the abraded skin was determined by external photon counting and/or by radiochemical analysis of the dissected application site and/or internal organs (Table A.12).

Ilyin *et al.* (1975) determined the retention of ^{85}SrCl$_2$ applied to 6.5 cm^2 areas of finely abraded and scratched skin on the distal extensor surface of the left arm of adult male human volunteers. At 30 min and 6 h, the experimental skin areas were thoroughly decontaminated. Several techniques were used to estimate ^{85}Sr absorption (six independent assessments in each of three subjects, $n = 18$). Retention on the skin was (62 ± 18) and $(43 \pm 18)\%$ at 30 min and 6 h, respectively. Abraded human skin appears to be significantly more permeable to ^{85}SrCl$_2$ than abraded rat skin (Table A.12).

Absorption of soluble ^{131}I$^-$ and ^{137}Cs$^+$ from abraded rat skin was ~80 % of the amount applied, 20 % less than from a deep puncture wound. Absorption of less-soluble hydrolysable multivalent cations (^{144}Ce^{3+}, ^{241}Am^{3+}, and ^{210}Pu^{4+}) was substantially less than from a deep puncture wound, but still much greater than from intact skin.

A.4.3 *Thermally-Burned Skin*

Solutions of some representative radionuclides (0.04 mL, 1,110 kBq, pH 1.5 to 2) were applied to 1 cm^2 areas of the shaved skin of rats immediately after inflicting thermal burns of Grade I (skin hyperemia), Grade II (epidermal necrosis and dermal edema), or Grade III (dermal necrosis) with a calibrated heat lamp (Ilyin, 2001; Ilyin and Ivannikov, 1979). Radionuclide absorption into the body at 1 d is summarized in Table A.11. Skin structure was examined histopathologically, and the distribution and status of ^{210}Po^{4+} on and in the burned skin were investigated autoradiographically.

A solution of ^{144}CeCl$_3$ (0.1 mL, 185 kBq, pH 5) was applied to a 3 cm^2 area of the intact shaved skin of rats or the shaved skin of rats that had been irradiated 36 h earlier with an ultraviolet lamp until erythema developed. Absorption of the ^{144}Ce^{3+} through the burned skin at 1 d (0.26 % of the amount applied) was about twice that through intact skin (0.15 %) (Grigoryan, 1966).

TABLE A.12—*Experimental conditions and absorption of soluble radionuclides applied to damaged (abraded) skin in rats and mice.*

Radionuclide	Applied to Abraded Skin		pH	Fraction Absorbed from Wound Site (percent of applied amount)		
	Bq	μg^a		1 h	4 h	24 h
Na^{131}I [b]	7.4×10^4	1.6×10^{-5}	—	75	80	80
^{137}CsCl [b]	7.4×10^4	2.3×10^{-2}	6–7	90	90	92
^{85}SrCl$_2$ [b]	7.4×10^4	8.3×10^{-5}	2	32	36	~35
^{60}CoCl$_2$ [c]	7.4×10^4	1.8×10^{-3}	—	53	—	—
^{144}CeCl$_3$ [b]	7.4×10^4	6.3×10^{-4}	3	—	—	~3.0
^{241}AmCl$_3$ [b]	7.4×10^4	6.2×10^{-1}	3	6.0	7.0	~6.0
^{210}Po(NO$_3$)$_4$ [d]	7.8×10^5	4.7×10^{-3}	1.5	—	—	2.5

[a] Calculated by using Equation A.4.
[b] Ilyin and Ivannikov (1979). All radionuclides: 37 to 111 kBq in 0.01 to 0.05 mL at probable pH range of 1 to 3; quoted in Ilyin (2001).
[c] Kusama et al. (1986).
[d] Ilyin et al. (1977); quoted in Ilyin (2001) and Ilyin and Ivannikov (1979).

The skin barrier was still functionally intact after a Grade I burn, and hyperemia by itself did not appear to increase the permeability of the superficial skin layers to the dissolved electrolytes. Nearly all of the applied $^{210}Po^{4+}$ was found as aggregates of alpha tracks associated with the keratinized layer of the epidermis, but some single tracks were found with the hair follicle ducts. Grade II burns appeared to have compromised the epidermal barrier; for example, absorption of $^{210}Po^{4+}$ and $^{241}Am^{3+}$ was somewhat greater than through intact skin. The distribution of $^{210}Po^{4+}$ alpha tracks was similar to that after a Grade I burn. The Grade III burns damaged the dermis as well as the epidermis, and the somewhat reduced radionuclide absorption may be attributed to entrapment of the radionuclides in the necrotizing tissue (Ilyin, 2001; Ilyin and Ivannikov, 1979; Ilyin et al., 1977).

A.4.4 Acid-Burned Skin

$^{241}Am(NO_3)_3$, $^{210}Po(NO_3)_4$, or $^{239}Pu(NO_3)_4$ in 0.03 to 10 mol L^{-1} HNO_3 were applied to areas of shaved skin on the lower back of rats. Absorption of the radionuclides into the body from 1 to 3 d was determined by radiochemical analysis of blood and internal organs. The experimental conditions and the absorbed fractions at 1 and 3 d are summarized in Table A.13. The histopathology of the nitric-acid-burned skin and the microdistribution of the radionuclides, determined autoradiographically, were described (Ilyin, 2001; Ilyin and Ivannikov, 1979; Ilyin et al., 1982; Weeks and Oakley, 1955).

A solution of $^{239}Pu^{4+}$ in 10 mol L^{-1} HNO_3 was applied to 1 cm^2 areas of the shaved intact skin of rats or skin that had been freshly punctured with a lancet, producing a wound 2 mm wide and 3 mm deep. Absorption of the $^{239}Pu^{4+}$ from the wounded skin was the same at post-exposure times from 1 h to 30 d as that from unwounded skin, suggesting that the strong acid rapidly cauterized the puncture wound (Weeks and Oakley, 1955).

There were no visible structural changes in the skin at 24 h after $^{241}Am(NO_3)_3$ was applied in 0.05 mol L^{-1} HNO_3, and the $^{241}Am^{3+}$ was located almost entirely on the surface of the epidermis with some penetration of hair follicles.

There was mild epidermal thickening with focal cell swelling within 24 h after application of $^{239}Pu(NO_3)_4$ in 0.1 mol L^{-1} HNO_3, and at 24 h, edema and epidermal cell vacuolization were evident. Although slightly damaged, the skin was considered still to present an effective barrier to penetration of the $^{239}Pu^{4+}$. Skin damage was evident within 1 h after application of radionuclides in 0.5 to

TABLE A.13—*Absorption of $^{241}Am(NO_3)_3$, $^{210}Po(NO_3)_4$, and $^{239}Pu(NO_3)_4$ from the intact or acid-burned skin of rats.*[a]

| HNO$_3$ (mol L^{-1}) | Absorbed Fraction at 1 and 3 d (percent of applied amount) | | | | | |
| | ^{241}Am(NO$_3$)$_3$[b] | | ^{210}Po(NO$_3$)$_4$[b] | | ^{239}Pu(NO$_3$)$_4$[c] | |
	1 d	3 d	1 d	3 d	1 d	3 d
0.03	0.014		0.013			
0.05	0.031					
0.10					0.017	0.017
0.10[d]					0.012[d]	0.016[d]
0.5	0.18		0.035			
1.0	0.22	1.15	0.01		0.058	0.079
2.5	0.14		0.0065	0.045	0.038	0.10
4	0.14		0.003			
8	0.32	2.0	0.002			
10					0.03	0.047

[a]Absorption determined by radiochemical analysis of blood and internal organs and tissues.

[b]Americium-241 and ^{210}Po (0.1 mL, 2,590 to 3,515 kBq) in HNO$_3$ applied to 4 cm^2 of shaved skin on lower back of rats (Ilyin, 2001; Ilyin and Ivannikov, 1979).

[c]Plutonium-239 (0.15 mL, 1,110 kBq, 485 µg) in HNO$_3$ applied to 6 cm^2 of shaved skin on lower back of rats (Ilyin, 2001; Ilyin et al., 1982).

[d]Plutonium-239 polymer in 0.1 mol L^{-1} HNO$_3$ (Ilyin, 2001; Ilyin et al., 1982).

1 mol L^{-1} HNO$_3$. Observed changes included epidermal thinning, nuclear lysis, and collagen fibril swelling in the upper one-third of the dermis. Autoradiographs of ^{241}Am^{3+} and ^{239}Pu^{4+} showed large aggregations of alpha tracks on the epidermal surface, less dense aggregates of tracks in hair follicles, s.c. tissue, and muscle connective tissue layers, and diffuse alpha tracks within the skin and s.c. muscle layers. Within 1 to 24 h, most of the alpha tracks from all three radionuclides investigated were concentrated in a layer of necrotic tissue 20 to 400 µm below the surface, providing evidence for their low mobility in the necrotic zone. However, there were some aggregates of alpha tracks associated with damaged hair

follicles. Absorption of $^{210}Po^{4+}$ and $^{239}Pu^{4+}$, applied in ≥ 2.5 mol L^{-1} HNO$_3$, was the same as, or less than, their baseline levels for undamaged skin. Rapidly developing tissue necrosis caused by the concentrated HNO$_3$ solutions may have created a barrier to radionuclide transport consisting of coagulated tissue fluid and denatured protein.

There was a trend, most prominent for $^{241}Am^{3+}$, towards continued absorption from the acid-burned skin and the absorbed fractions of all three radionuclides at 3 d were greater than at 1 d. At 5 d after radionuclide application in ≥ 2.5 mol L^{-1} HNO$_3$, nearly all of the alpha tracks from $^{241}Am^{3+}$ were restricted to massive clumped aggregates in the necrotic zone. As had been observed after intradermal injection of $^{239}Pu(NO_3)_4$ in 0.2 mol L^{-1} in swine (Appendix A.2.3; Cable et $al.$, 1962), between 15 and 30 d after application of $^{239}Pu^{4+}$ in 10 mol L^{-1} HNO$_3$, an eschar separated that included both damaged skin and underlying muscle. The final scar consisted of fibrous tissue covered with a thin layer of regenerated epidermis with no dermal appendages. The few alpha tracks observed were contained within macrophages in the deepest layer of the atrophic skin.

A.5 Conditions that Alter Retention of Dissolved Radionuclides in Wounds

The studies used to define the "base case" retention of soluble radionuclides in deep puncture wounds were limited to those in which small volumes of dilute solutions of radionuclides were i.m. injected, mainly in rats. The amount of radionuclide plus stable carrier deposited was ≤ 5 µg, and radionuclide concentrations were low in both the injection media and at the wound site. The concentration of H$^+$ in the injection medium was usually sufficient to ensure that the radionuclide was in solution when injected but not great enough to cause more than transient local tissue damage. Tables A.2 and A.7 contain data for studies of 27 soluble radionuclides i.m. injected in rats that were not used to define "base case" retention, because they did not meet those criteria. In those cases, wound retention classification was assigned, shown in lower case letters, in Tables A.2 and A.7, based on the similarity of the individual retention pattern to the behavior of the assigned retention category.

A.5.1 *Increased Local Concentrations of Deposited Radionuclides*

Wound retention is increased and prolonged by increasing the local concentration, particularly of radionuclides that hydrolyze at pH ≤ 7.4, form stable complexes with fixed tissue constituents, or precipitate as insoluble compounds with tissue fluid constituents (Appendix B). Increasing the local radionuclide concentration facilitates compound formation, more complete hydrolysis with formation of larger aggregates and/or polymers, and binding to tissue constituents.

A.5.1.1 *Weakly- and Moderately-Retained Radionuclides.* The basic data set (Table A.2) contains some examples of weakly-retained radionuclides that do not hydrolyze at physiological pH or form insoluble compounds or stable complexes with bioligands. The wound retention patterns could still be classified as weak for $^{137}Cs^+$, $^{85}Sr^{2+}$, or $^{58}Co^{2+}$ when they were i.m. injected in rats with as much as 17 to 41 µg of stable element carrier (Table A.7; Morrow *et al.*, 1968), and for $^{71}GeO_3^{2-}$ when it was i.m. injected with 1 mg of stable germanium as GeO_3^{2-} (Table A.2).

The basic data set also includes examples of radionuclides that do not hydrolyze at pH 7.4, but were cleared more slowly from a wound when the mass injected was >5 µg. Carrier-free $^{111}Ag^+$ was moderately retained, but it was strongly retained when injected with 1 mg of stable Ag^+ (Table A.2), possibly due to the precipitation of insoluble chloride or carbonate and/or complexation with free sulfhydryl side chains of tissue proteins. Carrier-free $^{140}Ba^{2+}$ was weakly retained (Table A.2), while $^{133}Ba^{2+}$ injected with 40 µg of stable Ba^{2+} was moderately retained (Table A.7), possibly due to precipitation of insoluble carbonate or sulfate and/or transient binding to tissue protein.

When carrier-free $^{64}Cu^{2+}$ was injected, it was weakly retained. Injection of $^{64}Cu^{2+}$ with 1 mg of stable Cu^{2+} increased the concentration at the wound site enough to exceed K_{sp} for formation of the hydroxide, and retention was augmented from weak to moderate.

Neptunium was i.m. injected as soluble $^{237}NpO_2NO_3$ (100 to 150 µg, pH 1.5). In mildly acidic solution NpO_2^+ is stable, and it probably was not hydrolyzed in the injection solution. In aqueous solution, NpO_2^+ behaves like a large divalent cation, and moderate wound retention would have been expected, if the mass injected had been smaller. However, in the wound at pH 7.4, K_{sp} for formation of NpO_2OH was just exceeded, and *in situ* hydrolysis of the large mass of NpO_2^+ probably contributed to its greater and more prolonged retention, which was classified as strong (Table A.2). Additionally, NpO_2^+ is more easily reduced to Np^{4+} in neutral than in acid solution (Musikas, 1976), and biological reductants such as organic acids in tissue fluid may have contributed to slow reduction to Np^{4+}, which is more readily hydrolyzed, complexed, and retained (Cunningham, 1954).

High-specific-activity $^{230}UO_2^{2+}$ (4×10^{-6} µg) was weakly retained at an i.m.-injection site. That weak retention pattern was not changed when as much as 37 µg of $^{233}UO_2^{2+}$ was injected, even though the local concentration of the larger injected mass of uranyl ion was sufficient to exceed K_{sp} for formation of $UO_2(OH)_2$ and to enhance local protein binding. Uranyl ion forms stable, renally filterable carbonate complexes at pH 7.4 by reaction with circulating HCO_3^- (Dounce, 1949; Gindler, 1973). The HCO_3^- concentrations in tissue fluid and plasma are nearly the same (0.25 mol L^{-1}; Gamble, 1954), and circulating HCO_3^- was apparently sufficient to counteract UO_2^{2+} hydrolysis by complexing and facilitating transport of the larger mass of $^{233}UO_2^{2+}$ from the injection site.

A.5.1.2 *Strongly-Retained Radionuclides.* Small masses (<5 µg) of the trivalent radionuclides were strongly retained at an i.m. wound site in rats. Injection of trivalent ^{51}Cr, ^{140}La, ^{143}Pr, or ^{147}Nd diluted with 1 mg of stable element carrier enhanced wound retention from strong to avid. The heavy trivalent lanthanides (^{166}Ho, ^{175}Yb, and ^{177}Lu) were injected only with 30 to 50 µg of stable carrier, and they were classified as avidly retained (Tables A.2 and A.7). The K_{sp} values of the hydroxides were exceeded in the case of the heavy lanthanides and closely approached for the lighter lanthanides injected with stable carrier, in both cases causing more complete hydrolysis and protein binding and greater and more prolonged retention.

Retention of $^{239}Pu^{4+}$ at an i.m. wound site has been measured in rats and hamsters injected with $^{239}Pu(NO_3)_4$ in small volumes (0.01 to 0.1 mL) of HNO_3 at pH 1 to 2; the amounts of plutonium deposited were 0.011 to 8.8 µg (Gray *et al.*, 1994; Harrison and David, 1977; 1978; Harrison *et al.*, 1977a; 1977b; 1978a; 1978b; Taylor, 1967; Taylor and Sowby, 1962; Volf, 1974a; 1974b; 1975). The data are shown in Figure A.1. Initial retention of $^{239}Pu^{4+}$, as judged by the fraction retained at 7 d, is positively correlated with the deposited mass (Section B.1), and the fraction retained after deposition of 0.011 µg (34 %) is about one-half of that retained after deposition of 8.8 µg (69 %). The rate of clearance of $^{239}Pu^{4+}$ from the wound site between 7 and 90 d is negatively correlated with the deposited mass, and the clearance rates of the smaller masses (0.022 to 0.48 µg) is 0.011 d^{-1}, almost three times faster than that for 8.8 µg, the largest mass (0.004 d^{-1}).

Even the smallest mass of Pu^{4+} i.m. injected (0.011 µg) is expected to hydrolyze in the neutral environment of the injection

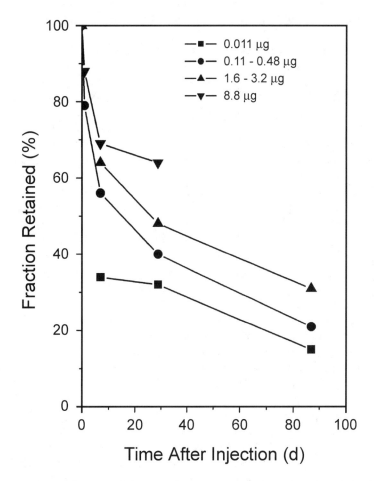

Fig. A.1. Influence of deposited mass on retention at an i.m.-injection site in rats and hamsters of $^{239}Pu(NO_3)_4$ administered in small volumes of dilute HNO_3, pH 1 to 2 (data sources cited in text and in Table A.1).

site. The hydrolysis products of Pu^{4+}, and those of the other tetra-positive ions, tend to aggregate and form cross-linked polymers, and the degree of plutonium hydroxide aggregation and polymerization increases with time and Pu^{4+} concentration (Hindman, 1954; Taylor, 1973a). As was suggested by Harrison *et al.* (1977b), increasing the mass of Pu^{4+} deposited in an i.m. puncture wound would be expected to accelerate hydrolysis, enhance the aggregation and polymerization of precipitated $Pu(OH)_4$, favor formation of larger and more insoluble polymers, and impede the dissolution and translocation of Pu^{4+} from the wound site.

A.5.2 *Radionuclides Injected as Soluble Complexes*

Retention at an i.m. wound site of multivalent cations that hydrolyze at physiological pH is greatly reduced by injecting them in solutions containing an excess of a stably binding complexing agent (*e.g.*, citrate ion). Retention at an i.m.-injection site in rats at 1 d after injection of ≤5 µg of tri- or tetravalent cations was reduced, on average, to ~11 % when they were injected in 0.08 mol L^{-1} sodium citrate, compared with ~75 % retained when the same amounts of those radionuclides were injected without a complexing species (Durbin *et al.*, 1957; Hamilton, 1948d; 1949b; 1949c; 1952; 1954a; 1954b; Harrison *et al.*, 1978a). The citrate complexes of most multivalent cations are sufficiently stable at physiological pH to reduce their affinities for OH^-, effectively suppressing hydrolysis and complexation with fixed tissue ligands at the wound site, at least as long as the local citrate concentration remains elevated.

A.5.3 *Special Case of the Oxidation States and Isotopes of Plutonium*

Plutonium merits special attention, because several plutonium isotopes are industrially important and the frequency of radiologically significant plutonium-contaminated wound accidents has exceeded that for all other radionuclides combined (Ilyin, 2001).

Three of the plutonium oxidation states are stable in neutral aqueous solution—Pu^{3+}, Pu^{4+}, and PuO_2^{2+}. The i.m. injection studies of plutonium in solution, summarized in Tables A.1 and A.2, include a range of injected masses from 0.04 ng of $^{238}Pu^{4+}$ to 8.8 µg of $^{239}Pu^{4+}$, 16 µg of $^{239}Pu^{3+}$ and 16 to 20 µg of $^{239}PuO_2^{2+}$. Data from the i.m. injection of soluble $^{238}Pu^{4+}$ and $^{239}Pu^{4+}$ (≤3.2 µg) were included in the data set used to define the wound retention of the strong category radionuclides. The i.m. injection studies in rats, in which large masses of plutonium (≥16 µg, pH 2 to 2.5) were administered, most likely as suspensions of colloidal hydroxide species, are described in Appendix B and discussed in Section 4.4.1.2 in the context of wounds containing insoluble forms of plutonium.

A.5.3.1 *Trivalent Plutonium.* The chemical properties of Pu^{3+} resemble those of its lanthanide analogues of similar ionic radius, Ce^{3+} and Pr^{3+}, most importantly in the solubilities of the hydroxides and the stabilities of complexes (Hindman, 1954). In the early study of Scott *et al.* (1948a) $^{239}Pu^{3+}$ (16 µg $^{239}PuCl_3$, 6.7×10^{-5} mol L^{-1}, pH 2.5) was probably in solution when injected (Tables A.1 and A.2). At the wound site, the K_{sp} for $Pu(OH)_3$ ($10^{-19.7}$)

was probably not exceeded, but microcolloidal hydrolysis products and complexes with fixed tissue protein were likely to have formed. The overall retention pattern in the wound was similar to that of ^{152,154}Eu (≤0.6 µg), the most strongly held lanthanide, suggesting that smaller injected masses of ^{239}Pu^{3+} will also be strongly retained.

Retention at the i.m.-injection site of rats injected with 16 µg of ^{239}PuCl$_3$ was analyzed using the wound model (Section 4, assuming radionuclide introduction into the soluble compartment) and Origin® software. The resulting wound retention curve (% ID), shown in Figure A.2, is:

$$R(t) = 14e^{-1.4t} + 70e^{-0.016t} + 16e^{-0.0003t}, \quad (A.14)$$

where t is days after injection. Initially, the wound retention of the Pu^{3+} resembled that of the avidly-retained radionuclides (Equation 4.5; Section 4.2.2.2.4), but its longer term behavior was more like that of the strongly-retained radionuclides (Equation 4.4; Section 4.2.2.2.3). The transfer rates of the wound model fits for ^{239}Pu^{3+} (16 µg i.m. injected in rats) shown in Table A.14 most closely resemble those for the smaller masses (≤5 µg) of the strongly-retained radionuclides, in particular ^{152,154}Eu.

A.5.3.2 *Hexavalent Plutonium.* Because of the early difficulties encountered in preparing unhydrolyzed ^{239}Pu^{4+} in media suitable for animal injection, less readily hydrolyzed ^{239}PuO$_2$$^{2+}$ (plutonyl ion) was used to investigate plutonium metabolism and toxicity in animals (Carritt *et al.*, 1947; Finkle *et al.*, 1947; Kisieleski and Woodruff, 1947; Painter *et al.*, 1946; Scott *et al.*, 1948a; Van Middlesworth, 1947). The amounts of ^{239}PuO$_2$$^{2+}$ i.m. injected in rats (16 to 20 µg at pH 2 to 2.5) were low enough to avoid hydrolysis in the injection media.

Retention data at the wound site in rats i.m. injected with 16 µg of ^{239}PuO$_2$Cl$_2$ (Scott *et al.*, 1948a) were analyzed by using the wound model (Section 4, assuming radionuclide introduction into the soluble compartment) and Origin® software. The wound retention curve (% ID), shown in Figure A.2, is:

$$R(t) = 66e^{-0.18t} + 34e^{-0.0028t}, \quad (A.15)$$

where t is days after injection. The first measurements of plutonium at the wound site were made at 4 d, and no fast-clearing initial component of retention could be identified.

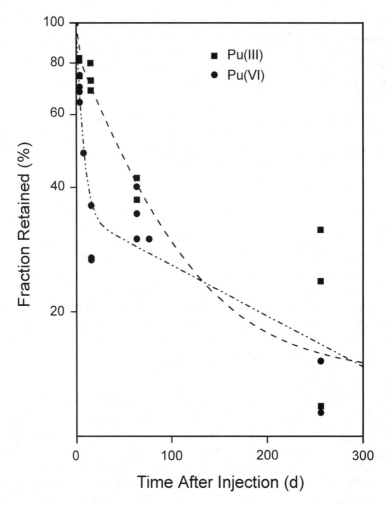

Fig. A.2. Retention at an i.m.-injection site in rats of plutonium injected as $^{239}PuCl_3$ (dashed line) or PuO_2Cl_2 (dash-dot line) [data of Scott *et al.* (1948a) shown in Table A.2].

The wound retention pattern of hexavalent plutonium is unlike that of any other multivalent cationic radionuclide studied. The major fraction (66 % of the amount deposited) was cleared from the wound site at a rate slower than the initial clearance rate (λ_1) of the strong category radionuclides (Equation 4.4), but faster than λ_2, the second rate constant of the retention equation for those radionuclides. The remaining 34 % of the plutonium deposited as PuO_2^{2+} was cleared more slowly, but at a rate about three times faster than the late clearance rate of the strong category radionuclides.

TABLE A.14—*Transfer rates (d⁻¹) obtained from the wound model for retention at an i.m.-injection site in rats of ≥16 μg of ²³⁹Pu in its three principal oxidation states.* [a,b]

Pathway	$^{239}\text{PuO}_2^{2+}$	$^{239}\text{Pu}^{3+}$	$^{239}\text{Pu}^{4+}$ [c]
Soluble to blood	0.20	0.25	0.062
Soluble to CIS	0.089	1.3	4.3
CIS to soluble	4.2×10^{-3}	0.10	0.35
CIS to PABS	0.0 [d]	6.5×10^{-3}	0.019
CIS to lymph nodes	2×10^{-5} [e]	2×10^{-5} [e]	1.9×10^{-3} [c]
PABS to soluble	0.0 [d]	2.6×10^{-5}	0.0
PABS to lymph nodes	2×10^{-5} [e]	2×10^{-5} [e]	4.2×10^{-5} [c]
Lymph nodes to blood	0.0	0.0	0.029 [c]

[a]Injected into soluble compartment of wound model (Section 4).
[b]Data of Scott *et al.* (1948a); Tables A.1, A.2, and B.1. $^{239}\text{Pu}^{3+}$ and $^{239}\text{PuO}_2^{2+}$ injected in solution; $^{239}\text{Pu}^{4+}$ injected as colloidal hydroxide.
[c]Wound model transfer rates taken from Figure 4.16; transfer rates associated with lymph-node compartment taken from dog study with plutonium colloid (Section 4).
[d]Three-compartment solution, assumes no transfer from the CIS to the PABS compartment.
[e]Fixed parameter value (see discussion in Section 4).

In contrast to other study radionuclides, the best wound model fit to the data for 16 μg of $^{239}\text{PuO}_2\text{Cl}_2$ i.m. injected in rats required only three parameters—the transfer rate from the soluble to blood compartments and the intercompartmental transfer rates between the soluble and CIS compartments (Table A.14). Although the transfer rates for PuO_2^{2+} are slower, similar to those for weak category radionuclides, the fraction of plutonium going to blood was twice that going to the CIS compartment. The rate of resolubilization and return of the plutonium from the CIS to the soluble compartment is slower, but the relative transfer of plutonium [(CIS to soluble) (soluble to CIS)⁻¹ = 0.047] is nearly the same as that of the strong category radionuclides, for which the relative transfer is 0.04.

Clearance of the plutonium deposited as PuO_2^{2+} appeared to be biphasic suggesting that two chemical processes were competing at the wound site. Although in solution in the injection medium,

$PuO_2(OH)_2$ may have formed in the wound site. The structures and stabilities of the plutonyl and uranyl biscarbonate complexes are nearly the same, and formation of soluble complexes may have initially suppressed PuO_2^{2+} hydrolysis and/or dissolved some of the $PuO_2(OH)_2$ allowing a fraction of the injected $^{239}PuO_2^{2+}$ to be transported from the wound to blood in soluble form (half-time ~4 d). Reduction of PuO_2^{2+} to Pu^{4+} is slow, but it can be accelerated in neutral solution by mild reducing agents like organic acids. The greater stabilities of the hydroxide and other complexes of Pu^{4+}, compared with those of PuO_2^{2+}, favor reduction of PuO_2^{2+} to Pu^{4+}. It is reasonable to postulate that the slower loss after 20 d of the plutonium injected as PuO_2^{2+} was the result of chemical processes that tend to reduce and immobilize it as $Pu(OH)_4$. However, early clearance of 16 µg of plutonium injected as $^{239}PuO_2^{2+}$ reduced the amount of plutonium remaining at the wound site at 20 d to ~5 µg (30 % of the amount deposited). The later rate of clearance of the fraction retained at the wound site was 0.0028 d^{-1}, similar to the implied rate (0.004 d^{-1}) for clearance from 7 to 30 d of 8.8 µg of $^{239}Pu^{4+}$ i.m. injected in 3 mol L^{-1} HNO_3 (compare Equations A.9 and A.15).

A.5.3.3 *Tetravalent ^{238}Pu and ^{239}Pu.* In the first direct comparison of soluble $^{238}Pu^{4+}$ and $^{239}Pu^{4+}$ i.m. injected in rats, retention of $^{239}Pu^{4+}$ was observed to be much greater than that of $^{238}Pu^{4+}$. However, the mass of ^{239}Pu injected (50 to 230 µg) was almost 1,000 times greater than that of $^{238}Pu^{4+}$ (0.5 to 0.23 µg) (Lafuma *et al.*, 1971; Morin *et al.*, 1972; 1973a; Nenot *et al.*, 1972a; 1972b). Retention of 0.011 µg (0.26 kBq) of $^{239}Pu^{4+}$ was compared to that of 4×10^{-5} µg (0.026 KBq) or 0.011 µg (7.3 KBq) of $^{238}Pu^{4+}$ after i.m. injection in rats. Retention was nearly the same for the small equal masses of the two plutonium isotopes and for the small masses with equal activities (Harrison *et al.*, 1977b). The authors concluded that the difference in retention of the two plutonium isotopes that had been observed earlier was caused almost entirely by the large difference in the mass of plutonium deposited in the wound, but that "radiolytic" effects of the more intense alpha activity of ^{238}Pu might be a factor in accelerating its clearance.

Figure A.3 displays the combined data from several studies of the retention at an i.m. wound site in rats and hamsters of $^{239}Pu^{4+}$ deposited at two low masses [0.011 µg (0.026 kBq) or 0.1 to 0.48 µg (0.26 to 1.1 kBq)] (Gray *et al.*, 1994; Harrison and David, 1977; 1978; Harrison *et al.*, 1977a; 1977b; 1978a; 1978b) and the combined data for two comparable masses of $^{238}Pu^{4+}$ [4×10^{-5} to 0.011 µg (0.026 to 7.3 kBq) or 0.05 to 0.23 µg (32 to 148 kBq)] (Gray *et al.*, 1994; Harrison *et al.*, 1977b; Lafuma *et al.*, 1971; Morin *et al.*,

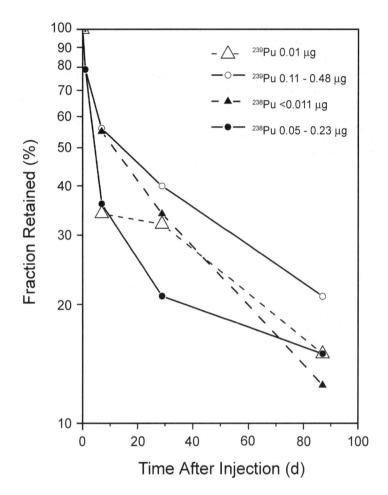

Fig. A.3. Comparison of the retention at an i.m.-injection site in rats of similar deposited masses of ^{238}Pu(NO$_3$)$_4$ and ^{239}Pu(NO$_3$)$_4$ administered in small volumes of HNO$_3$, pH 1 to 2: 0.01 µg ^{239}Pu (light dashed line); ≤0.011 µg ^{238}Pu^{4+} (dark dashed line); 0.11 to 0.48 µg ^{239}Pu (solid line); 0.05 to 0.23 µg ^{238}Pu (solid line). [Data from Gray *et al.* (1994), Harrison and David (1977; 1978), Harrison *et al.* (1977a; 1977b; 1978a; 1978b), Lafuma *et al.* (1971), Morin *et al.* (1972; 1973b), Nenot *et al.* (1972a; 1972b), and Stradling *et al.* (1993; 1995b).]

1972; 1973b; Nenot *et al.*, 1972a; 1972b; Stradling *et al.*, 1993; 1995b). Retention at the i.m. wound site is generally similar for the smaller masses of the two plutonium isotopes (≤0.011 µg), for which the activity is ≤7.3 kBq. However, when similar, but 10-fold greater masses of the plutonium isotopes are deposited, wound retention of

$^{239}Pu^{4+}$ is greater after the first day than that of $^{238}Pu^{4+}$. In the studies using the larger masses, the ^{238}Pu alpha activity was, on average, 130 times greater than that of ^{239}Pu, and the results support the view that the high specific alpha activity of ^{238}Pu contributes to its somewhat more efficient clearance from the wound site.

All of the individual data sets for wound retention of $^{238}Pu^{4+}$ and <5 µg of $^{239}Pu^{4+}$ i.m. injected in solutions of HNO_3 at pH 1 to 2 met the criteria for inclusion in the class of strongly-retained radionuclides (Table A.5).

Appendix B

Insoluble Radionuclides Deposited in Experimental Wounds: Sources and Data

Only a few studies provide the kinetic data needed to analyze wound retention (*e.g.*, serial measurements of the radionuclide content of the wound site, and/or of the major draining lymph nodes, tissues, blood, and excreta) of radionuclides implanted in wounds in forms that are insoluble (colloids, polymers, particles, contaminated microspheres, metallic fragments). Descriptions of the experiments and implanted sparingly soluble forms and summaries of the wound retention data are provided for each study.

B.1 Insoluble Forms of Plutonium

B.1.1 *Colloidal Plutonium in Puncture Wounds*

B.1.1.1 *$^{239}PuCl_4$ or $^{239}Pu(NO_3)_4$ Injected Intramuscularly in Rats.* In four studies ≥16 μg of $^{239}Pu^{4+}$ was i.m. injected in rats, as follows:

- 16 μg of $PuCl_4$ (37 kBq) in 1 mL of HCl, pH 2.5 (Scott *et al.*, 1948a);
- 16 μg of $Pu(NO_3)_4$ (37 kBq) in 0.5 mL of HNO_3, pH 1.5 (Morin *et al.*, 1972; 1973b);
- 25 μg of $Pu(NO_3)_4$ (58 kBq) in 0.1 mL of HNO_3, pH 1.5 (Lafuma *et al.*, 1971); and
- 240 μg of $Pu(NO_3)_4$ (555 kBq) in HNO_3, pH 1.5 (Nenot *et al.*, 1972a).

The wound retention data from those studies are collected in Table B.1 and plotted in Figure B.1.

203

TABLE B.1—*Retention at the wound site of i.m. or s.c. injections of hydrolyzed $^{239}Pu^{4+}$ in rats and rabbits at days after injection.*

Time (d)[a,b]	Fraction Retained at Wound Site (percent of injected amount) at Time t (days post-injection)									References
	1	4	6–8	14–16	28–32	50–64	90–112	256–280	365	
^{239}Pu mass (µg)										
Colloidal $^{239}Pu^{4+}$, i.m. in rats										
1.6×10^1		84, 96		95		75		74		Scott et al. (1948a)
1.6×10^1	98			98	90		74			Morin et al. (1972; 1973a)
2.5×10^1	95				90	72	65			Lafuma et al. (1971)
2.4×10^2	99		98	91	89, 91	77	74			Nenot et al. (1972a)
Colloidal $^{239}Pu^{4+}$, s.c. in Rats										
9.2×10^1	86, 88		85	85						McClanahan and Kornberg (1967)
Colloidal $^{239}Pu^{4+}$, i.m. in Rabbits[b,c]										
5.7×10^1	95		85		72	56	54			Taylor (1969)
1.05×10^2			92		93	66, 70	72	47	77	Taylor (1969)

[a]Time intervals shown accommodate data generated in the different experiments.
[b]Means of timed groups of rats; means of timed groups of rabbits for days 8 and 112, otherwise individual rabbits.
[c]Wound retention normalized to 100 % material recovery (text; Appendix B.1.4).

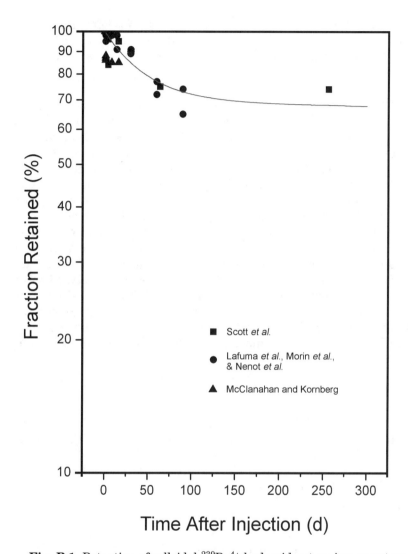

Fig. B.1. Retention of colloidal ^{239}Pu^{4+} hydroxide at an i.m. puncture wound site (% *ID*) in rats; data used in model development $R(t) = 31e^{-0.022t} + 69e^{-0.00008t}$. French studies: 16 µg ^{239}Pu(NO$_3$)$_4$ (Morin *et al.*, 1972; 1973a); 25 µg ^{239}Pu(NO$_3$)$_4$ (Lafuma *et al.*, 1971); 240 µg ^{239}Pu(NO$_3$)$_4$ (Nenot *et al.*, 1972a); and Scott *et al.* (1948a) 16 µg ^{239}PuCl$_4$. Shown for comparison: s.c. injection in rats of 92 µg ^{239}Pu(NO$_3$)$_4$ (McClanahan and Kornberg, 1967).

B.1.1.2 *^{239}Pu(NO$_3$)$_4$ Injected Subcutaneously in Rats.* Rats were s.c. injected with 92 µg of Pu(NO$_3$)$_4$ (210 kBq) in 0.1 mL of HNO$_3$, pH 2 (McClanahan and Kornberg, 1967). Wound retention data are given in Table B.1 and plotted in Figure B.1.

B.1.1.3 *Summary.* In each of the above studies the molar concentration and pH of the Pu^{4+} preparation indicate that the injected plutonium was probably a suspension of colloidal plutonium hydroxide. More acidic Pu^{4+} solutions and/or solutions containing smaller masses of Pu^{4+} ($\leq$5 µg) were classified as strongly retained at an i.m. wound site in rats. However, as might be expected, retention of the larger masses of colloidal plutonium hydroxide is more tenacious than that of the other tetravalent radionuclides (in solution at trace concentrations) that were classified as avidly retained.

The wound retention data of the timed groups from the four studies in rats of i.m. injection of a large mass of colloidal Pu^{4+} hydroxide (16 to 240 µg) in rats were combined and analyzed using the wound model (Section 4), assuming initial deposition into the soluble compartment, and nonlinear regression fitting with the Origin® software. The wound retention curve (% *ID*) shown in Figure B.1 is described in Equation B.1, where *t* is days after injection:

$$R(t) = 31e^{-0.022t} + 69e^{-0.00008t}. \tag{B.1}$$

B.1.1.4 *^{239}Pu(NO$_3$)$_4$ Injected Intramusculary in Rabbits.* Twelve adult rabbits were i.m. injected in an upper foreleg with a freshly prepared, neutralized solution of ^{239}Pu(NO$_3$)$_4$ (0.00083 or 0.0017 mol L^{-1}), which was almost certainly a colloidal suspension (Taylor, 1969). The rabbits were injected in two groups. One group received, on average, 57 µg of plutonium (130 kBq), and the other group received on average 105 µg of plutonium (240 kBq). The dosage for each rabbit was adjusted by injecting 0.1 mL of a plutonium preparation per kilogram of body weight. The rabbits were killed at post-injection intervals from 1 to 365 d. The report included radio-analytical results for the plutonium content of the injected leg, and of the liver, kidneys, spleen, lungs, testes, adrenals and whole skeleton (estimated from the plutonium concentrations of several bones).

The different injected volumes and the uncertainties inherent in delivering a precisely known amount of a colloidal suspension in a given volume suggest that satisfactory material balances would have been difficult to achieve. For example, the reported plutonium contents of the injected legs of two rabbits (one killed at 8 d, the other at 28 d) were >100 % of the amount injected, and the reported recoveries of plutonium (in injected leg plus measured tissues and skeleton) of four rabbits were >100 % of the injected amount.

However, information is available to refine the estimates of total plutonium recovery for each rabbit. The plutonium content of the unanalyzed soft tissues, assuming no significant uptake in local lymph nodes, is estimated to be 0.09 times the plutonium content of all measured soft tissues, based on complete distributions of plutonium and continuous collections of excreta for three adult rabbits i.v. injected with ^{237,238}Pu^{4+} citrate and killed at 100 d.[4] Data are also available for plutonium excretion by rabbits i.v. injected with ^{239}Pu(NO$_3$)$_4$ (periodic collections from 1 to 42 d; Finkle et al., 1947). Those data were used to estimate the small fractions of the plutonium absorbed from the i.m. wound that were excreted by each rabbit; estimated plutonium excretion ranged from 0.07 to 4.3 % of the injected plutonium at 1 and 280 d, respectively. A reasonable estimate was obtained for the plutonium recovery for each rabbit by summing the reported plutonium contents of its injected leg, skeleton, and measured soft tissues and the estimates of plutonium in the unmeasured soft tissues and cumulative excretion. The values shown in Table B.1 for retention of plutonium at an i.m. wound site in rabbits are the reported values normalized to 100 % material recovery (i.e., multiplied by the ratio of the recovered mass of plutonium to the injected mass).

The two-component exponential wound plutonium retention curve (% ID) shown in Figure B.2 was obtained by using the wound model with the assumption of initial deposition into the CIS compartment (Section 4) and fitting with Origin® software. The equation of the fitted curve, where t is days after injection, is:

$$R(t) = 44e^{-0.025t} + 56. \qquad \text{(B.2a)}$$

The long-term clearance rate of a large mass of colloidal Pu^{4+} from an i.m. wound site in the rabbits was not distinguishable from zero, and so was set to zero in Equation B.2. However, the terminal zero slope of the retention curve generated by the wound model for the rabbits may be an artifact created by the variable and somewhat uncertain plutonium dosage and the considerable variability in the retention patterns of the small number of rabbits, each of which contributed only one retention-time datum. Those data can be described equally well by sequential log-linear regression

[4]Durbin, P.W. and Jeung, N. (2003). Personal communication (Lawrence Berkeley National Laboratory, Berkeley, California).

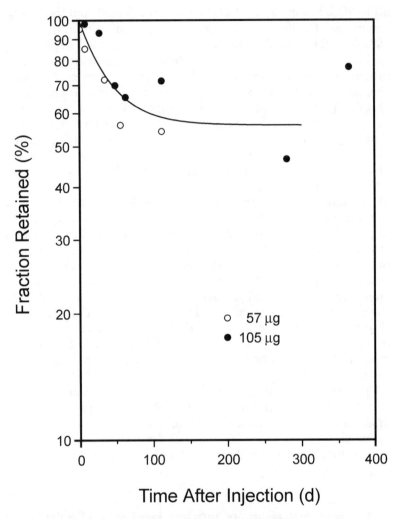

Fig. B.2. Retention of colloidal $^{239}Pu^{4+}$ nitrate at an i.m. wound site in rabbits (Equation B.2); 57 or 105 µg $^{239}Pu(NO_3)_4$ (Taylor, 1969).

analysis over three time intervals (0 to 1 d, 1 to 49 d, 35 to 365 d), which yields a three-component negative exponential equation with a defined early clearance component and a non-zero terminal slope:

$$R(t) = 5e^{-1.3t} + 31e^{-0.022t} + 64e^{-0.00012t}, \qquad \text{(B.2b)}$$

where t is days after injection. The parameters of the second and third components of Equation B.2.a are consistent with those of the two components of Equation B.1 that described retention of ≥16 μg of colloidal Pu^{4+} in an i.m. puncture wound in rats.

B.1.1.5 *"Polymeric-Plutonium" Injected Intramuscularly in Rats.* Rats were i.m. injected with 1.3 μg (3 kBq) of a prepared Pu^{4+} hydroxide polymer ("polymeric plutonium"; Lindenbaum and Westfall, 1965) to investigate tumor induction by local alpha irradiation (Brues *et al.*, 1965; 1966). Retention of the plutonium at the i.m. wound site was measured in a few rats killed at six months and in rats that died or were necropsied 1.5 to 2 y after the plutonium injection. The i.m.-injection sites contained ~80 % of the injected polymeric plutonium at six months and 38 to 75 % (midrange, 56 %) at 1.5 to 2 y. Those two somewhat uncertain data points, 80 and 56 % retention at 180 and 640 d, respectively, imply that 92 % of the injected 1.3 μg of polymeric plutonium was being cleared from the i.m. wound site at a rate of 0.0008 d^{-1}.

Male and female rats were i.m. injected in a thigh muscle with a $^{239}Pu^{4+}$ preparation designated "plutonium-citrate polymer" [6 to 7.2 μg, 14 to 17 kBq in 0.1 mL of saline, pH 6.5 (Bazhin *et al.*, 1984)]. Retention of plutonium at the wound site was measured from 4 h to 512 d to provide internal dosimetry for a study of local and systemic cancer induction. The results were reported only as ranges of five of six parameters of a three-component exponential equation, as follows: A_1 (20 to 21 %), A_2 (29.5 to 37.6 %), A_3 (41.7 to 44.4 %), λ_2 (6.0 to 6.5 × 10^{-3} d^{-1}), λ_3 (2.5 to 6 × 10^{-4} d^{-1}). An initial clearance rate, λ_1, was not defined, but the text implies that, similarly to soluble $Pu(NO_3)_4$ (Appendix A.1.4.1), the first component, A_1, was exhausted in 1 d. If A_1 were reduced to 1 % of its initial value in 1 d, λ_1, its rate constant, would be 4.6 d^{-1}. Retention of the polymeric plutonium at the wound site (% *ID*) can be reasonably estimated by assigning λ_1 = 4.6 d^{-1}, assigning the mid-range values to the other five parameters and normalizing total retention to 100 % at $t = 0$:

$$R(t) = 21e^{-4.6t} + 35e^{-0.0063t} + 44e^{-0.00042t}, \tag{B.3}$$

where t is days after injection.

The authors indicated that their polymeric plutonium was likely to have been a mixture of readily absorbed $^{239}Pu^{4+}$ citrate and tenaciously-retained polymerized $^{239}Pu(OH)_4$. If the fraction absorbed during the first day (~20 %) was the soluble plutonium citrate complex, the first term of Equation B.3 may be ignored, and only retention (% *ID*) of the sparingly soluble polymeric plutonium fraction (~80 %) considered. In that case, Equation B.3 is reduced to:

$$R(t) = 44e^{-0.0063t} + 56e^{-0.00042t}.$$ (B.4)

The rate of early loss from an i.m. wound site in rats of the smaller mass (6.6 µg) of polymeric plutonium is only one-fourth that of larger masses (≥16 µg) of colloidal Pu^{4+} injected in rats and rabbits, indicating the difficulty with which polymerized Pu^{4+} is solubilized and/or physically translocated (by macrophages) from a wound site. The final slow rate constant of the retention curve for 6.6 µg of polymeric plutonium i.m. injected in rats (Equations B.3 and B.4) is similar to those obtained for larger masses (≥16 µg) of colloidal Pu^{4+} i.m. injected in rats (Equation B.1) and rabbits (Equation B.2a), suggesting that biological responses at the wound site eventually dominate the clearance process, nearly independently of the mass of plutonium deposited or the history of the plutonium hydroxide polymer (injected as such or formed *in situ*).

B.1.1.6 *Colloidal* $^{239}Pu(NO_3)_4$ *Injected Subcutaneously in Dog Paws.* $^{239,240}Pu(NO_3)_4$ was s.c. injected just above the metacarpals of the left forepaw of male beagle dogs. Hereinafter this mixture of plutonium isotopes is designated simply as plutonium. The published numerical data and curve of plutonium retention at the wound site, based entirely on external photon measurements (*in vivo* counting), indicated rapid clearance, particularly in the first few days, with plutonium retention at 1, 30 and 365 d of 65, 53 and 18 % of the injected amount, respectively (Bistline, 1973; Bistline *et al.*, 1972; 1976; Lebel *et al.*, 1976). Retention of similar amounts of $Pu(NO_3)_4$ (16 to 25 µg in HNO_3 pH 1.5 to 2.5) at an i.m.-injection site in rats and rabbits, determined by radiochemical analysis of the dissected injection site, was, at the post-injection intervals noted above, on average, 96, 90 and 65 % of the amount injected, respectively (Table B.1; Figure B.2). The disparities are too great to be explained by species differences or structural and/or functional differences in the wounded tissues.

According to the *in vivo* measurements, the major draining lymph node [left superficial cervical lymph node (LSCLN)] contained ~25 % of the injected plutonium at 10 d and 7 % at 365 d. However, radiochemical analyses of the tissues of these dogs accounted for ≤2.1 % of the injected plutonium in the LSCLN and left axillary lymph nodes (LAXLN) at any time from 13 to 365 d (Table B.2; Bistline, 1973). Furthermore, only small fractions of Pu^{4+} in solutions that were i.m. injected in rats accumulated only transiently in the regional lymph nodes (Harrison *et al.*, 1978b).

TABLE B.2—*Distribution and excretion of s.c.-injected colloidal Pu^{4+} in dogs, based on radiochemical analysis of tissues and excreta.*[a,b]

Plutonium[d] Injected	Group 1 (13 d)	Group 2 (30 d)	Group 3 (59 d)	Group 4 (92 d)	Group 5 (185 d)	Group 6 (365 d)
	Percent of Injected Plutonium (mean ± SD)[c]					
	32 µg (73 kBq)	31 µg (71 kBq)	32 µg (74 kBq)	15 µg (34 kBq)	52 µg (118 kBq)	2.9 µg (6.6 kBq)
Liver	3.5 ± 3.0	2.7 ± 2.4	2.3 ± 1.8	3.6 ± 1.3	3.1 ± 3.2	9.2 ± 1.6
Spleen	0.18 ± 0.17	0.65 ± 0.64	0.11 ± 0.04	0.16 ± 0.03	0.16 ± 0.14	0.25
Kidneys	0.05 ± 0.04	0.06 ± 0.10	0.13 ± 0.09	0.12 ± 0.09	0.02 ± 0.02	0.03 ± 0.03
Blood volume	0.12 ± 0.06	0.14 ± 0.04	0.09 ± 0.05	0.04 ± 0.01	0.04 ± 0.03	0.06 ± 0.04
Soft tissues	0.49 ± 0.19	0.54 ± 0.32	0.71 ± 0.24	0.81 ± 0.12	1.4 ± 0.2	1.3 ± 0.17
Skeleton	3.9 ± 1.8	4.9 ± 2.6	8.5 ± 2.6	8.2 ± 1.6	19 ± 2.5	11 ± 2.3
Whole body	9.0 ± 5.3	9.0 ± 5.3	12 ± 4.0	13 ± 2.8	24 ± 3.7	22 ± 2.8
Lymph nodes	1.2 ± 1.0	2.1 ± 0.45	1.5 ± 1.1	1.3 ± 0.74	1.1 ± 0.59	0.12 ± 0.09
Excreta 0 – 13 d	3.2 ± 1.9	5.9 ± 4.2	6.7 ± 4.0	7.1 ± 5.4	9.3 ± 5.7	2.4 ± 2.2
Excreta ≥14 d		0.73	1.4	1.4	2.3	11
Recovered[e]	13 ± 2.0	18 ± 8.4	21 ± 7.1	23 ± 7.1	37 ± 8.4	35 ± 1.7
Injected paw[f]	87	82	79	77	63	65

[a]Plutonium (0.1 mL of 0.0012 mol L^{-1} Pu^{4+}) in 0.004 mol L^{-1} HNO$_3$ at pH 2.4, s.c. injected in left forepaw. Solubility calculations and dosing solution behavior indicate that these were colloidal suspensions of ^{239}Pu^{4+} hydrolysis products, except for Group 6, in which the smaller amount of plutonium (2.9 µg) may have been in solution when injected.
[b]Bistline, R.W. (2000). Personal communication (Abilene, Kansas).
[c]Four dogs per group. SD = [Σ dev^2 (n − 1)$^{-1}$]$^{1/2}$.
[d]Plutonium dosage [micrograms (kilobecquerel)] for each dog in each group based on contemporaneous assay of dosing solution.
[e]Sum of recovered plutonium in whole body, lymph nodes, and excreta.
[f]Retention of plutonium in injected paw is 100 % (injected dosage) minus injected plutonium recovered (percent).

B.1.1.6.1 *Reanalysis of plutonium retention at the wound site.* Reanalysis of the wound retention data from this study of s.c.-injected $Pu(NO_3)_4$ in the paws of dogs was prompted by disagreement with the reported retention of similar amounts of colloidal Pu^{4+} in puncture wounds in rats and rabbits and the internal disagreement between the results of the *in vivo* and radiochemical measurements of the plutonium content of the lymph nodes. The log books containing the serial *in vivo* counting data and the radiochemical analyses of plutonium in blood, urine and tissue specimens of the individual dogs were obtained from Bistline.[5] Material transmittal forms provided by the Rocky Flats Division of the Dow Chemical Company (Golden, Colorado) described the composition of the Pu^{4+} preparation as $^{239,240}Pu(NO_3)_4$ (0.001 mol L^{-1} Pu^{4+}) in 0.004 mol L^{-1} HNO_3, with a measured pH of 2.4. Under those conditions, the ion product $(Pu^{4+})(OH^{-4})$ exceeds K_{sp} for Pu^{4+} hydroxide, and the plutonium preparation injected was probably a colloidal suspension of Pu^{4+} hydroxide. Achievement of consistent dosing with a colloidal suspension is technically difficult, and the best estimate of the average plutonium dosage for the four dogs in each of the six timed groups was considered to be assay of the Pu^{4+} stock suspension made on the same day that each group was injected [range 2.9 to 52 µg (6.6 to 118 kBq) of plutonium, Table B.2].

Starting at 2 h after the Pu^{4+} implant, blood samples were drawn several times during 8 h, daily for the first week, three times during the second week, and starting on day 28, on three consecutive days every 30 d thereafter. Urine was collected on the same schedule, starting at 24 h. The six groups of four dogs each were killed at intervals from 13 to 365 d after the plutonium injection. The ^{239}Pu was determined radiochemically in the tissue samples taken at necropsy and in the blood and urine specimens. The injected paws were not analyzed.

The activity in the injected paws and LSCLN had been monitored *in vivo* with a wound counter on the same schedule as the blood sampling. The wound counter was a 5 cm diameter × 0.4 cm thick NaI(Tl) crystal with a thin beryllium window, set to detect 10 to 20 keV x rays, ~90 % of which were contributed by plutonium isotopes at the start of the study. "The detector was calibrated with a sample of the implant material with the proper ratio of uranium (plutonium daughters) and neptunium (^{241}Am daughter) L-shell x rays, and all counts were corrected for tissue absorption" (Bistline *et al.*, 1972). However, no injection phantoms were

---

[5]Bistline, R.W. (2000). Personal communication (Abilene, Kansas).

prepared, and no details of the method used to determine tissue absorption were published or stored with the collected experimental records.

B.1.1.6.2 *Estimation of* $^{239}Pu^{4+}$ *retention in the injected paws based on material recovery.* Retention of plutonium in the injected paws can be estimated as the difference between 100 % injected and the sum of the plutonium recovered in the radiochemically analyzed tissues at death and total plutonium excretion estimated from $t(0)$ to death. It was assumed that the radiochemical analyses of the plutonium in blood, urine and tissue specimens were accurate and that the contemporaneous assay of the plutonium dosing suspension for each timed group represented the best estimate of the average amount of plutonium injected into the paws of the four dogs in that group. The group designations, length of studies, and the plutonium dosages [micrograms (kilobecquerel)] are shown in Table B.2.

Tissue plutonium analysis, reported for 24 dogs, included LSCLN and LAXLN (shown combined in Table B.2), liver, spleen, kidneys, one femur, and several small tissues and glands (*e.g.*, eyes, testes). The plutonium content of the whole skeleton was taken as 31.6 times that in one femur (Atherton *et al.*, 1958). The plutonium in five major tissues (blood, liver, spleen, kidneys, whole skeleton) had been measured or could be calculated, and the plutonium in the unanalyzed bulk soft tissues of dogs (mainly muscle, pelt, GI tract, fat) was taken as 6 % of the plutonium in the five major tissues combined (Painter *et al.*, 1946; Stover *et al.*, 1959).

In this study, whole blood was sampled for convenience, although circulating plutonium is associated with plasma constituents (Stover *et al.*, 1959). The radiochemical analyses were reported as plutonium concentrations in whole blood (dpm mL^{-1}). The plutonium in the blood volume (% *ID*) was calculated using the body weight of each dog and the mean blood volume of dogs, 90 mL kg^{-1} (Altman and Katz, 1961):

$$\text{blood Pu} = 100 \, [\text{Pu in blood sample (dpm mL}^{-1})] \times \quad \text{(B.5)}$$
$$(90 \text{ mL blood kg}^{-1}) \, [\text{body weight (kg)}] \, [\text{Pu injected (dpm)}]^{-1}.$$

Urine specimens (24 h) were collected daily for the first 7 d, on days 8, 10 and 13, and on three consecutive days every 30 d thereafter, starting on day 28. Total urinary plutonium excretion was estimated for each dog by summing (1) the measured daily urinary plutonium from days one through six, (2) the calculated total urinary plutonium for days 7 to 13 [seven times the average measured urinary plutonium (dpm d^{-1}) in the interval], and (3) total urinary plutonium excretion in the interval 14 d to death, which was estimated by fitting all of the daily urinary plutonium data from day 13 to death for each dog to one or two exponential terms by log-linear regression analysis and integrating over the interval. Because no fecal samples were analyzed, total plutonium excretion was estimated as 3.1 times the total urinary plutonium excretion from $t(0)$ to 13 d, and 2.6 times total urinary plutonium excretion estimated from day 13 to death (Painter *et al.*, 1946; Stover *et al.*, 1959).

Retention of plutonium at the s.c. wound sites of the six groups of dogs shown in Table B.2 was calculated as 100 % injected minus the plutonium recovered in the tissues and the estimated plutonium excretion. Log-linear regression analysis of the four estimates of wound plutonium content obtained between 59 and 365 d suggested that 79 % of the deposited plutonium was released at a rate of 0.00066 d^{-1}, where t is days after injection.

Only small fractions of the plutonium translocated from the s.c. wound site were recovered in the regional lymph nodes at death. Lymph-node plutonium, which was greatest at 65 d (1.2 %), had declined to 0.12 % by 365 d. The small amounts of plutonium recovered in the lymph nodes of these dogs agree with the observations of Schallberger *et al.* (1976), who injected aliquots of the same colloidal Pu^{4+} hydroxide suspensions s.c. into dog paws and found that during the first 4 h after the injection nearly all of the plutonium entering the regional nodes (afferent lymph) was in the form of soluble complexes in the cellular fraction.

About 10 % of the injected plutonium was cleared from the wound to blood in the first hours to days after the s.c. injection of ≤15 μg of a colloidal suspension of Pu^{4+} (Table B.3). Nearly that same amount of plutonium, 12.5 %, could be accounted for in the analyzed tissues and excreta of the dogs killed at 13 d (Table B.2). During the year after the injection, continuous slow transfer from the wound site to blood supported a low blood level, a low level of plutonium excretion, and gradual accumulation of plutonium in all of the sampled tissues except lymph nodes and kidneys.

B.1.1.6.3 *Estimation of plutonium retention in injected paws by simulation modeling of serial blood plutonium data.* The large systematic collection of blood plutonium data, starting at 2 h after the plutonium implants, provided a way to examine that early phase of wound clearance and to obtain independent estimates of the fraction and clearance rate of the last identified component of wound retention. The study assumptions included the following: (1) the cellular fraction of whole blood can be regarded as a passive diluent, (2) a single fixed rate constant can be assigned to represent clearance of plutonium that has entered the circulation from the wound site to tissues and excretion (blood to systemic transfer rate in the wound model shown in Section 4.4.1), and (3) circulatory feedback of plutonium from tissues to blood was neglected.

The measured serial blood plutonium concentrations, expressed as dpm mL^{-1}, for each of the 24 dogs in this study were converted to plutonium in the blood volume by using Equation B.5. Blood plutonium, mean ± SD, was calculated for each of the six four-dog groups at each sampling time. The mean blood plutonium levels of the five groups of dogs injected with 15 to 52 µg of plutonium did not differ significantly from one another at any of the 15 sampling times for which there were data for three or more groups, and all of those data are shown in Table B.3. The mean blood plutonium for the four dogs in Group 6 (2.9 µg of plutonium injected, right-hand columns of Table B.3) was significantly greater than the means for the dogs that received ≥15 µg of plutonium at sampling times during the first 24 h after the plutonium injection. Thereafter, the blood plutonium levels appeared to be independent of the amount of plutonium injected.

In order to use the blood plutonium data to estimate retention at the wound site, a single rate was assigned to the plutonium clearance from blood to tissues and excretion following its transfer from the wound to the circulation. Clearance of $^{239}Pu^{4+}$, injected as a citrate complex, from the plasma volume of dogs during the first year after i.v. injection (% *ID*) is described by a five-component exponential equation, where t is days after injection:

$$\text{plasma } ^{239}\text{Pu} = 29e^{-150t} + 13e^{-5.3t}$$
$$+ 57e^{-0.9t} + 1.3e^{-0.1t} + 0.1e^{-0.004t}, \tag{B.6}$$

(Stevens and Bruenger, 1972; Stover *et al.*, 1959; 1962). The first term is assumed to represent intravascular mixing and escape of $^{239}Pu^{4+}$ citrate into extracellular fluid. The second and third terms appear to represent several processes, mainly plutonium deposition in the target tissues, its excretion, and its return from extracellular water as soluble ^{239}Pu citrate and/or transferrin complexes. The fourth and fifth terms are believed to represent plutonium recycle back into the circulation from the tissues.

Entry of plutonium into the circulation from a wound deposit is much slower than after an i.v. injection, thus the first term in Equation B.6 is not relevant, because the plutonium is transported away from the wound already mixed with lymph and tissue fluid (Schallberger, 1974; Schallberger *et al.*, 1976). Terms two and three

TABLE B.3—*Kinetics of plutonium in blood and urine of dogs s.c. injected in a forepaw with colloidal Pu(NO₃)₄ at pH 2.4.*[a]

Time After Injection (d)	Number of Dogs	Percent of Injected Plutonium			
		15 to 52 μg Plutonium (Groups 1–5)		2.9 μg Plutonium (Group 6)[b]	
		Blood Volume ± SD[c,d,e] (%)	Urine ± SD[d,e] (% d⁻¹)	Blood Volume ± SD[c,d] (%)	Urine ± SD[d,e] (% d⁻¹)
0.083	20	6.6 ± 1.7		23 ± 1.8[f]	
0.17	20	7.7 ± 1.9		20 ± 1.5[f]	
0.25	20			23 ± 1.7[f]	
0.33	20	7.4 ± 2.4		22 ± 1.8[f]	
1	20	5.1 ± 1.4	1.2 ± 1.1	11 ± 1.0[f]	0.46 ± 0.73
2	20	2.4 ± 1.2	0.21 ± 0.18	2.8 ± 1.5	0.087 ± 0.074
3	20	1.4 ± 0.5	0.15 ± 0.18	1.5 ± 0.9	0.064 ± 0.031
4	20	1.0 ± 0.5	0.12 ± 0.17	1.2 ± 0.7	0.062 ± 0.033
5	20	0.56 ± 0.3	0.035 ± 0.026	1.1 ± 0.4[f]	0.043 ± 0.019
6	20	0.49 ± 0.2	0.032 ± 0.026	0.43 ± 0.3	0.029 ± 0.011
8	20	0.31 ± 0.2	0.019 ± 0.012	0.46 ± 0.2	0.026 ± 0.015
10	20	0.25 ± 0.1	0.018 ± 0.009	0.21 ± 0.05	0.023 ± 0.011

13	20	0.24 ± 0.1	0.014 ± 0.011	0.28 ± 0.1	0.019 ± 0.012
29 – 31	16	0.16 ± 0.1	0.012 ± 0.008	0.20 ± 0.1	0.015 ± 0.009
55 – 65	12	0.089 ± 0.08	0.008 ± 0.003	0.096 ± 0.04	0.014 ± 0.004
85 – 95	8	0.074 ± 0.06	0.007 ± 0.003	0.059 ± 0.02	0.016 ± 0.015
120 – 130	4	0.11 ± 0.03	0.006 ± 0.002	0.077 ± 0.05	0.016 ± 0.007
155 – 165	4	0.09 ± 0.03	0.005 ± 0.002	0.079 ± 0.03	0.017
185 – 187	4	0.044 ± 0.03		0.012 ± 0.07	0.017 ± 0.005
219 – 221				0.038 ± 0.02	0.012 ± 0.005
248 – 250				0.051 ± 0.04	0.009 ± 0.003
276 – 278				0.053 ± 0.02	0.006 ± 0.002
304 – 306				0.062 ± 0.02	0.009 ± 0.002
336 – 338				0.067 ± 0.03	0.008 ± 0.005
365				0.056 ± 0.04	

[a] Serial blood and urine plutonium data for individual dogs were obtained from experimental records [Bistline, R. W. (2000) personal communication (Abilene, Kansas)].

[b] Data for group of four dogs injected with 2.9 μg of plutonium.

[c] Plutonium in blood volume (percent of injected amount) calculated by using Equation B.5.

[d] $SD = [\Sigma\ dev^2\ (n-1)^{-1}]^{1/2}$.

[e] Spaces are blank when no data were taken.

[f] Mean is significantly greater than corresponding mean for dogs injected with 15 to 52 μg of plutonium (t-test, $p \le 0.01$; Mack, 1967).

are not likely to be distinct. The last two terms were considered to contribute negligibly to the total amount of plutonium circulating, compared with the amount of plutonium, albeit small, continuously entering from the wound site. Neglect of circulatory feedback will underestimate wound retention. The rate constant of the third and dominant component of Equation B.6, 0.9 d^{-1} was assigned as the rate, blood to systemic, at which dog plasma is cleared of plutonium that has entered the circulation from a wound deposit.

The wound model (Section 4) was implemented by using as input the combined blood plutonium data sets from the dogs of Groups 1 through 5 (15 to 52 μg of plutonium) and separately for the four dogs of Group 6 (2.9 μg of plutonium). It was assumed in both cases that the plutonium was initially deposited in the soluble compartment and that the rate of exit from the blood to systemic was 0.9 d^{-1}. The three-component exponential equations of the two wound retention curves generated by the model (% ID) (Figure B.3) were obtained by nonlinear regression fitting software (Origin®) where t is days after injection:

$$R(t) \ (\geq 15 \ \mu g \ Pu) = 11e^{-9.0t} + 6.5e^{-0.048t} + 82e^{-0.00077t}, \qquad (B.7)$$

$$R(t)(2.9 \ \mu g \ Pu) = 23e^{-26t} + 8e^{-0.05t} + 69e^{-0.00076t}. \qquad (B.8)$$

The simulation model calculation of wound retention was repeated, using as input the combined blood plutonium data for the five groups of dogs given ≥15 μg of plutonium (Table B.3) and the estimates of wound plutonium retention and lymph-node plutonium content for all six groups of dogs (Table B.2). The overall fits to those three data sets are plotted against the model-generated curves in Figure B.4. The three-component exponential equation of the wound retention curve (% ID) based on the combined blood, wound site, and lymph-node data sets was obtained by using the wound model (Section 4) and fitting of the predicted kinetics curve (Origin® software), where t is days after injection:

$$R(t) = 15e^{-3.1t} + 7.8e^{-0.056t} + 77e^{-0.00073t}. \qquad (B.9)$$

The shapes of the two retention curves are generally similar, as are the structures of their respective equations, except that some of the smaller mass of plutonium (2.9 μg), which may have been in solution when injected, was initially cleared more efficiently from the s.c. wound site to blood.

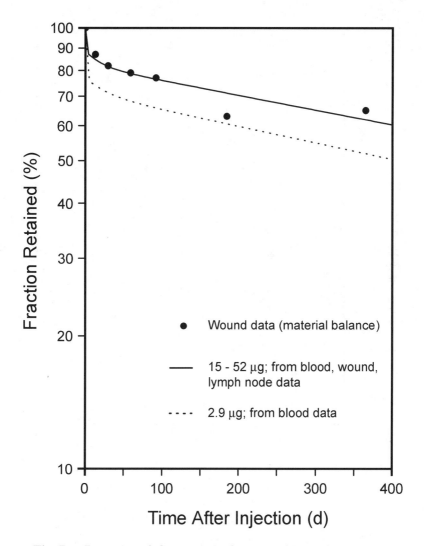

Fig. B.3. Retention of plutonium in the paws of dogs after s.c. injection of colloidal Pu^{4+} hydroxide. Data points for wound plutonium were estimated from analysis of material recovery (Table B.2). The upper curve was obtained by simulation modeling of serial blood plutonium data from 20 dogs injected with ≥15 μg of plutonium (Table B.3; Equation B.7). The lower curve was obtained by simulation modeling of the blood plutonium data from four dogs injected with 2.9 μg of plutonium (Table B.3; Equation B.8).

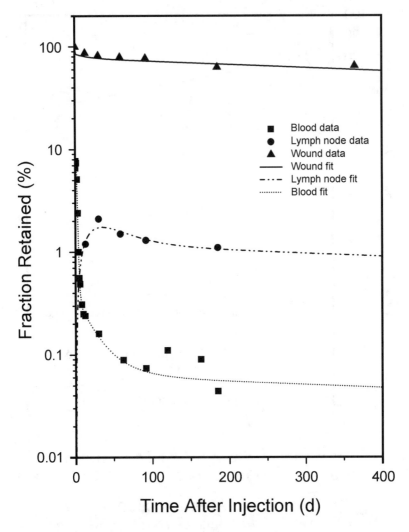

Fig. B.4. Estimated plutonium content of s.c. wound site, lymph nodes, and blood volume generated by the wound retention model (Section 4). Input data points shown are mean blood plutonium values for 20 dogs s.c. injected in a paw with of ≥ 15 μg of a colloidal suspension of Pu^{4+} [$Pu(NO_3)_4$ at pH 2.4] (Table B.3), and the estimated wound plutonium retention and lymph-node plutonium content obtained from calculation of material recoveries of plutonium in 24 dogs injected with ≥ 2.9 μg of $Pu(NO_3)_4$ at pH 2.4 (Table B.2).

B.1.1.6.4 *Late retention of plutonium in the injected paws.* Three methods were used to reexamine the radioanalytical data from Bistline's (1973) study of s.c.-injected colloidal Pu^{4+} in dogs. Two methods, based on material recovery and on simulation modeling of the blood plutonium data, yielded essentially the same result for retention of deposits ≥15 μg of plutonium at the s.c. wound site. A fraction of the injected plutonium, ~13 %, was cleared from the s.c. wound site to blood, tissues and excretion within a few hours. A smaller fraction, ~7 %, was transported away from the wound site in ~60 d. The major fraction, ~80 %, was cleared with a half-time, on average, of ~1,000 d.

A study of the late effects of colloidal Pu^{4+} [$Pu(NO_3)_4$, pH 2.4] s.c. injected in the paws of eight dogs included radiochemical analysis of the injected paws, regional lymph nodes, skeleton, liver, and spleen (Dagle *et al.*, 1984). The reported amount of plutonium injected was 20 ± 10 μg. At 5 y, the injected paws and the analyzed tissues were reported to contain 15.9 and 14 %, respectively, of the injected plutonium. Based on the studies of i.v.-injected monomeric Pu^{4+} citrate in dogs, Equation C.2, which describes urinary plutonium excretion of the dogs s.c. injected with ≥15 μg of colloidal Pu^{4+} hydroxide from 10 to 185 d, may be assumed to continue describing urinary plutonium excretion for 5 y, and the fecal to urinary plutonium excretion ratio of 2.6 may be assumed not to change in that interval (Stover *et al.*, 1959; 1962). Plutonium excretion in 5 y can be estimated as the sum of the amount calculated for 1 to 365 d (13.4 %, from Table B.2) plus the amount predicted from 365 d to 5 y obtained by integration of Equation C.2, that is, 4.2 % of plutonium excreted in the urine and ~15 % total plutonium excretion. Total plutonium excretion in 5 y is estimated to be ~28 % of the amount injected. Thus, at 5 y ~58 % of the plutonium reported to have been injected (16 % in the injected paws, 14 % in the analyzed tissues, 28 % excreted) can be accounted for. However, the inability to account for as much as 40 % of the injected plutonium suggests that the plutonium dosage may have been less than that reported by Dagle *et al.* (1984).

Injection data for those eight dogs (identified by colony number) were included with the records of the studies of $PuNO_3$ in dogs provided by Bistline.[6] The last group of dogs in Bistline's (1973) study was injected in July of 1970, 17 months before the injection of the eight long-term dogs reported by Dagle *et al.* (1984), and there is no record of receipt of a new $Pu(NO_3)_4$ shipment.[6] Therefore, it is

[6]Bistline, R.W. (2000). Personal communication (Abilene, Kansas).

reasonable to assume that the plutonium injected into the dogs studied by Dagle *et al.* (1984) was drawn from the same stock source as the $Pu(NO_3)_4$ used in Bistline's (1973) studies. That hydrolyzed plutonium preparation (0.001 mol L^{-1} Pu^{4+}, pH 2.4) would, on long standing, have tended to sorb progressively onto the walls of the containers, reducing the amount left in solution/suspension and making reproducible dosing difficult. The initial, $t(0)$, external measurements of the plutonium in those dogs indicated an average plutonium dosage of 9.9 ± 4.8 µg (22.6 ± 11 kBq), about one-half of that reported by Dagle *et al.* (1984).

If a smaller amount of plutonium, as little as 9.9 µg, had been injected, the fraction of plutonium in the injected paw, and the analyzed tissues at 5 y would have been 31 ± 12 and 28 ± 4.6 % of the injected amount, respectively, and whole-body plutonium retention would be ~59 % of the injected amount. If 28 % of the injected plutonium had been excreted in 5 y (see above) nearly 90 % of the injected plutonium could be accounted for.

Equation B.9 predicts that 77 % of colloidal Pu^{4+} s.c. injected in the dog paw was cleared at a rate of 0.00073 d^{-1}. Long-term clearance rates, based on 77 % associated with the slowest-clearing compartments are 0.0009 d^{-1} for the reported wound plutonium retention of 15.9 % at 5 y and 0.0005 d^{-1} for an estimated wound plutonium retention of 31 % at 5 y. The midrange value of those two "bounding" estimates of λ_3 agrees well with the slowest wound plutonium clearance rate obtained from modeling the combined wound, lymph-node, and blood plutonium data from the dogs s.c. injected in a paw with ≥2.9 µg of colloidal Pu^{4+} hydroxide and followed for as long as 365 d (Tables B.2 and B.3).

B.1.2 *Very Small Particles of $^{239}PuO_2$ Injected Intramuscularly in Rats*

Minute particles of $^{239}PuO_2$ (1 nm diameter) were i.m. injected in rats (0.01 µg of ^{239}Pu in ≤0.05 mL of water) (Harrison *et al.*, 1978b). Retention at the wound site, translocation to local lymph nodes and tissues, and excretion were measured at 7 and 28 d. Retention of the injected ^{239}Pu at the wound site was 27 and 17 % at 7 and 28 d, respectively, about the same as that of 0.011 µg of $^{239}Pu(NO_3)_4$ in solution (Table A.2). In addition to dissolution, clearance from the wound site of the ^{239}Pu injected as tiny oxide particles included translocation of presumably intact particles that were small enough to pass through the glomerular filter (Smith *et al.*, 1977).

Tissue distribution of the translocated [239]Pu similar to that of i.m.-injected [239]Pu(NO$_3$)$_4$ and a lack of accumulation of the [239]Pu in the local lymph nodes are good evidence for the solubility and filterability of these minute particles.

B.1.3 Air-Oxidized [239,240]PuO$_2$ Particles Implanted Subcutaneously in Dog Paws

Aqueous suspensions of PuO$_2$ particles were s.c. implanted in the paws of dogs to determine plutonium translocation from the wound site, localization of the transported fraction in the regional lymph nodes and other tissues and excretion from the body, and the effect of CaNa$_3$-DTPA therapy on plutonium clearance from the wound site and the tissues. The properties of the air-oxidized PuO$_2$ particles were as follows: ~98 % [239,240]Pu by weight, 2,200 ppm [241]Am, estimated to be 7 μm geometric median diameter (79 % of particles <25 μm in diameter). The dry PuO$_2$ powder (1 mg per vial) was suspended in water and shaken, and aliquots of "~0.25 mL" were withdrawn with a needle and syringe and delivered into the s.c. tissue above the metacarpals of the left forepaw of 40 male beagle dogs (Johnson, 1969; Johnson *et al.*, 1970a; 1970b; 1972).

Twenty of the dogs were treated with CaNa$_3$-DTPA by i.v. injection (25 mg kg^{-1}) on 10 d during the first two weeks starting 2 h after the PuO$_2$ implant and on three consecutive days every 30 d thereafter, starting 30 d after the implant. Blood samples were drawn and urine samples (24 h) were collected from all dogs on the same schedule as the CaNa$_3$-DTPA treatments. A few fecal samples were collected and analyzed during the first 60 d. The activity in the injected paw and the first major draining lymph node (LSCLN) was monitored by *in vivo* counting with a 3.8 cm × 1.5 mm NaI(Tl) crystal detector, and all photons with energies ≥10 keV were recorded. The schedule of *in vivo* counting was the same as that for collection of blood and excreta and CaNa$_3$-DTPA treatments.

Pairs of CaNa$_3$-DTPA-treated and untreated dogs were killed at intervals from 14 to 364 d after implant, and tissue specimens were taken for radiochemical analysis of plutonium and americium. The analyzed samples included blood, urine, feces, the injected paw, the LSCLN and the LAXLN, liver, kidneys, spleen, several small tissues, one femur, and several other bone samples. Nearly half of the injected paws were lost during chemical digestion.

The dense PuO$_2$ particles settled rapidly, and the amount implanted in each dog could not be controlled. A whole-body *in vivo* measurement of the 60 keV gamma rays of the [241]Am daughter at

8 to 10 d after the implant was used to estimate the implant dosage for each dog. The average plutonium implant was stated in several publications to be from 73 to 94 μg (166 to 215 kBq) with relative standard deviations of ~50 %. In addition to the difficulties encountered in implanting known amounts of plutonium, there were technical difficulties with the *in vivo* measurements of both the wound site and the LSCLN. The detected photons included both the weakly penetrating uranium L-shell x rays (13 to 22 keV) emitted following the alpha decay of the plutonium isotopes and the penetrating gamma rays (60 keV) of [241]Am. Formation and destruction of scar tissue and nodules also changed the structure of the wound site, adding to the uncertainty in detection of the x rays.

In spite of those handicaps, some practical conclusions were drawn by normalizing the *in vivo* measurements at the wound site and LSCLN for each dog to its value at 60 and 120 d, respectively, and by presenting the radiochemical data for plutonium and americium as plutonium/americium ratios for individual excreta and tissue samples of individual dogs. Neither of those procedures required knowledge of the absolute amounts of PuO_2 or americium implanted. Translocation to the major local lymph nodes (LSCLN and LAXLN) of the plutonium implanted as insoluble PuO_2 particles was substantial. Only small amounts of plutonium or americium accumulated in other tissues or were excreted during the year of observation, implying that little of the plutonium or its accompanying [241]Am was solubilized and that both nuclides were translocated together to and trapped within the local lymph nodes as particles. The $CaNa_3$-DTPA regimen did not significantly change the retention of either the plutonium or americium at the wound site or in the LSCLN, compared with the untreated dogs, but it significantly enhanced the excretion of americium.

B.1.3.1 *Reanalysis of Plutonium Distribution and Excretion.* The detailed radioanalytical data for plutonium in the blood, tissues and excreta of the individual dogs were reported in the appendices of Johnson's (1969) thesis. Those data can be used to estimate retention of the insoluble air-oxidized PuO_2 particles s.c. implanted in the paws of the dogs and the distribution and excretion of the plutonium translocated from the wound site. The plutonium recovery for each dog was assumed to be the sum of the measured plutonium in the injected paw, regional lymph nodes (LSCLN and LAXLN), bones, tissues, and the calculated total plutonium excretion from injection to death. The radiochemical analyses of the air-oxidized PuO_2 in the tissue and excreta samples were considered to have been accurate.

Complete plutonium analyses were reported for 19 dogs, specifically, the plutonium in the injected paw, major draining lymph nodes, liver, one femur, spleen, kidneys, some small soft tissues, blood, urine, and a few feces samples. The americium, but not the plutonium, content of the injected paw was reported for three dogs with otherwise complete plutonium analyses. The plutonium in the paws of these dogs was estimated from their americium content and the mean ratio of the alpha activities of the other 19 fully analyzed paws. The LSCLN of one dog was taken for histopathology, and the plutonium in that tissue was estimated from the smooth curve of all LSCLN values.

The plutonium concentration in liver (dpm g^{-1}) was reported for all 22 dogs included in this data reanalysis, and total plutonium in liver was calculated as total liver weight (grams) times the measured plutonium concentration. Liver weights of two dogs were estimated from the mean weight of the other 20 dogs (383 ± 92 g). The plutonium content of one femur was available for all 22 dogs, and total skeleton plutonium was taken as 31.6 times the plutonium content of one femur (Atherton *et al.*, 1958). The plutonium in the unanalyzed bulk soft tissue was taken as 6 % of that in the liver, skeleton and spleen combined (Painter *et al.*, 1946; Stover *et al.*, 1959).

Total urinary plutonium excretion of each untreated dog was estimated by summing: (1) the measured daily urinary plutonium from 1 through 7 d; (2) urinary plutonium in the interval from 8 to 30 d, estimated from the mean of the measured plutonium in samples taken in that interval times the 22 d in the interval; and (3) total urinary plutonium from 30 d to death, estimated by fitting all of the daily plutonium urine data to one exponential, $Ae^{-\lambda t}$, by log-linear regression analysis and integrating over the interval. There was too much scatter in the data to justify use of more than one exponential term. For the eight untreated dogs, was on average 7×10^{-3} d^{-1}.

Estimation of total urinary plutonium excretion of the DTPA-treated dogs required some additional assumptions. Urinary plutonium excretion remains elevated above the undisturbed level for several days after a CaNa$_3$-DTPA injection (Volf, 1978). Urinary plutonium during the 8 to 30 d after the implant was estimated as the mean of the three lowest daily plutonium urine values times the 22 d in the interval plus the sum of the higher values, corrected for the baseline rate. Johnson (1969) noted that urinary plutonium was lowest on the first day of each 3 d monthly excreta collection and CaNa$_3$-DTPA treatment sequence. For eight CaNa$_3$-DTPA-treated dogs that exhibited a well defined decline in urinary plutonium excretion rate from 30 d to death, the first day value of each treatment and collection sequence was fitted by log-linear regression analysis to one exponential term, which was integrated over the interval, yielding an "undisturbed" subtotal of urinary plutonium excretion after 30 d. Total late urinary plutonium excretion was estimated by adding to that subtotal the sum of all of the urinary plutonium values for the second and third days under $CaNa_3$-DTPA treatment, corrected for the baseline level. There was no apparent decline in the late urinary plutonium excretion baseline rates of three $CaNa_3$-DTPA-treated dogs. For these dogs, total urinary plutonium excretion from 30 d to death was estimated as the mean of all its urinary plutonium values for the first day of each collection sequence times the number of days from 30 d to death plus the sum of all the corrected plutonium values for the second and third collection days.

Most of the fecal samples that were analyzed for plutonium were collected in the first 30 d after injection. The fecal to urinary excretion ratio (FU^{-1}) was independent of post-implant time for both $CaNa_3$-DTPA-treated and untreated dogs. The mean value of FU^{-1} for untreated dogs was 2.5 (65 same-day collections from individual dogs). Chelation therapy with $CaNa_3$-DTPA promoted mainly urinary plutonium excretion (Volf, 1978), and that was reflected in a plutonium FU^{-1} ratio of 0.56 for the $CaNa_3$-DTPA-treated dogs (66 same-day collections from individual dogs). Total plutonium excretion by untreated dogs was estimated to be 3.5 times the total urinary plutonium excretion and that for the $CaNa_3$-DTPA-treated dogs to be 1.6 times their total urinary plutonium excretion.

B.1.3.2 *Estimation of Plutonium Retention at the Subcutaneous Wound Site.* Radiochemical analysis of plutonium and/or americium in the injected paws was reported for the 22 dogs listed in Table B.4. Based on the calculated plutonium recoveries for those dogs (sum of measured plutonium in injected paw, analyzed tissues, and calculated total excretion from injection to death), the mean amount of plutonium implanted in these 22 dogs was $1.3 \times 10^7 \pm 1.6 \times 10^7$ dpm [94 ± 116 µg (216 ± 263 kBq)], in agreement with the revised PuO_2 implant dosage reported by Johnson *et al.* (1972). The reanalyzed tissue distribution and excretion data, expressed as percent of recovered plutonium, are shown in Table B.4 for eight untreated dogs and 14 $CaNa_3$-DTPA-treated dogs with data sets suitable for inclusion in this reanalysis.

During the year after implantation of the air-oxidized PuO_2 particles, the preponderance of the implanted plutonium remained at the s.c. wound site in the paw. Clearance was inefficient and slow. The recalculated data for plutonium retention in the injected paw and the accumulation of plutonium in the regional lymph nodes, expressed as percent of recovered plutonium, are plotted in Figure B.5. The reanalysis verified Johnson's (1969) original conclusions that there were no discernible effects of the CaNa$_3$-DTPA treatments on retention of plutonium in the wound or on its translocation into and/or away from the regional lymph nodes. The three data sets, the estimated wound site, lymph node, and systemic plutonium (plutonium in tissues and excreta) for the 22 individual dogs (Table B.4) were fitted simultaneously using the wound model with initial deposition into the PABS compartment (Section 4). The model generated the curves shown in Figure B.5 for clearance of plutonium from the wound site and accumulation of plutonium in the local lymph-nodes and systemic compartments. The equation of the curve for plutonium retention at the wound site is, where t is days after injection:

$$R(t) = 8.5e^{-0.05t} + 91.5e^{-0.0003t} \text{ % of recovered amount.} \qquad \text{(B.10)}$$

B.1.3.3 *Translocation of Plutonium from the Subcutaneous Wound Site.* Nearly all of the plutonium translocated from the s.c. wound site was trapped in the regional lymph nodes (Figure B.5). The equation that describes plutonium accumulation in the local lymph nodes (*LN*) is, where t is days after injection:

$$LN(t) = 17.7(1 - e^{-0.0076t}) \text{ % of recovered amount.} \qquad \text{(B.11)}$$

During the first 30 d, transport of plutonium away from the wound site and/or local lymph nodes to other tissues and excretion accounted for <0.5 % of the recovered plutonium, and during the first year after the implant only ~1.5 % of the recovered plutonium was in tissues other than lymph nodes or had been excreted. The equation that describes plutonium translocation to tissues and excretion [systemic (*Sys*)] is, where t is days after injection:

$$Sys(t) = 2.1(1 - e^{-0.0056t}) \text{ % of recovered amount.} \qquad \text{(B.12)}$$

B.1.3.4 *Long-Term Retention and Distribution of PuO$_2$ Particles.* Ten dogs were given s.c. implants of air-oxidized PuO$_2$ particles (79 % < 25 μm diameter) and held for long-term clinical observation

TABLE B.4—*Distribution of recovered plutonium in dogs s.c. implanted with 7 μm air-oxidized PuO₂ particles.*[a]

Time After Implant (d)	Dog	Plutonium Recovered (10^6 dpm)	Fraction of Recovered Plutonium (%)[b]						
			Paw	LSCLN	LAXLN	Liver	Skeleton	Other Tissues	Excreta
			Untreated						
15	1991	7.3	92	4.4	2.9	0.01	0.10	0.02	0.09
120	1633	19	96	3.8	<0.001	0.15	0.11	0.003	0.14
139	1353	3.3	84	15	<0.001	0.094	0.46	0.007	0.85
150	0925	14	97	3.0	<0.001	0.14	0.09	0.007	0.15
270	1367	9.0	88	(11)[c]	0.034	0.85	0.13	0.009	0.51
	0792	4.8	77	22	—	0.89	0.16	0.029	0.71
360	1688	1.8	62	37	0.001	0.059	0.19	0.024	1.2
	1689	3.3	95	4.5	<0.001	0.046	0.23	0.014	0.66
			DTPA-Treated						
15	2179	8.0	99	1.2	—	0.011	0.068	0.002	0.14

30	2666	28	92	8.0	0.003	0.011	0.087	0.003	0.38
60	1403	17	83	17	0.001	0.014	0.12	0.004	0.23
90	2894	19	93	6.6	0.012	0.054	0.10	0.037	0.44
120	1008	2.0	86	12	0.001	0.50	0.35	0.02	1.8
	1696	12	90	9.3	<0.001	0.093	0.18	0.004	0.32
150	1429	13	92	7.2	0.003	0.088	0.15	0.017	0.37
	2963	71	95	2.8	<0.001	2.4	0.03	0.007	0.10
180	2761	(6.3)[d]	80	12	6.9	0.33	0.18	0.024	0.55
	1990	(9.2)[c]	89	8.6	0.65	0.44	0.22	0.067	0.57
210	2100	(5.4)[c]	73	26	<0.001	0.45	0.12	0.006	0.74
	1803	6.5	91	8.4	<0.001	0.084	0.19	0.002	0.79
270	2447	4.1	88	11	<0.001	0.20	0.15	0.038	1.4
360	2315	3.0	84	15	0.04	0.14	0.31	0.018	1.3

[a] Reanalyzed data from Appendix Tables B2, B3 and B4 of Johnson (1969).
[b] See text for explanation of calculations used to estimate total liver plutonium, total skeleton plutonium, and total plutonium excretion.
[c] See text for explanation of calculations used to estimate these four missing plutonium radioanalyses.

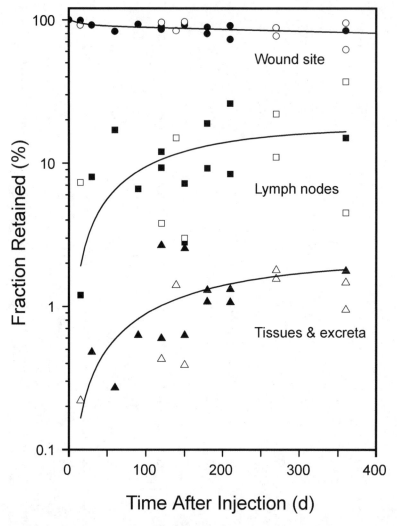

Fig. B.5. Retention of plutonium at the s.c. wound site in the paws of dogs after implantation of an aqueous suspension of air-oxidized PuO_2 particles (7 μm GMD), plutonium accumulation in the regional lymph nodes, and transfer of plutonium to tissues and excreta (systemic) (data of Johnson, 1969). (closed symbols) dogs treated with $CaNa_3$-DTPA; (open symbols) dogs not treated with chelator; (circles) plutonium retention at the s.c. wound site; (squares) plutonium accumulation in regional lymph nodes; (triangles) plutonium accumulation in tissues (mainly liver and bone) and excreted. From top to bottom, the solid curves correspond to Equation B.10 for the wound site, Equation B.11 for the lymph nodes, and Equation B.12 for tissues and excreta, respectively.

(Dagle *et al.*, 1984). The date of the implants, the source and size of the PuO_2 particles, and the methods of preparing and injecting the aqueous particle suspensions, combined, indicate that these air-oxidized PuO_2 particles were from the same batch used by Johnson (1969). The reported amount of plutonium deposited was 153 ± 7 µg (350 ± 16 kBq). The method used to determine the dosage given to each dog was not described, but the same difficulties discussed in Appendix B.1.3 would have been encountered in delivering an accurately known amount of PuO_2 to each dog.

Retention of plutonium at 8 y post-implant in the injected paws and the distribution at death of plutonium in the regional lymph nodes, liver, spleen, and skeleton of nine of those dogs (one dog died of pneumonia 1 y after the PuO_2 implant) were reported. The average amount of plutonium retained in the injected paws 8 y after implant was 32 ± 18 µg (33.5 to 166 kBq, 20.9 ± 11.4 %) of the reported amount injected. Radiochemical analysis of the plutonium in the paws and other tissues is considered to have been reliable (Keough and Powers, 1970), and dissolution of the air-oxidized PuO_2 is assumed to have been complete. However, there is no mention of correction of the reported amounts of plutonium in the paws or lymph nodes for tissue (and its plutonium) removed for histopathology. Without those corrections, the total amounts of plutonium in those important specimens could have been seriously underestimated. The reanalyzed data of Johnson (1969) for 22 dogs given s.c. implants of similar air-oxidized PuO_2 particles and killed from 15 to 360 d, predict that at 8 y the wound site would contain at least 37 % of the amount of plutonium implanted (Equation B.10).

The mean plutonium content of the regional lymph nodes at 8 y, 6.5 ± 5.8 % of the reported implant dosage, is about one-half of that estimated to have accumulated in those lymph nodes during the first year after the PuO_2 implant (Table B.4 and Figure B.5). The plutonium in liver, spleen and skeleton at 8 y was reported to be 4.8, 0.18, and 1.0 % of the implant dosage, respectively. Those tissue plutonium levels are substantially greater than were estimated at 360 d from recalculation of Johnson's (1969) data (Table B.4). Such a time-dependent increase in tissue plutonium may be regarded as evidence of continuous, albeit slow, transport away from the wound site and regional lymph nodes.

If Equation 4.6, which describes urinary plutonium excretion of untreated dogs in Johnson's (1969) study from 1 to 360 d, continues to describe urinary plutonium excretion for 8 y, plutonium excretion in urine for the interval 1 to 8 y is predicted by integration to be ~1 % of the implanted plutonium, and urinary plus fecal plutonium excretion would be ~3.5 %. The sum of the estimated plutonium excretion from 1 to 365 d (~1 %, Table B.4) and that for the interval 1 to 8 y (~3.5 %) predicts a total excretion in 8 y of ~4.5 % of the implanted amount.

The total recovery of plutonium in the analyzed tissues, was, on average, 33 % of the reported implant dosage, and 4.5 % can be accounted for by excretion, for a total plutonium recovery of ~37.5 %. There is no evidence from investigations in animals or humans of the distribution and elimination of various plutonium preparations (ranging in initial solubility from soluble Pu^{4+} injected as the citrate complex to inhaled highly insoluble PuO_2) for sequestration over long times of more than a minor fraction (5 to 10 %) of the systemic plutonium burden in tissues other than the portal of entry, local lymph nodes, liver, spleen, and skeleton (ICRP, 1986). It is reasonable to conclude that the amount of PuO_2 actually implanted in the dog paws was less than was reported.

The best estimate of the average dosage of plutonium s.c. implanted as air-oxidized PuO_2 particles in the paws of 22 of the dogs in Johnson's (1969) study of the kinetics of s.c.-implanted PuO_2 is 94 ± 116 µg of plutonium (Appendix B.1.3.2, Table B.4). As noted above, the source and injected volumes of the air-oxidized PuO_2 particles s.c. implanted in the paws of the dogs kept for long-term clinical observation were likely to have been the same as those described by Johnson (1969). If the plutonium dosages implanted in both studies were, on average, 94 ± 166 µg, a revised estimate of plutonium recovery would be 61 %. Distribution of the recovered plutonium would be as follows: injected paw, 36.4 %; lymph nodes, 10.8 %; liver, 8.3 %; skeleton, 1.7 %; spleen, 0.3 %, estimated total excretion, 4.5 %. Equation B.10 predicts that 91.5 % of plutonium s.c. implanted in the dog paw as air-oxidized PuO_2 particles (7 µm GMD) will be cleared at a rate of 0.00031 d^{-1}. Long-term clearance rates based on 91.5 % in the slowest-clearing compartment at $t(0)$ would be 0.0005 and 0.00032 d^{-1}, respectively, for the reported wound plutonium retention of 20.9 % at 8 y and the estimated wound plutonium retention of 36.4 % at 8 y. The latter estimate of λ_3 agrees with the slowest wound plutonium clearance rate obtained from simultaneous modeling of the wound, lymph node and systemic plutonium data from the 22 dogs given air-oxidized PuO_2 particle implants and followed for 365 d (Equation B.10).

B.1.4 *High-Fired $^{239,240}PuO_2$ Particles Implanted Subcutaneously in Dog Paws*

The properties of the PuO_2 particles were as follows: 99.6 % ^{239,240}Pu by weight; 360 ppm ^{241}Am; 0.7 µm GMD (68 % of particles

<1 μm diameter); heat treated (850 °C, 100 h). The dry PuO_2 powder (~1 mg per vial) was suspended in 1 mL of physiological saline with vigorous shaking, and 0.25 mL portions were withdrawn with a needle and syringe and injected into the subcutis about the metacarpals of the left forepaw of 45 male beagle dogs (Bistline, 1973; Bistline et al., 1972; 1976; Lebel et al., 1976). The amount of plutonium implanted in the paw of each dog was reported to be 323 μg (740 kBq) (Bistline et al., 1972). That reported dosage is 30 % greater than would have been delivered (250 μg), if the 1 mg of PuO_2 in each vial had been uniformly and stably dispersed in 1 mL of water. These small dense particles settle fairly rapidly, so it is likely that the amounts implanted were actually <250 μg.

Twenty-three of the 45 dogs were treated with $CaNa_3$-DTPA (25 mg kg^{-1}) on 10 occasions during the first two weeks, starting at 2 h after the implant and immediately after drawing the blood samples on three consecutive days starting at 30 d, and every 30 d thereafter. The untreated and $CaNa_3$-DTPA-treated dogs were killed in groups of three or four from 14 to 365 d after the PuO_2 implant to obtain tissue specimens. Several tissues (including the injected paw, regional lymph nodes, liver, and femur) and the blood and urine samples (collected on the same schedule as the $CaNa_3$-DTPA treatments) were analyzed radiochemically for plutonium.

The plutonium activity in the injected paw and the major draining LSCLN was monitored externally with a wound counter four or five times on the day of the implant between $t(0)$ and 8 h, and thereafter on the same schedule as the sampling of blood, collection of urine, and $CaNa_3$-DTPA treatment. The wound counter was set to detect only low energy x rays (10 to 24 keV).

The published curves of plutonium retention at the wound site, based on the wound counting and expressed as fractions of unspecified individual implant dosages, depict unexpectedly rapid clearance of plutonium, with retention of only 50 and 10 % at 50 and 300 d, respectively (Bistline, 1973; Bistline et al., 1972). Those authors commented that the apparently rapid clearance of the smaller high-fired particles of PuO_2 was at odds with the greater and more prolonged retention of 7 μm GMD air-oxidized PuO_2 particles that had been observed in the same animal model (Johnson, 1969). The sizes of both of these polydisperse PuO_2 preparations are within the range that can be accumulated by macrophages (Snipes, 1989), and the patterns of retention of these two insoluble forms of particulate PuO_2 can be expected to be similar. Furthermore, the published curves of plutonium retention in the injected paw and plutonium accumulation in the LSCLN account from only 60 % of the nominal plutonium implant dosage at 50 d and only 20 % at 300 d. Reanalysis of the fate of the plutonium s.c. implanted in the paws of dogs as larger air-oxidized particles of PuO_2 shows that transport of the implanted plutonium to tissues other than the LSCLN and loss from the body by excretion account for only a few percent of the plutonium implanted (Table B.5; Johnson, 1969). These discrepancies are likely to have been mainly the result of the difficulties inherent in controlling and quantifying the amount of the inhomogeneous PuO_2 suspensions delivered to the paw of each dog, and inadequate standardization of the wound counting procedure.

B.1.4.1 *Reanalysis of Plutonium Retention at the Subcutaneous Wound Site and Accumulation in Regional Lymph Nodes.* R.W. Bistline kindly provided all of the original records of this study for reexamination. Unfortunately, there was a systematic error in the radiochemical procedure for plutonium that was not recognized until all of the samples had been processed. All of the analyzed tissue, blood and urine samples had been wet digested with hot concentrated HNO_3-$HClO_4$, which is insufficient to dissolve high-fired PuO_2 completely. Paraphrasing Cunningham (1954): In contrast to PuO_2 prepared by gentle ignition (air oxidized), which can be dissolved in hot nitric acid, strongly ignited PuO_2 (high-fired) is inherently difficult to dissolve, and addition of hydrofluoric acid or fusion with potassium pyrosulfate is required for its complete dissolution. Although a ^{236}Pu tracer was added to each sample before digestion, it could not faithfully trace the fate of the insoluble refractory PuO_2, because complete isotopic mixing was not achieved. Consequently, the radiochemical data, particularly for plutonium in the injected paws and local lymph nodes, were considered not useful for this reanalysis.

Given that the individual dog's PuO_2 implant dosages varied and were not accurately known, and that many of the radiochemical analyses of plutonium in the tissues were probably unreliable, reanalysis of this potentially valuable data set required an approach that did not depend on knowledge of the actual amount of plutonium implanted in the paw of each dog.

The entire study was completed in one calendar year; Group 1 was introduced first and killed last at 357 d, and the other five groups were entered into the study and killed at appropriate times during the year. The wound counting records show that during that year the counting rate of the 1 µg plutonium detector calibration standard was stable; the standard deviation of its mean counting rate was 5.6 % for 110 measurement sessions. Each dog could be considered to be an individual accident case with a documented set

TABLE B.5—*In vivo counting of injected paw and regional lymph nodes (LSCLN) of dogs s.c. implanted with 0.7 μm GMD particles of high-fired PuO₂, and not treated with DTPA.*

		Fraction of $w(0)$ (% ± SD)[a,b]	
t(d)	Number of Dogs[c]	Paw	LSCLN
1	21	109 ± 11	0.6 ± 0.4
2	21	102 ± 14	1.0 ± 0.8
3	21	99 ± 5	1.5 ± 1
4	21	96 ± 5	2.2 ± 2
5	21	98 ± 6	2.4 ± 2
6	21	96 ± 8	2.9 ± 2
8	21	95 ± 9	3.0 ± 2
10	21	93 ± 11	3.6 ± 2
13	21	95 ± 8	4.1 ± 3
30 – 35[d]	8	82 ± 10	5.4 ± 2
45 – 49	7	80 ± 11	8.3 ± 8
64 – 69	8	76 ± 16	9.9 ± 10
77	4	82 ± 20	8.0 ± 4
101 – 104	8	74 ± 10	11 ± 11
134 – 139	8	82 ± 14	12 ± 12
162	4	77 ± 6	6 ± 1
182	4	91 ± 16	15 ± 9
216	4	88 ± 10	15 ± 10
286	4	77 ± 15	21 ± 13
328	4	81 ± 18	22 ± 13
357	4	73 ± 18	20 ± 8

[a]Wound counts of each dog normalized to 100 % of its own $w(0)$ value (see text) derived from original laboratory records of Bistline, R.W. (2000) personal communication (Abilene, Kansas).

[b]$w(0)$ set equal to mean *in vivo* counts of (paw + LSCLN) measured on days three, four and five post-implant.

[c]Number of dogs contributing data at time t.

[d]Data for $t \geq 30$ d are averaged *in vivo* counts for three consecutive days.

of external measurements of the wounded paw and local lymph nodes. The trends of plutonium retention at the wound site and accumulation in the LSCLN of each dog could be examined independently of the amount of PuO_2 implanted.

Penetration and spreading of the bulk of these small polydisperse PuO_2 particles would have been restricted initially to a small volume of extracellular fluid immediately surrounding the implant site (Matsuoka *et al.*, 1972). After subsidence of temporary local edema created by the injection of 0.25 mL of saline, perhaps within 4 to 8 h, and during the earliest stages of the tissue reactions to the foreign bodies and the alpha radiation, perhaps as long as two weeks, the geometrical relationships of the implanted particles to the enclosing interstitial space may be considered to be reasonably constant. It was assumed that during the first days after the PuO_2 implant:

- the injected paw and the LSCLN combined (paw + LSCLN) contained close to 100 % of the plutonium implanted;
- for the anatomically well defined wound site and LSCLN, the intensity of the externally detected low energy photon was constantly proportional to the amount of plutonium present;
- the detection efficiencies for the L-shell x rays were nearly the same for plutonium in the paw and LSCLN; and
- there was little change in the absorption of the x rays by overlying tissue of the individual dogs during their study times.

The data taken at each external wound counting session were normalized to the daily count rate of the 1 µg plutonium standard and recorded as equivalent plutonium (μg_e):

$$\text{wound equivalent Pu} = [\text{wound (cpm)} - \text{bkgd (cpm)}]$$
$$[\text{standard (cpm)} - \text{bkgd (cpm)}]^{-1}. \qquad \text{(B.13)}$$

The serial wound monitoring data for plutonium in the injected paw, the LSCLN, and their sum (paw + LSCLN) expressed as μg_e plutonium, were tabulated individually for each dog. The external count rates of the paws of 80 % of the dogs increased from their $t(0)$ values to maxima of ~1.2 times the $t(0)$ value on day one or two, but by days three to five, the initial fluctuations in the wound count rates of the paws of most of the dogs had subsided, and the sum of the count rates (paw + LSCLN) for each dog was stable through day 13. The mean sum (paw + LSCLN) μg_e plutonium on days three, four and five was adopted as the initial 100 % plutonium value for each dog, termed $w(0)$, and all other measurements for that dog were expressed as percent of $w(0)$. The amounts of plutonium implanted, as measured by $w(0)$, were variable. The mean $w(0)$ for all 45 dogs in the study was $15.4 \pm 8.6 \mu g_e$ of plutonium, and the largest $w(0)$ for an individual dog ($37.6 \mu g_e$) was 22 times that for the dog with the smallest $w(0)$ ($1.5 \mu g_e$).

B.1.4.2 *Plutonium Retention in the Injected Paw and Accumulation in Regional Lymph Nodes.* The reanalyzed data for retention of plutonium in the injected paw and accumulation of plutonium in the local LSCLN are presented in Table B.5; note that only the eight dogs in Groups 1 and 2, killed at 360 and 180 d, respectively, contributed data after 80 d. Even though the DTPA treatment had no discernible effect on retention of the plutonium in the wounded paw, only results from the 22 untreated dogs were used in the data analysis. The data sets for the estimates of wound site and lymph-node plutonium (Table B.5) were modeled simultaneously with the estimated blood plutonium (Table B.3) using the wound model (Section 4) and Origin® software, assuming initial deposition into the PABS compartment. The model output for the two body compartments generated the curves shown in Figure B.6 for clearance of the plutonium from the wound site and accumulation of plutonium in the local lymph nodes. The equation of the curve for plutonium retention at the wound site is:

$$R(t) = 4.3e^{-0.13t} + 95.7e^{-0.0006t} \% \text{ of } w(0), \tag{B.14}$$

where t is days after implant.

Equation B.14, which describes wound retention of plutonium implanted as small high-fired PuO_2 particles, is similar to Equation B.10, which describes retention of plutonium implanted as larger air-oxidized PuO_2 particles, except that only one-half as much plutonium from the smaller, more refractory high-fired PuO_2 particles appears to be cleared soon after implantation, and the long term clearance rate of the smaller high-fired PuO_2 particles appears to be somewhat faster. Neither study included any measurements beyond 1 y after implant, both data sets contained considerable scatter, and analyses required several assumptions. All of those factors make it difficult to decide whether the differences are apparent or real.

Transfer of plutonium from the injected paws to the LSCLN was immediately evident in most of the dogs (Figure B.6). The amounts

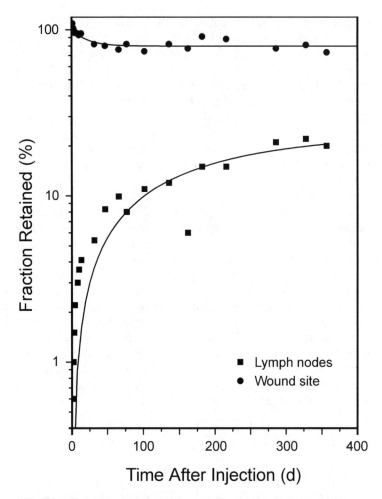

Fig. B.6. Retention of plutonium at the s.c. wound site in the paws of dogs after implantation of an aqueous suspension of high-fired PuO_2 particles (0.7 μm GMD) and accumulation in the regional lymph nodes. Retention of plutonium, estimated by serial *in vivo* counting data, is expressed as percent of $w(0)$ (see text). The curves correspond to Equations B.14 and B.15, respectively.

of plutonium transferred to the LSCLN of individual dogs varied, both within and between the groups of dogs given the high-fired PuO_2 particle implants (Table B.5). Lymph-node accumulation of PuO_2 occurred in two phases, with rapid accumulation during the first 30 d followed by slower net uptake during the remainder of the year (Figure B.6). The equation that describes plutonium uptake in the local lymph nodes (LN) is:

$$LN(t) = 7.7(1 - e^{-0.038t}) + 79.4(1 - e^{-0.00022t}) \% \text{ of } w(0), \quad \text{(B.15)}$$

where t is days after implant.

B.1.5 *Plutonium Metal Discs Implanted Subcutaneously in Rats and Rabbits*

Plutonium metal discs (1 mm diameter, on average 0.1 mm thick, 1.9 mm^2 surface area) were s.c. implanted in the left upper quadrant of the abdomen of eight rabbits (1,085 ± 380 µg plutonium) and three rats (717 ± 97 µg plutonium) (Lisco and Kisieleski, 1953). One rabbit died 2 d after the implant of acute enterocolitis of unknown origin. The remaining animals were observed for their lifespans. The implant sites were examined regularly by palpation and radiography. Excreta were collected for the first 56 to 70 d and at 105 and 280 d. At necropsy, liver, spleen, kidneys, lungs, testes, and several bones were taken for radioanalysis and histopathology. The isolated implant sites were dissected, and examined visually and radiographically (Appendix B.6.3). The amount of plutonium implanted in each animal, its time of death, estimated plutonium absorption, and published excretion data are shown in Table B.6.

Plutonium was not detectable in the excreta of either species during the first 70 d after the implants. Peak plutonium excretion by the rats was observed at 105 d, and it had declined substantially by ~280 d. Between 122 and 305 d, plutonium was detectable in a few samples of rabbit urine, but plutonium was not detected in any fecal samples from the rabbits at any time. The liver and bones of all the animals that survived 260 d or longer contained measurable amounts of plutonium. Absorption of plutonium was estimated by summing the amounts of plutonium recovered in the tissues and bones of each individual animal (Table B.6). Reported absorption in the rabbits (0.52 ± 0.37 % absorbed, 99.48 ± 0.34 % retained at the implant site) was about three times that absorbed by the rats (0.18 ± 0.10 % absorbed, 99.82 ± 0.10 % retained). Total plutonium absorption in the rats was underestimated, possibly by as much as 40 %, because plutonium excretion was not taken into account. The rat liver efficiently clears plutonium to excretion, and turnover of trabecular bone in the continuously growing rat skeleton releases some skeletal plutonium to excretion and redistribution (Scott *et al.*, 1948a; Simpson *et al.*, 1950; Taylor *et al.*, 1961).

Transfer of those small fractions of the implanted plutonium to the tissues and excreta are evidence of the solubilization of a small fraction of the implanted plutonium. In neither species was plutonium absorption well correlated with the amount of plutonium

TABLE B.6—*Absorption and excretion of ^{239}Pu in rats and rabbits after s.c. implantation of plutonium metal wire fragments (Lisco and Kisieleski, 1953).*

Time After Implant (d)	Implant (μg)	Absorption[a] (%)	Urinary Excretion[b,c] (% d^{-1})	Fecal Excretion[b,c] (% d^{-1})
Rabbits				
2[d]	1,800	0	na	na
260	1,000	0.16	nd	nd
340	1,330	0.63	nd	nd
516	670	0.22	na	na
623	770	0.76	na	na
710	1,140	1.20	na	na
738	1,250	0.37	na	na
1,048	720	0.27	na	na
Rats				
105	—[e]	—[e]	2×10^{-5} [f]	$8.8. \times 10^{-4}$ [f]
280	—[e]	—[e]	6.3×10^{-6} [f]	6.4×10^{-5} [f]
356	800	0.28	na	na
484	610	0.18	na	na
580	740	0.09	na	na

[a]Absorbed fraction (percent), based on analysis of selected tissues and implant site.
[b]No analysis.
[c]Not detectable using available methods; thus, is less than the reported excretion rates for rats at the same implant times.
[d]Cause of death acute enterocolitis.
[e]Excretion data only.
[f]Average excretion rate based on 717 ± 97 μg plutonium implanted.

implanted, the time between implant and death, or the surface area of the implant site at death. However, the decline in plutonium excretion by the rats after 70 d and encapsulation of the fragmented and corroded plutonium metal by mineralizing fibrous tissue combine to indicate that plutonium absorption occurred mainly during the first year after the implants.

If some plutonium particles (most likely a mixture of hydrous plutonium oxides) were small enough to be phagocytized and transported to local lymph nodes, plutonium retention at the wound site would be slightly less than the published estimates. However, the fibrous capsule that formed around the implanted plutonium metal and its corrosion products would constitute a barrier to lymphatic transport of plutonium-laden macrophages.

The data from this study are not sufficient for analysis with the wound model. However, the overall time-dependent plutonium absorption pattern for plutonium wire s.c. implanted in the rabbits resembled uranium absorption from DU metal wafers i.m. implanted in rats (Appendix B.3.4), in particular Rat 102 (see Table B.9 in Section B.3.4.2). The transfer rates obtained for Rat 102, which included transfer of particles to lymph nodes and subsequent release of solubilized uranium from lymph nodes to blood, were used as starting values to simulate plutonium absorption by the rabbits. The transfer rates were adjusted until the calculated plutonium absorption curve was an acceptable visual fit to the data (Figure 4.23; Table 4.10). The data for the three rats were not sufficient for simulation modeling, but their plutonium absorption pattern closely resembled that of uranium absorption by Rat 86, and the wound model transfer rates for that rat were used to obtain a surrogate plutonium retention equation for the plutonium wire s.c. implanted in rats. Reasonable wound plutonium retention equations for s.c.-implanted plutonium metal fragments in rabbits and rats are, where t is days after implant:

$$R(t)_{\text{rabbit}} = 0.5e^{-0.0089t} + 99.5e^{-2.8 \times 10^{-6}t} \% \qquad (B.16)$$

and

$$R(t)_{\text{rat}} = 0.14e^{-0.009t} + 99.86e^{-1.6 \times 10^{-6}t} \% \qquad (B.17)$$

of the implanted amount.

Those estimated plutonium wound retention equations predict that after 365 d there will be little additional plutonium absorption, deposition in tissues, or excretion. Although the data from this study are insufficient to demonstrate the validity of the assumptions underlying Equations B.16 and B.17, long-term release of plutonium from the wound site is likely to be very slow, and nearly all of the plutonium retained at 1 y would be expected to be retained indefinitely. Continuous alpha irradiation may accelerate necrosis of the inner aspect of the fibrous capsule surrounding the plutonium implant (Appendix B.6.5) causing it to thin, as was found at late times in cases of thorotrastoma (Appendix B.6.6) and to allow sporadic escape of a few PuO_2 particles from the wound site.

B.2 Small Particles of Insoluble Radiolabeled Compounds Injected Intramuscularly in Rats

In a study of the mechanisms of clearance of insoluble dusts from the lungs, Morrow et al. (1968) compared the lung clearance patterns of eight insoluble radiolabeled compounds with their retention at an i.m. or s.c. wound site in rats. The radiolabeled solids listed in Table B.7 were prepared by mixing the radiolabel with a solution of the appropriate carrier cation, precipitating the desired compound, and washing the particles by dialysis against water. The sizes of the particles in the aqueous suspensions were not reported, but when aerosolized for the inhalation studies, the activity median diameters were 0.49 to 0.54 μm (σ_g 2.0 to 2.3). The pH of the injected suspensions was close to neutral, since some of these solids dissolve in acid. The mass of metal ion deposited in 0.05 mL of suspension was estimated to have been ≥16 μg in all cases. Samples of the same radiolabeled suspensions used to inject the rats were dispersed in blood serum to determine ultrafilterability. Retention of the radiolabel in the injected leg was monitored repeatedly by in vivo counting with a small collimated NaI(Tl) crystal of the energetic gamma rays of the radiolabels.

The compounds injected as suspensions are listed in Table B.7 in the order of their increasing retention at the i.m. wound site. That is also roughly the order of their decreasing ultrafilterability from serum, confirming the correlation of low aqueous solubility with prolonged retention at an i.m. wound site. All of the solids injected as aqueous suspensions are variably soluble in acid, and it is reasonable to consider that all could be slowly dissolved in the mildly acidic medium within macrophage phagolysosomes (pH 4.5 to 5.5, depending on species).

Retention half-times at an i.m.-injection site exceeded 100 d for suspensions of $^{110}AgO\text{-}AgI$, $^{51}Cr\text{-}Fe(OH)_3$, and $^{59}Fe_2O_3$ and 200 d for $^{65}Zn_3(PO_4)_2$ and $^{51}Cr_2O_3$. These five compounds dissolve slowly in dilute acid. The interatomic distances between the metal ion and the oxygens of the oxides of the small trivalent cations, Cr^{3+} and Fe^{3+}, are short, and bonding is strong, making them quite resistant to attack by dilute acid. Three suspensions of compounds that are insoluble in pure water were less tenaciously retained at an i.m. wound site. ^{203}HgO is sparingly soluble in pure water (solubility limit ~3×10^{-4} mol L^{-1}), but its retention pattern was nearly

TABLE B.7—*Comparison of retention at an i.m.-injection site in rats and ultrafilterability from serum of suspensions of small particles of selected radiolabeled compounds insoluble in water (Morrow et al., 1968).*

Radiolabeled Compound[a]	Clearance Rates from i.m.-Injection Site (d^{-1})[b]	Ultrafilterable from Serum (%)[c]
^{203}Hg-HgO	1.4/0.09	2.0
^{54}Mn-MnO$_2$	0.6/0.05	4.4
^{113}Sn-Sn$_3$(PO$_4$)$_2$	0.012	1.7
^{110}Ag-Ag$_2$O-AgI[d]	$<7 \times 10^{-3}$	0.2
^{51}Cr-Fe(OH)$_3$	$<4.3 \times 10^{-3}$	2.5
^{65}Zn-Zn$_3$(PO$_4$)$_2$	$<3.5 \times 10^{-3}$	1.1
^{51}Cr-Cr$_2$O$_3$	$<3.5 \times 10^{-3}$	0.2
^{59}Fe-Fe$_2$O$_3$	$<5 \times 10^{-3}/<1.4 \times 10^{-3}$	0.5

[a]Prepared by mixing radiolabel with stable carrier cation in solution, precipitation of desired solid, purification by dialysis against water.
[b]When two half-times are shown (a/b), retention was clearly biphasic.
[c]Ultrafiltration through cellophane tubing, mean pore size 45 nm.
[d]Questionable composition.

the same as that of soluble ^{203}Hg(acetate)$_2$ (Table A.7), indicating efficient dissolution of the oxide *in vivo*. The retention patterns of ^{54}MnO$_2$ in suspension and soluble ^{54}MnCl$_2$ were essentially the same (Table A.7), suggesting efficient reduction of MnO$_2$ to soluble Mn^{2+} *in vivo*. ^{113}Sn$_3$(PO$_4$)$_2$ decomposes in acid, and it appears to have been dissolved at a moderate rate *in vivo*, presumably within the lysosomes of macrophages.

B.3 Insoluble Forms of Uranium

B.3.1 *Suspensions of Uranium Oxides Injected Intramuscularly in Rats and Rabbits*

Beiter *et al.* (1975) investigated retention at an i.m. wound site of ^{235}UO$_3$ and ^{235}UO$_2$, neither of which is soluble in water. That study was a follow-up to their intercomparisons of lung clearance rates and retention in i.m. puncture wounds of some representative soluble and insoluble compounds (Morrow *et al.*, 1968;

Appendices A.1.4.5 and B.2). Particles of $^{235}UO_3$ and $^{235}UO_2$ were i.m. injected into one hind leg of three to seven rats in 0.1 mL of aqueous suspensions containing 4 mg of ^{235}U. One rabbit was i.m. injected with 0.4 mL of the $^{235}UO_2$ suspension (17 mg of ^{235}U). The mass median diameter of the $^{235}UO_3$ particles was 2.4 μm and that of the $^{235}UO_2$ particles was 1 μm. Starting at 1 d after the injections, retention of ^{235}U in the injected legs and accumulation of ^{235}U in the uninjected legs were monitored for 14 weeks by frequent measurement *in vivo* of the 25 to 210 keV photons. The measured ^{235}U content of the uninjected leg was used to correct the measurements of the injected leg for ^{235}U content not associated with the wound site. The timed data for wound retention of $^{235}UO_2$ from the rabbit and the individual rats, read from Figure 4 of Beiter *et al.* (1975), are shown in Table B.8. Retention of $^{235}UO_3$ after the first day was biphasic with clearance rates of 0.16 and 0.016 d^{-1}. The authors identified only one clearance rate from the combined data for less-soluble $^{235}UO_2$, 4.4×10^{-3} d^{-1}.

The reconstructed data sets shown in Table B.8 for wound retention of $^{235}UO_2$ in the rabbit and the three rats were reanalyzed by using the wound model and Origin® software, with input into the PABS compartment (Section 4). The resulting wound retention equations (% *ID*) for particulate $^{235}UO_2$ are as follows:

$$\text{rat: } R(t) = 48e^{-0.023t} + 52 \tag{B.18}$$

and

$$\text{rabbit: } R(t) = 37e^{-0.027t} + 63, \tag{B.19}$$

where t is days after injection.

The deposited amounts of both uranium oxides were apparently small enough and/or their rates of solubilization and/or transfer to local lymph nodes were slow enough to avoid acute renal toxicity. The rapid clearance of $^{235}UO_3$ from the site of deposition agrees with its greater solubility in blood serum than in pure water and also with its more rapid clearance from the lungs after inhalation (Beiter *et al.*, 1975). In dilute acid, UO_3 decomposes rapidly to UO_2^{2+}, a reaction that apparently can be accomplished in the macrophage lysosomes. Once converted to UO_2^{2+}, extracellular fluid bicarbonate is available to complex the solubilized uranium and facilitate its transport away from the wound site. It also appears that a fraction of a large mass (4 mg) of more inert $^{235}UO_2$ can be dissolved slowly or transported to local lymph nodes (not sampled).

TABLE B.8—*Percent of i.m.-injected $^{235}UO_2$ particles retained at wound site in rats and a rabbit.*[a]

Time After Injection[b] (d)	Rats[c] (4 mg)	Rabbit[d] (16 mg)
1	98	100
5	99, 81	93
10 – 20	82, 80	86
20 – 30	93, 68	91
30 – 40	95, 81	78
40 – 50		80, 76
50 – 60	80, 72, 61	67, 66
60 – 80	76, 64, 61	68
80 – 100	86, 44	70
100 – 110	84, 64, 48	

[a]Timed data read from Figure 4 of Beiter *et al.* (1975).
[b]Time intervals accommodate measurements made on different schedules.
[c]Three rats; fewer than three rats measured on some days.
[d]One rabbit.

B.3.2 *Dry UO_2 Particles Implanted Subcutaneously in Rats*

Dry UO_2 powder was s.c. implanted in rats to investigate the deposition and toxicity of the uranium solubilized and translocated from the implantation site (De Rey *et al.*, 1984). Weighed amounts of powdered UO_2 prepared at high temperature were s.c. implanted on the backs of rats *via* a small skin incision [1.6, 8, 80, and 160 mg per rat (*i.e.*, 10, 50, 500 and 1,000 mg kg^{-1}, respectively), in 160 g rats]. The implant sites were examined by light and electron microscopy in rats killed from 3 to 72 h after the implants. All of the rats implanted with ≥50 mg kg^{-1} of UO_2 died within 6 d. Neither toxicity nor the local tissue response appeared to depend on initial particle size (4 to 40 μm diameter); electron microscopy showed that the UO_2 particles distributed throughout the intercellular spaces of the implantation site were smaller than when they were implanted. The presence after 6 h of electron-dense deposits in the cells and renal tubular lumina and the increasing degree (with both dosage and time) of proximal tubular necrosis provide evidence for the dissolution of a small but toxic fraction of the deposited UO_2. The presence of uranium in bones and teeth (determined by x-ray scanning) is additional evidence for some UO_2 dissolution. Rats injected parenterally with soluble uranium salts survive dosages ≤ 0.6 mg kg^{-1}, and all are sick or dead at dosages ≥ 1 mg kg^{-1} (Haven and Hodge, 1949). The results of this study imply early solubilization and absorption of at least (1 mg kg^{-1}) (50 mg kg^{-1})$^{-1}$, that is, ~2 % of the uranium implanted as UO_2.

B.3.3 *Dry UO_2 Powder Implanted Subcutaneously in Rabbits*

A 3 cm skin incision was made in rabbits, and dry UO_2 powder [10, 20, or 40 mg (*i.e.*, 3.3, 6.7, and 13.3 mg kg^{-1}, respectively), in 3 kg rabbits] was implanted between the skin and the superficial muscle layer. The animals were observed for 30 d. At 7 d, there was only slight erythema and edema at the wound site for all dosage levels; at 25 d, healing was complete, but regrowth of hair was incomplete, and the skin above the scar slightly thickened. At necropsy at 30 d, there was no grossly visible indication of inflammation or irritation in the healing wounds that was not referable to the operative trauma. Black UO_2 powder was clearly visible in the fascia beneath the skin, but there was no thickening or erythema of the tissues surrounding the particles. On average, 91 ± 8.3 % of the deposited uranium was recovered in the tissues at or surrounding the wound site, but that value was within the limits of error of the fluorometric analytical method used. The author concluded, based on the chemical analysis and the absence of a toxicological response, that there was no significant dissolution and/or absorption of the uranium implanted as UO_2 powder (Allen, 1949). Rabbits injected parenterally with soluble uranium salts all survived at dosages <0.1 mg kg^{-1} and all died at dosages ≥ 0.1 mg kg^{-1} (Haven and Hodge, 1949). The absorption of solubilized uranium would have had to be at least: (0.1 mg kg^{-1}) (13.3 mg kg^{-1})$^{-1}$ (*i.e.*, 0.75 % of the amount implanted) to have elicited a toxic response among the rabbits that received the largest amount of UO_2 powder.

B.3.4 *Depleted Uranium Metal Fragments Implanted Intramuscularly in Rats*

A number of U.S. veterans of the Persian Gulf War were wounded with DU fragments as a result of "friendly fire" incidents in which Abrams tanks and Bradley fighting vehicles were struck by DU antiarmor munitions (AEPI, 1995). Because of their number, size and/or location, many of these DU fragments were surgically inoperable, and some of the wounded veterans have been left with localized deposits of metallic uranium. Long-term excretion of uranium has been observed in these veterans 6 to 11 y after their wounding with DU shrapnel, with levels averaging ~1 µg uranium per gram creatinine (Section 3.2; McDiarmid et al., 2000; 2004; Squibb et al., 2005). To evaluate the potential long-term health effects from embedded DU fragments, their biokinetics, toxicity and carcinogenicity were investigated. Although those studies focused on biological effects (Appendix B.6.4), they provide information on the biokinetic behavior of DU fragments in muscle wounds (Hahn, 2000; Hahn et al., 2002; Pellmar et al., 1999, McClain et al., 2001).

Adult male Wistar rats were each implanted with four cleaned DU metal fragments in the form of cylindrical pellets (2 × 1 mm diameter), or small (2.5 × 2.5 × 1.5 mm) or large (5 × 5 × 1.5 mm) square wafers, with total initial surface areas of 6.3, 110, and 320 mm^2, respectively. The implants were placed surgically in the biceps femoris muscle of each rat, two on each leg, and the animals were followed for lifespan. Periodic radiographs of selected rats defined the gross morphologic appearance of the DU implants and the surrounding tissue. The uranium content of the kidneys and the eviscerated carcass (minus the implant sites) was determined at death (Hahn, 2000; Hahn et al., 2002).

Sprague-Dawley rats were implanted with small cylindrical DU metal pellets (2 × 1 mm diameter). Dosing was varied by implanting 4, 10 or 20 DU pellets and adding inert tantalum fragments so that each rat received 20 metal implants; the maximum surface area of 20 DU implants was 31.4 mm^2. Rats were killed serially at 1 d and 1, 6, 12 and 18 months after implant. Urine samples (24 h) were collected at each sampling time (Pellmar et al., 1999).

B.3.4.1 *Urinary Uranium Excretion.* In the study of Hahn et al. (Hahn, 2000; Hahn et al., 2002), 24 h urine samples were collected from six rats that had been implanted with four large (5 × 5 × 1.5 mm) DU wafers with a total weight of 2.6 ± 0.1 g of DU. The urine sampling schedule was as follows: daily from –2 to 7 d, then twice weekly to 28 d, weekly to 88 d, twice a month to 564 d, and monthly to 664 d. The daily uranium excretion increased steeply during the first 30 d after the DU implantation, in some rats by as much as two orders of magnitude, and the daily urinary excretion rate was greatest at ~90 d post-implant, ranging from 3 × 10^{-3} to 1 × 10^{-2} % d^{-1} of the implanted DU. The average daily urinary uranium excretion rate was 2.4×10^{-3} % d^{-1} during the first 150 d, and it decreased to $\sim 1 \times 10^{-3}$ % d^{-1} for the remainder of the study. In comparison, peak daily urinary uranium excretion in the study of Pellmar et al. (1999) was observed at six months after implantation. However, no urine samples were taken between one and six months, and the exact time of maximum urinary uranium excretion is uncertain in that study, but it is clearly later than was observed by Hahn et al. (Hahn, 2000; Hahn et al., 2002). The difference in the urinary uranium excretion patterns may be due to the differences in the initial surface areas of the implants and their number (i.e., as many as 20 of the 2×1 mm cylindrical pellets) (surface area 31.4 mm^2) used by Pellmar et al. (1999) versus four $5 \times 5 \times 1.5$ mm square wafers (surface area 320 mm^2) used by Hahn et al. (Hahn, 2000; Hahn et al., 2002), as well as differences in the rates and degrees of corrosion of the DU metal surfaces and disintegration of the DU fragments and the rates of fibrotic encapsulation.

In general, the data from both studies showed that the biokinetics of uranium in the kidneys, the principal initial deposition site for systemic soluble uranium, reflect the kinetics of release of solubilized uranium (presumably UO_2^{2+}) from the wound site to blood. Pellmar et al. (1999) observed maximum kidney uranium concentrations at six months after implant, followed by a decrease to 60 to 70 % of the maximum concentrations at 18 months. Concomitantly, urinary uranium excretion also peaked at six months after implant. A similar temporal comparison between urinary uranium excretion rate and kidney content cannot be made in the study of Hahn et al. (Hahn, 2000; Hahn et al., 2002), because no kidney uranium data were obtained during the first year post-implant. However, after 1 y, the kidney uranium content was positively correlated with the amount of DU implanted, and there was a slight indication of decreasing kidney uranium content during the second year, corresponding to the observed slow decline in the urinary uranium excretion rate.

B.3.4.2 *Retention at the Wound Site of Uranium Implanted as Depleted Uranium Metal Fragments.* The frequent collection of urine over the lifespans of six rats each implanted with four large DU metal wafers provides the data needed to calculate the pattern of retention within the wound site of uranium deposited in the form of DU metal fragments. The tabulated urine data were expressed both as gram uranium per day and as the fraction of the total implanted DU excreted in urine per 24 h, fraction per day (Hahn, 2000). For the purposes of this Report, the mean urinary uranium on days two, one and zero is considered to be the background uranium excretion contributed by soluble uranium in the diet and drinking water. The average daily excretion of uranium in urine for these three days for the six rats was equivalent to $0.56 \pm 0.39 \times 10^{-6}$ d^{-1} of the average DU implant. The background daily urinary uranium, calculated individually for each rat, was subtracted from the reported uranium content of each of its urine samples. The data were then recast in terms of percent of the total implanted DU per day (% d^{-1}). Urinary uranium levels exceeded twice the background level by 3 to 5 d after the implants. Urinary uranium excretion during the intervals between collections, urine uranium (t_1 to t_2), percent of implant, was accounted for by linear interpolation (i.e., as the average daily urinary uranium excretion rate on the day just before) ($t_1 - 1$) and the day just after ($t_2 + 1$) each unmeasured interval times the number of days in the interval. Cumulative urinary uranium excretion was calculated by summing the urinary uranium excretion (measured and interpolated) from the time of implant to the time of sampling or death.

Total absorption from the wound site of solubilized uranium (systemic uranium) at any time after the DU implant is the sum of the total amount of uranium excreted in the urine up to that time plus the amounts of uranium present at that time in the tissues, mainly kidneys and carcass. Hahn et al. (2002) provided mean values at death for kidney uranium content ($4.1 \pm 2.1 \times 10^{-3}$ % of the implanted DU) and for the eviscerated carcass (mainly bone) minus the injection sites ($4.7 \pm 4.3 \times 10^{-2}$ % of the implanted DU). On average, for the six rats with lifespan urine collections, total urinary uranium was (92 ± 5) % of the total amount of implanted uranium that could be accounted for in urinary excretion, kidneys, and carcass. Because some tissues were not analyzed, a rounded value of 90 % was adopted to convert the timed values for cumulative urinary uranium to timed values of total systemic uranium, where urinary uranium = 0.9 (systemic uranium). Systemic uranium can be considered to be the amount of uranium solubilized and cleared from the wound site (i.e., the amount absorbed). The results of those calculations are summarized in Table B.9, which presents the cumulative uranium absorption from the wound site containing the DU fragments, expressed as percent of the amount of DU metal implanted, as a function of time after the implant for the six individual rats.

Urine collections from three of the rats were stopped before the end of the 662 d study period. Total uranium absorption at 662 d was estimated for those rats by linear extrapolation of the trend in their uranium absorptions during the last 12 weeks (Rats 96 and 97) or last 28 weeks (Rat 100) in which urine was collected from

TABLE B.9—Cumulative absorption of uranium from DU metal wafers implanted in thigh muscle of rats.[a,b]

Time After Implant (d)[b]	Cumulative Uranium Absorption (percent of implant)						Systemic[c]	SD[c]
	Rat 86	Rat 90	Rat 96	Rat 97	Rat 100	Rat 102		
5	0.00036	0.00029	0.00016	0.0012	0.00039	0.00086	0.00011	0.0014
10	0.0062	0.0040	0.0047	0.009	0.0061	0.0097	0.0066	0.0023
20	0.016	0.033	0.017	0.035	0.024	0.029	0.026	0.0080
32	0.022	0.067	0.028	0.11	0.052	0.058	0.056	0.032
60	0.029	0.17	0.082	0.22	0.11	0.11	0.12	0.067
88	0.054	0.23	0.24	0.40	0.24	0.19	0.226	0.11
116	0.081	0.29	0.31	0.47	0.32	0.23	0.28	0.13
158	0.12	0.51	0.43	0.68	0.54	0.30	0.43	0.20
200	0.14	0.58	0.49	0.76	0.64	0.35	0.49	0.22
256	0.16	0.66	0.55	0.83	0.86	0.39	0.58	0.27
298	0.18	0.69	0.57	0.89	0.99	0.41	0.62	0.30
354	0.19	0.75		0.93	1.15	0.42	0.69	0.38
396	0.21	0.81			1.29	0.46	0.69	0.47

452	0.23	0.89			1.40	0.50	0.76	0.51
508	0.24	0.93			1.53	0.52	0.80	0.56
550	0.26	0.97			1.63	0.52	0.84	0.60
592	0.27	1.01				0.53	—	—
662	0.28	1.05	(0.86)[d]	(1.17)[d]	(1.87)[d]	0.54	0.96	0.55

[a]Summary of data for systemic absorption of solubilized DU calculated from the data of Hahn. *et al.* (Hahn, 2000; Hahn *et al.*, 2002) from daily urinary uranium excretion rates of individual rats and the average terminal uranium content of kidneys and eviscerated carcass (see text).

[b]Only about one-half of the full data sets for the six individual rats is shown here.

[c]Composite fit to the systemic absorption, with its standard deviation.

[d]Values obtained from linear extrapolation of cumulative uranium absorption data for the last 12 weeks (Rat 96, Rat 97) or 28 weeks (Rat 100) before death.

them. Those extrapolated values are shown in parentheses in Table B.9. The urine data demonstrate a slow but persistent release to blood of a small fraction of the uranium implanted as DU metal wafers. The mean fraction of the DU implanted that was released from the wound site and absorbed into the blood in 662 d was (0.96 ± 0.55) % of the implanted DU. Despite the significant disintegration and surface corrosion of the DU wafers, which with time substantially increased their specific surface area, there was no long-sustained release of solubilized uranium reaching the blood. The urinary uranium excretion rate increased during the first 90 d after the DU implants, but the rate stabilized and then slowly declined during the remainder of the study. The connective tissue capsules that formed around each fragment would have impeded the mechanical transport of phagocytized particles of corrosion products (a mixture of hydrous uranium oxides) and diffusion of soluble UO_2^{2+} ions. The thickening of the capsules with time would be expected to further reduce the rate at which uranium could reach the draining lymph nodes or the blood. Mineralization of the necrotic debris on the inner aspects of the capsule walls suggests that solubilized uranium was being further immobilized within the capsule, possibly by precipitation as uranyl phosphate (Appendix B.6.4; Henge-Napoli *et al.*, 1994).

The systemic uranium data sets for the six rats implanted with DU wafers and followed for continuous urinary uranium excretion (Table B.9) were analyzed individually using the wound model (Section 4), with input into the fragments compartment, to generate the wound uranium retention curves shown in Figure B.7. The parameters of the six corresponding wound uranium retention equations, obtained using the Origin® software, are shown in Table B.10, as are the mean parameter values:

$$R(t) = 0.5e^{-8.6 \times 10^{-3}t} + 99.48e^{-6.5 \times 10^{-6}t} \text{ \%} \qquad \text{(B.20)}$$

of the implanted amount.

The detailed structures of the individual wound retention curves vary as might be expected, since each curve is the net result of several chemical and biological processes occurring in the four implant sites and their draining lymph nodes in each rat. How ever, the wound uranium retention curves reveal a common pattern; early release of a small fraction of the implanted uranium, (0.50 ± 0.24) % (Equation B.20), with a half-time of ~80 d followed by the nearly imperceptible release of the remaining 99.5 % of the implanted DU (average half-time of 292 y). The experimental

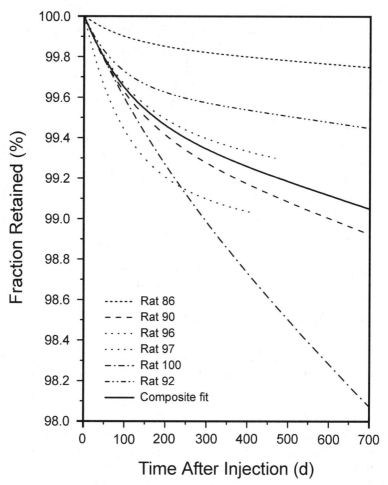

Fig. B.7. Retention of uranium at the wound site in rats i.m. implanted with DU metal wafers. Individual curves for six rats (identified by number) were obtained using the wound model (Section 4) to analyze their systemic uranium data (Table B.10).

observations indicate prolonged residence of the DU metal fragments and their corrosion products at the wound site, with potential risk for both radiation- and chemically-induced biological effects at the implant sites.

In addition to the implant sites, kidneys, and suspected neoplasms, some tissues were examined visually at necropsy and prepared for histopathology. At necropsy, the lumbar and popliteal nodes draining the DU implant sites appeared gray in color. Microscopically, they contained black UO_2 particles confined within

TABLE B.10—*Parameters of two-component exponential wound uranium retention curves in individual rats i.m. implanted with wafers of DU metal.*[a,b]

Rat Number	A_1 (%)	λ_1 (d^{-1})	A_2 (%)	λ_2 (d^{-1})
86	0.14	9.0×10^{-3}	99.86	1.6×10^{-6}
90	0.55	7.9×10^{-3}	99.43	7.6×10^{-6}
96	0.55	8.0×10^{-3}	99.43	3.5×10^{-6}
97	0.85	9.8×10^{-3}	99.13	3.3×10^{-6}
100	0.57	4.5×10^{-3}	99.41	2×10^{-5}
102	0.35	1.2×10^{-2}	99.63	2.9×10^{-6}
Mean	0.50	8.6×10^{-3}	99.48	6.5×10^{-6}
±SD	0.24	2.5×10^{-3}	0.24	6.9×10^{-6}

[a]Wound uranium retention equations of DU of the form $R(t) = \sum_i A_i e^{-\lambda_i t}$,
where t is days after implant (based on data given in Table B.9).
[b]$A_1 + A_2$ <100 %, because 0.023 % of the implanted DU was estimated to be associated with the local lymph nodes and outside of the wound at death.

macrophages. The amounts of uranium in those lymph nodes were not determined.[7] The size of the lymph nodes and their modest uranium content suggested that much <1 % of the implanted uranium was retained as UO_2 particles in the local lymph nodes at the end of the study.

The wound model (Section 4) accommodates transfer of particles to draining lymph nodes. Such transfer was taken into account by making reasonable estimates of the rates of input of UO_2 particles to lymph nodes and the rate of dissolution of the uranium confined within lymph-node macrophages. The calculated average uranium content of the lymph-node compartment at the end of the study (662 d) was (0.023 ± 0.02) % of the implanted uranium, which for 2.6 g of DU implanted is ~600 g, an amount large enough to have been seen in the tissue sections.

[7]Hahn, F.F. (2003). Personal communication (Lovelace Respiratory Research Institute, Albuquerque, New Mexico).

B.4 Insoluble Particles of Mixed Composition

B.4.1 *Mixed Oxide Particles Injected Intramuscularly in Rats*

A saline suspension of particles of strongly ignited (1,750 °C) industrial MOX nuclear fuel $(Pu,U)O_{1.96}$ was i.m. injected in rats (Paquet *et al.*, 2003). The MOX preparation was, by weight, 74 % UO_2, 26 % PuO_2, and <0.1 % ^{241}Am; each rat was given 130 μg of plutonium, 370 μg of uranium, and <0.4 μg of ^{241}Am. Size was not reported, but the maximum particle diameter was likely to have been ≤5 μm (Eidson, 1980a; Stanley *et al.*, 1982). At 8 d, the fractions of the deposited nuclides cleared from the wound site and their estimated initial wound clearance half-times were as follows: plutonium, 3.1 %, 176 d; americium, 19.8 %, 25 d; uranium, 64.5 %, 5.4 d. The plutonium leaving the wound site was translocated to the carcass (mainly bone) and liver, and a small fraction was excreted. The americium exiting the wound site was translocated to the liver and bone, and a small fraction was excreted. The uranium was translocated from the wound site to the kidneys and bone, and ~36 % of the deposited uranium was excreted, mainly in the urine. The local lymph nodes were not analyzed. However, the differences between the estimated radionuclide contents of the whole skeleton (20 times that of one femur) and the carcass (minus liver and kidneys) were <3 % of the injected amounts of the three constituent radionuclides, suggesting little translocation of intact MOX particles to regional lymph nodes in 8 d.

The fraction of the plutonium that initially dissolved in the i.m. wound was about the same as it was *in vitro* in a simulated serum ultra filtrate, while the americium, and to a greater degree, the uranium, were initially dissolved more efficiently *in vivo* (Eidson, 1980a). Changes in the surface chemistry of the MOX particles caused by adsorption of atmospheric H_2O and CO_3^{2-} (Eidson, 1980b) were likely to have been important contributors to the initial rapid dissolution of its components, especially the UO_2, both *in vitro* (Eidson, 1980a) and at the i.m. wound site, and to the relatively efficient initial dissolution of $^{235}UO_2$ particles deposited in an i.m. wound in rats (Appendix B.3.1; Beiter *et al.*, 1975).

Later dissolution of the plutonium and americium components of the MOX preparation in serum ultra filtrate was essentially the same as for $PuO_2 \cdot AmO_2$ mechanically mixed with UO_2, while the presence of the less-soluble PuO_2 in the MOX solid solution apparently impeded late dissolution of the UO_2 component, compared with that of the UO_2 admixed with PuO_2 (Eidson, 1980a). If the dissolution rates *in vivo* give useful guidance about the late clearance of the MOX components from an i.m. wound, the residues of each retained at 8 d after injection can be expected to be cleared slowly, at an average rate of ~6 × 10⁻⁵ d⁻¹ (Eidson, 1980a).

B.4.2 *Minispheres Contaminated with Plutonium and Amercium Implanted Subcutaneously in Rats*

Particles (minispheres) contaminated with plutonium isotopes and ^{241}Am were collected from a former nuclear weapons test site at Maralinga, Australia (Harrison *et al.*, 1990; 1993). In all, eight atmospheric nuclear weapons tests were conducted at that site in 1956 and 1957, of which six were surface or tower bursts (Perkins and Thomas, 1980). Under the intense temperature conditions of nuclear fission explosions variable amounts of plutonium isotopes were mixed with a variety of melted and/or vaporized materials, which upon cooling, returned to the ground as local fallout. The radioactive contamination of some particles of local weapons test fallout exists as a thin shell that condensed on the surfaces of cooling particles, but particles of materials that were vaporized and intimately mixed with vaporized fission products, radioactive weapons residues, and neutron activation products trapped those radionuclides as they cooled, and they are contaminated rather uniformly (Freiling, 1961; Glasstone, 1962).

As shown in Table B.11, minispheres with six different chemical compositions were identified by x-ray analysis for this study. Particles composed mainly of aluminum (light alloy 2/1), carbon steel (ferromagnetic 1/5), or high impact polystyrene (plastic 25) are considered to have originated from strongly heated or melted construction materials; those composed mainly of UO_2 (U317) from vaporized weapons debris; and those composed mainly of limestone (oxide 8/1) or clay (organic 8/5) from vaporized soil constituents that were sucked up into the stem, dirt cloud, and fireball of the surface and tower-burst nuclear explosions.

Average particle diameter was 1 mm with a range of 0.5 to 2 mm; on average, the surface area was 3.1 mm², with a surface to volume ratio of ~60 cm⁻¹. The median plutonium and americium contents (kilobecquerel) of the individual particles of each specific composition are also shown in Table B.11.

For each of the six particle composition categories, 12 rats were implanted with one particle inserted surgically under the skin of the ventral surface of a hind paw. Those rats were killed in groups of six at 30 and 180 d to determine the distributions of the nuclides in the tissues. No excreta were collected. Some additional rats were implanted with particles and held for 1 y or longer. They were used

TABLE B.11—*Translocation from s.c. implants in rat paws of ^{239}Pu and ^{241}Am contaminants of minispheres composed of nuclear weapons test debris.*[a]

Particle Material[b]	Sample Code[c]	Nuclide	Median Activity (kBq)	Total Translocated Fraction (%) [d,e]		Fraction of Amount Translocated to Specific Tissues in 180 d (%)[f]	
				30 d	180 d	Tissues	Lymph Nodes
Aluminum	Light alloy (2/1)	^{239}Pu	48	0.073	0.44	30	0.9
		^{241}Am	2.4	0.05	0.25	36	0.4
Polystyrene	Plastic (25)	^{239}Pu	8.2	0.19	0.32	52	0.4
		^{241}Am	1.2	0.12	0.12	46	0.3
Carbon Steel	Ferro-magnetic (1/5)	^{239}Pu	16	0.04	0.18	51	0.2
		^{241}Am	0.9	0.038	0.13	90	6.2
Limestone	Oxide (8/1)	^{239}Pu	39	0.019	0.008	74	1.3
		^{241}Am	6.2	0.011	0.016	89	3.8
UO_2	Uranium (U317)	^{239}Pu	50	0.004	0.005	81	1.2
		^{241}Am	4.8	0.005	0.004	70	0.9
Clay	Organic (8/5)	^{239}Pu	390	0.0013	0.0046	20	1.4
		^{241}Am	26	0.0024	0.0012	38	3.1

[a]Calculated from the data of Harrison et al. (1990).
[b]Main chemical constituents of particles.
[c]Author's original sample code designation.
[d]Sum of nuclide recovered in all tissues, lymph nodes, and the injected leg proximal to the implant in the paw.
[e]Difference from 100 % is fraction in the injected leg proximal to the implant in the paw.
[f]Includes data from rats killed at 7, 90 and 365 d (Harrison et al., 1990).

primarily to determine the tissue response to the particles and to prepare autoradiographs of the tissue surrounding the implants as described in Appendix B.6.3.

Tissues taken at necropsy included inguinal and iliac lymph nodes, the implanted paw, liver, both femora, the remainders of both hind legs, and the residual carcass. The tissues were dry and wet ashed, and the implant sites were further treated with concentrated hydrofluoric acid and HNO_3 to obtain complete dissolution of the particles. Preparation of the dissolved samples for separate determination of plutonium and americium by alpha spectrometry is described. The radiochemically measured activity ratio of plutonium to [241]Am (ingrown from decay of [241]Pu) ranged from 6:1 to 19:1. Because the particle sizes and the concentrations of plutonium and americium in the individual particles of each specific material varied, it was necessary to use each rat as its own control and to express the radioanalytical results as fractions (percent) of the total amounts of plutonium and americium recovered.

The tissue distribution data for plutonium and americium at 30 and 180 d are summarized in Table B.11. The fractions of the implanted actinides (percent of recovered plutonium and [241]Am) translocated from the wound site are slightly underestimated, because account was not taken of hepatobiliary excretion and rapid loss of some of the initial bone deposit, which are important features of actinide biokinetics in rats (Finkle *et al.*, 1947; Scott *et al.*, 1948a; 1948b; Taylor *et al.*, 1961).

The average fractions of plutonium and americium translocated from the minispheres in 180 d were, respectively, 0.31 and 0.17 % of the implanted amounts from the particles composed mainly of construction materials and 0.006 and 0.007 % from the particles composed mainly of UO_2 or soil constituents. Translocation of both plutonium and americium at 180 d did not depend on the actinide concentrations in the particles; correlations were weakly negative. The chemical compositions and thermal histories of the minispheres appeared to be important factors underlying the solubilization of their contained actinides. Both nuclides were more tightly held in the minispheres composed mainly of soil constituents (limestone, clay) or UO_2, which contained the greatest concentrations of the nuclides, indicating that those particles were more uniformly contaminated.

Substantial fractions of the small amounts of the plutonium and americium translocated (≥20 %) were located in the tissues (liver, bones and carcass), but in some cases, more than one-half of both nuclides translocated from the implant site was associated with the tissues of the leg proximal to the implanted paw. The authors considered that only the fractions of the nuclides translocated to the tissues had been dissolved. They attributed the substantial fractions of translocated nuclides retained in the implant leg to movement, perhaps by lymphatic drainage of undissolved material, but that does not appear to be the most likely explanation. The fractions of the plutonium and americium translocated from the various minispheres to the draining lymph nodes were quite small; the degree of fragmentation of the minispheres that were studied autoradiographically was not remarkable; substantial alpha activity in the vicinity of the minispheres at the implant site was associated with tissue structures (Appendix B.6.3). Combined, these observations suggest that the nuclides were being leached from the solid minispheres in soluble form as chemical species that could be bound by local tissue constituents or complexed and transported in tissue fluid, and were not being moved with intact insoluble particles small enough to be phagocytized.

The translocated fractions measured at 180 d were greater than those measured at 30 d in 8 of the 12 comparisons available (shown in Table B.11), indicating progressive solubilization of the actinides associated with the particles. In four cases, the translocated fractions at 180 d were the same or slightly less than those measured at 30 d. However, those discrepancies were likely to have been experimental artifacts; both the sizes and compositions of the particles varied within each particle composition category. In these cases only small amounts of actinide had been translocated at either sampling time, and the standard errors of the mean actinide contents of the tissue samples were large.

The data from this study were not adequate for analysis with the wound model. However, the patterns of plutonium and americium absorption from the fallout particles composed mainly of structural materials were similar to each other, and both resembled the absorption of uranium in rats implanted with wafers of DU metal (Appendix B.3.4). Simulation modeling was used to estimate an equation that describes the combined retention of the plutonium and americium in those fallout particles at the s.c.-implant site. Transfer rates for absorption of uranium from implanted DU metal were used as starting parameter values in the wound model (Section 4), and they were varied until acceptable fits were obtained to both the systemic and lymph-node data (Table B.11). The equation for combined retention of plutonium and americium at the implant site is, where t is days after implant:

$$R(t)_{\text{Pu,Am}} = 0.24e^{-0.02t} + 99.76e^{-3.3 \times 10^{-8}t}, \tag{B.21}$$

for the fallout minispheres composed mainly of structural materials.

The amounts of plutonium and americium translocated from the minispheres composed mainly of UO_2 or soil constituents were so small and their absorption patterns were so variable that clearance of the actinides from the implant site after 30 d is uncertain. A reasonable estimate of the retention at the implant site of plutonium and americium combined in fallout particles composed mainly of UO_2 or soil constituents is, where t is days after implant:

$$R(t)_{Pu,Am} = 100e^{-3.5 \times 10^{-7} t}. \qquad (B.22)$$

It must be recognized that the data are not adequate to define the long-term clearance rates for these particles. Thus, the values quoted in Equation B.21 (3.3×10^{-8} d^{-1}) and Equation B.22 (3.5×10^{-7} d^{-1}) should be regarded as uncertain, but nonetheless very small.

B.5 Colloidal ^{232}ThO$_2$ "Thorotrast"®

Thorotrast® is an aqueous colloidal suspension of nanometer-sized particles of strongly heated ^{232}ThO$_2$ stabilized with colloidal dextran (a starch derivative). It was used clinically as a radiographic contrast medium from about 1930 to 1955 (Carrigan, 1967; IAEA, 1964). Nearly all of the mass of the standard Thorotrast® suspension is ^{232}Th (25 % by weight), but most of the activity is contributed by the chain decay of its alpha-emitting progeny (Dudley, 1967). Preparation of Thorotrast® involved high-temperature calcination (550 °C) of thorium oxalate for several hours to produce ThO$_2$; strongly ignited ThO$_2$ is one of the most refractory substances known, and it is dissolved only by long heating in concentrated acids (Carrigan, 1967; Katzin, 1957).

Reticuloendothelial cells throughout the body accumulate i.v.-injected Thorotrast®. For example, the distribution of ^{232}Th in the whole body of a patient 36 y after i.v. injection of Thorotrast® was liver, 45 %; bones and marrow, 34.6 %; spleen, 13.3 %; lymph nodes, 2.8 %; rest of tissues, 4.5 %; and a cervical Thorotrast® granuloma contained 3.5 % of the total ^{232}Th recovered (McInroy et al., 1992).

The reported size of the ThO$_2$ particles of Thorotrast® ranges from ~7 nm (Grampa, 1967; Kathren and Hill, 1992; Riedel et al., 1983) to ~150 nm (Carrigan, 1967; Hyman and Paldino, 1967). The effective size of the particles after the Thorotrast® suspension (ThO$_2$ plus dextran) has mixed with the blood serum has not been determined. The lack of prompt renal filtration and the efficient uptake in the reticuloendothelial cells in the bone marrow as well as those in the liver and spleen suggest that initially the effective size of the circulating particles is on the order of 10 nm (Berliner, 1973; Dobson et al., 1949; Tessmer and Chang, 1967).

With time the Thorotrast$^®$ particles become aggregated within the phagocyte lysosomes, particularly in the Kupfer cells of the liver (Hampton and Rosario, 1967; Tessmer and Chang, 1967). For all practical purposes (see above) the phagocytized ThO$_2$ is not dissolved. The "stored" Thorotrast$^®$ may be released to new generations of phagocytes, transported by macrophages within a s.c.- or i.m.-injection site and to regional lymph nodes, or become involved within fibrous connective tissue (da Horta, 1967b; Faber, 1962; McInroy et al., 1992; Tessmer and Chang, 1967). Very little ^{232}Th i.v. injected as Thorotrast$^®$ particles is excreted. Hursh (1967) determined that ~0.5 % of ^{232}Th i.v. injected as Thorotrast$^®$ in two patients was excreted in the first three weeks and that the long-term excretion rate was ~3.5×10^{-4} % d^{-1}, implying a half-time in the body longer than 500 y.

As a positive radiation control in a study of the local effects of i.m.-implanted DU metal (Appendix B.3.4), Hahn et al. (2002) i.m.-injected Thorotrast$^®$ (115 Bq alpha at each site) in the femoris biceps muscle of each hind leg of rats. The injected ThO$_2$ was determined radiographically to be localized initially in a tiny sphere of tissue, but with time the radiopaque ThO$_2$ migrated and dispersed within the muscle tissue apparently along the fascial planes of the muscle tissue. ThO$_2$-laden macrophages infiltrated the connective tissue between the muscle fiber bundles. The major draining lumbar and popliteal lymph nodes contained microscopically identifiable ThO$_2$ particles, but the amounts that had migrated were not determined.[8]

Unfortunately, none of the investigations of "wounds" contaminated with Thorotrast$^®$, neither the human cases of Thorotrast$^®$ granulomas nor the animal experiments, provide quantitative information about retention of the ^{232}ThO$_2$ deposited at the wound site. However, they demonstrate that, when s.c. or i.m. deposited, some of these small refractory particles can be transported within macrophages from the original deposition site to regional lymph nodes and within the wounded tissue mass.

[8]Hahn, F.F. (2003). Personal communication (Lovelace Respiratory Research Institute, Albuquerque, New Mexico).

B.6 Late Effects in Wounds
Containing Insoluble Radionuclides

B.6.1 *Air-Oxidized $^{239}PuO_2$ Particles Implanted Subcutaneously in Dog Paws*

The main purposes of this study were to identify and assess the late biological effects of sustained alpha irradiation at the site of an implant of 350 kBq of PuO_2 in 0.25 mL of saline and in the regional lymph nodes draining the site, and also to trace the status and effects of the plutonium that migrated from those locations (Dagle *et al.*, 1984). The tissues known to accumulate soluble plutonium (mainly liver and skeleton) and the tissues with important reticuloendothelial components that accumulate particles (mainly liver, spleen, and bone marrow) were of special interest (Bair *et al.*, 1973; ICRP, 1972; Vaughan, 1973).

Variable hair loss and dermal thickening at the injection site, observed in two dogs 1 y after the PuO_2 implant, were common by 5 to 8 y. Focal atrophy and scarring of the subcubitis were seen at the injection sites of all dogs with PuO_2 implants, and local tissue damage was extensive and severe. Atrophy of dermal adnexal tissue was seen in six of the eight dogs that came to necropsy. Autoradiographs showed pronounced accumulations of overlapping plutonium aggregates (observed as alpha track stars) concentrated in the central areas of the scars; there were few single alpha tracks. No neoplasms or microscopic evidence suggesting neoplastic changes were seen in the tissues in and around the implant sites.

The regional lymph nodes were greatly reduced in size, and in five dogs nothing remained except scar tissue. The scar tissue consisted of small knots of dense collagen with mature fibroblasts in the cortical areas, enclosing hypocellular medullary areas containing large alpha track stars associated with hemosiderin granules.

At 8 y, some of the plutonium implanted as air-oxidized PuO_2 particles was found in the radiochemically analyzed tissues other than the wound site and regional lymph nodes. Nearly all of the plutonium demonstrated autoradiographically in liver, spleen and kidneys was present as particles or aggregates. The amounts of plutonium translocated to the liver were sufficient to cause significant tissue damage, exemplified by adenomatous hyperplasia and accumulations of hemosiderin, and to induce multiple hepatomas in one dog. The amount of plutonium apparently solubilized and translocated to the bone surfaces was sufficient to induce multiple osteosarcomas in one dog.

B.6.2 *High-Fired $^{239}PuO_2$ Particles in Lymph Nodes*

Small (0.7 μm GMD) particles of high-fired $^{232}PuO_2$ similar to those studied by Bistline (1973) were s.c. implanted in the hind paws of dogs to investigate the progression of damage and late effects in the regional (popliteal) lymph nodes (Dagle *et al.*, 1975). Four weeks after the implants, the lymph nodes contained small irregular areas that were obliterated by reticular cells, macrophages, fibrous connective tissue, and diffuse neutrophil infiltration; the remainder of the tissue was intact with normal morphology. Between 8 and 32 weeks, scar tissue, which had replaced large areas of these lymph nodes, encapsulated volumes as large as 0.5 cm in diameter. The scar tissue was composed of dense fibrous tissue streaked with strands of collagen in an eosinophilic matrix; that matrix, which became progressively less cellular towards the center, also contained foci of hemorrhage and arterial necrosis. Adjacent to the scar tissue, the most damaged nodes contained increased numbers of reticular cells and macrophages that obliterated areas of both the nodal cortex and medulla. In some cases, scar tissue had obliterated and replaced all of the normal structure of the node.

Electron micrographs showed that the plutonium accumulated in the popliteal nodes only as phagocytosed particles within the phagolysosomes. The plutonium particles were polygonal, had smooth or slightly serrated borders, and although generally electron opaque, were occasionally less dense at the periphery. The plutonium particles were distinct and not enveloped by hemosiderin. The association of plutonium particles and hemosiderin in macrophages is believed to be the result of phagocytosis of multiple kinds of particulate material by the same macrophages. Similarly, the aggregation of plutonium particles within macrophages was attributed to the gathering of smaller individual particles during rephagocytosis after the deaths of the previous generation of macrophages.

B.6.3 *Plutonium Metal Wire Implanted Subcutaneously in Rats and Rabbits*

Adult rats and rabbits were observed for as long as 1,048 d after s.c. implantation of tiny pieces of ^{239}Pu metal wire (1 mm diameter, 0.04 to 0.12 mm thick, 0.61 to 1.33 mg plutonium) (Appendix B.1.5; Lisco and Kisieleski, 1953). Serial x rays showed that the pieces of plutonium wire disintegrated rapidly into smaller fragments and granules, greatly increasing the surface area of the plutonium implants; at necropsy, the plutonium metal implants had corroded into tiny fragments coated with oxide and coarse to fine green-black granules of hydrous plutonium oxides. The area of tissue reaction surrounding the plutonium implants in the rabbits increased from 3×3 mm at 2 d to $(33 \pm 25) \times (16 \pm 10)$ mm at death. The areas of tissue involvement at the plutonium implant sites in the rats were smaller, $(3.8 \pm 0.8) \times (3 \pm 0.5)$ mm at death.

Apart from the difference in size, the plutonium implant sites in the rats and rabbits changed similarly with time. The serial x rays showed that at 14 d the piece of plutonium wire had broken up into smaller fragments that were confined to an area that was still small, but larger than that initially occupied by the piece of plutonium wire implanted. Later x rays demonstrated the presence of smaller granules embedded in localized but gradually increasing volumes of progressively more dense calcifying soft tissue. Over time, there were substantial changes in the size, density, and general configuration of those tissue masses in four of the seven long-surviving rabbits. In the other three rabbits and the rats, the plutonium implant sites remained relatively small, stationary, well circumscribed, and localized.

At necropsy the implant sites in both species were well-defined masses of firm consistency resembling calcified plaques; they adhered firmly either to the derma or the underlying muscle. The implant sites in two of the rabbits were described in more detail. At death at 260 d, the smaller implant site (9×5 mm) showed a few green-black granular deposits just beneath the surface of the slightly elevated central portion. The corresponding x rays showed coarse radiopaque granules scattered throughout about two-thirds of the tissue mass at the implant site with a few granules scattered in the periphery of the remainder. The larger implant site from the rabbit that died at 623 d (53×24 mm) adhered tightly to the underlying abdominal muscle; there was gradual dispersal of the granular material, so that at death the granules were more concentrated in the upper portion, while lesser concentrations of granules were scattered throughout the rest of the calcified tissue mass.

The plutonium implant sites in the rats remained smaller but were grossly similar to those in the rabbits. The absence of a more vigorous widespread tissue response in the rats was regarded by the authors as "striking." The lesions in the rats consisted of a central ovoid portion containing a few green-black granules that were visible through the surface layer of tissue. At each end of the oval there were foci of calcified material. The central portion (3×3 mm) appeared to contain nearly all of the plutonium metal shards and granular corrosion products.

The implant site in the rabbit that died 2 d after the implant showed no grossly visible evidence of an inflammatory reaction, which led the authors to suggest that plutonium metal *per se* is not a tissue irritant.

B.6.4 *Depleted Uranium Metal Fragments Implanted Intramuscularly in Rats*

Small wafers of DU metal were implanted surgically in the muscle of the hind legs of rats (Appendix B.3.4; Hahn *et al.*, 2002). The radiographic appearance of the fragments changed markedly during the first year. At 21 d, small dense outgrowths extended from the previously sharp edges of the fragments, making them appear larger than at implantation. At 1 y, the fragments had lost their edge sharpness, and at death, their radiographic profiles were often 50 % larger than originally, due to surface corrosion and fibrous capsule formation. The capsular tissue adhered to the fragments, and a layer of black granular material was left on the inner surface of the capsules. The capsules were histologically characterized by fibrosis, inflammation, degeneration and demineralization, with shards of black material, presumably uranium, embedded in the fibrous tissue. Chronic inflammatory cells and particle-laden macrophages were frequently scattered throughout the capsule wall. The interface of the fibrous tissue of the capsule with the implant was often devitalized and necrotic. The lumen of the capsules contained necrotic and proteinaceous debris, acute inflammatory cells, and varying amounts of black shards and particles and particle-laden macrophages. Osteosarcomas and soft tissue tumors such as malignant fibrous histiocytomas and fibrosarcomas, were noted in some of the animals, all associated with the capsules surrounding the implant sites.

B.6.5 ^{239}Pu and ^{241}Am *in Subcutaneous Tissue After Implantation of Contaminated Minispheres*

Histological sections and autoradiographs were prepared of the s.c.-implant sites of some rats killed 1 y or longer after insertion of ^{239}Pu-plus ^{241}Am-contaminated minispheres (~1 mm mean diameter) composed mainly of aluminum, polystyrene, or carbon steel. In all cases, the minispheres were encapsulated with fibrous tissue, which was surrounded by collections of polymorphonuclear cells and macrophages. The autoradiographs of the implant sites containing minispheres of the materials noted above suggest some fragmentation at the metallic surfaces, which would have slightly accelerated plutonium and americium dissolution from the increased surface areas. The hair follicles close to the polystyrene minispheres contained alpha activity. Alpha activity was associated with macrophages and polymorphonuclear cells of the fibrotic tissue surrounding the aluminum minispheres and with hair follicles and sebaceous glands throughout the sections. The fibrotic tissue surrounding the carbon steel minispheres contained many single alpha tracks and aggregates of tracks (stars), and alpha activity was spread throughout the sections with notable concentrations in hair follicles, sebaceous glands, and blood vessels (Harrison et al., 1990; 1993).

B.6.6 *Deposited $^{232}ThO_2$ Particles (Thorotrast®)*

The pathological effects of Thorotrast® arise mainly in the organs of greatest deposition—liver, spleen, and bone marrow (Abbatt, 1967; da Horta, 1967a; Faber, 1962; Faber and Johansen 1967; Dahlgren, 1967b). However, there are also severe late appearing consequences of the accidental deposition of Thorotrast® in the s.c. tissues adjacent to an intravascular injection site, most often the carotid artery in the neck (da Horta, 1967b; Faber, 1962; Stougaard et al., 1984; Tauber, 1992). The extravasated Thorotrast® induced formation of dense locally invasive fibrotic masses (Thorotrast® granulomas) that encapsulated the $^{232}ThO_2$. Some of those Thorotrast® granulomas eventually gave rise at their edges to local malignant neoplasms. Some of the extravasated ThO_2 migrated locally, transported within macrophages, contributing to the progressive expansion and extension of the granulomas and involvement of adjacent structures (da Horta, 1967b).

Induction of sarcomas in reticuloendothelial tissues was investigated in rabbits injected in an ear vein with varying amounts of Thorotrast®. Fibrosarcomas developed slowly at the injection site in a few of the animals. Thorium was present within all of those tumors (Johansen, 1967).

Chinese hamsters were i.v. injected with Thorotrast® to investigate radiation-induced liver cancer. The injections were made into the surgically exposed jugular vein through the leading edge of the pectoralis muscle. Locally invasive fibrosarcomas developed in the cervical region adjacent to the injection site. Tumor incidence was positively correlated with Thorotrast® dosage; 54 % of the hamsters injected with the largest amount of Thorotrast®, 7.4 Bq g^{-1} body weight, developed tumors. Most of the tumors contained aggregated ThO_2, located mainly within macrophages (Guilmette et al., 1989).

Hahn *et al.* (2002) i.m.-injected Thorotrast® in the legs of rats and followed them for their lifespan (Appendix B.5). The ThO_2 particles were not encapsulated nor was there inflammation at the injection sites, and no fibrotic or proliferative local lesions were seen. Malignant soft tissue tumors developed at 23 % of the injected sites in the legs of the rats treated with Thorotrast®.

Appendix C

Translocation of Radionuclides from Wounds

This Appendix provides brief descriptions of the experimental evidence that was used to develop the transport model for radionuclides in contaminated wounds.

C.1 Demonstrations of Transport of Radionuclides Deposited in Aqueous Solution

Transport of soluble and relatively insoluble radionuclides from wounds has been repeatedly demonstrated indirectly by the correlation of the tissue distributions of the translocated radionuclides and those observed after parenteral injection. Transport of slowly dissolved radionuclides from a wound has also been demonstrated indirectly by the correlation of the tissue distributions after injection of hydrolyzable uncomplexed radionuclides and those same radionuclides injected as soluble complexes, as for example, with citrate ion (ICRP, 1959; 1972).

C.1.1 *Chemical Studies*

C.1.1.1 *Initial Transport of Pu^{4+} in Lymph.* Studies in dogs have quantified the transport of soluble and/or colloidal Pu^{4+} in lymph. Two dogs were s.c. injected in a hind paw with $^{239}Pu(NO_3)_4$ (Schallberger, 1974; Schallberger *et al.*, 1976). Details were not reported, but it is likely that the experimental conditions were the same as those in the contemporaneous studies of Bistline (1973) and Dagle *et al.* (1984), in which dogs were s.c. injected in a paw with a colloidal suspension of $Pu(NO_3)_4$ at pH 2.4 (Appendix B.1.1.6). Under continuous anesthesia, starting immediately after the plutonium injection, all lymph that would have entered the popliteal node (afferent lymph) was collected from one dog of the pair at 30 min intervals for 4 h, and lymph leaving that node (efferent lymph) was similarly collected from the second dog. The acellular (fluid) fraction of the afferent lymph collected during the 4 h of the experiment contained 1,000 times more of the injected plutonium than the cellular fraction. The fluid fraction of the efferent lymph contained 40 times more of the injected plutonium than the cellular fraction. The study was not repeated, and the afferent and efferent lymph were collected from different dogs, so only generalizations are possible. However, the data suggest that some of the plutonium transported to the lymph node in the afferent lymph may have been weak complexes with albumin or low molecular weight bioligands, which dissociated in the node and was, at least temporarily, retained there. The plutonium in the fluid portions of the lymph samples was not separated into protein-bound and low molecular weight fractions, but transferrin was found to be the dominant plutonium-binding protein in both afferent and efferent lymph. The plutonium-transferrin complex was apparently sufficiently stable to pass through the lymph node unchanged.

C.1.1.2 *Renal Clearance of Plutonium Injected Subcutaneously in Dog Paws as Colloidal $^{239}Pu(NO_3)_4$.* Renal clearance provides information about the status of metal ions in the blood plasma, that is, as filterable low molecular weight complexes, nonfilterable protein complexes, or minute particles. Solubilized plutonium cleared from a wound to blood is expected to be either in the form of the nonfilterable transferrin complex (90 to 95 %) or in the form of filterable low molecular weight complexes with small bioligands like citrate ion (Popplewell *et al.*, 1975). In that case, its renal clearance should be similar to that of i.v.-injected soluble Pu^{4+} citrate in the same species (Stevens *et al.*, 1968; Stover *et al.*, 1959; 1968). Very small renally filterable particles (nanoparticles) such as those investigated by Harrison *et al.* (1978a) would be expected to be more efficiently cleared from blood to urine than plutonium that is in large part bound to nonfilterable protein. Larger, nonfilterable particles that enter the circulation would be expected to be scavenged by reticuloendothelial cells in liver, spleen, and bone marrow and not to pass through the glomeruli into the urine.

Stover *et al.* (1959) published pairs of logarithmic equations describing the kinetics of plutonium in the plasma volume and the daily urinary excretion of beagle dogs during the intervals 1 to 22 d and 22 to 1,460 d after an i.v. injection of monomeric Pu^{4+} citrate.

Renal clearances of plutonium were 7.5 and 9 % of the plutonium in the plasma volume per day, respectively, as calculated from the ratios of the integrals of those pairs of equations ($\text{urine}_1/\text{plasma}_1$) and ($\text{urine}_2/\text{plasma}_2$).

The method of Stover *et al.* (1959) was used to analyze the blood and urine plutonium data from five groups of dogs s.c. injected in the paw with 15 to 52 µg of colloidal $^{239}\text{Pu(NO}_3)_4$ at pH 2.4 [as described in Appendix B.1.1.6 (Bistline, 1973)]. The blood and urine plutonium data (Table B.3) are plotted in Figure C.1. Those 20 dogs provided data for as long as 185 d, and plutonium was readily detected in the later blood and urine samples. The four dogs of Group 6 were followed for 365 d, but they received about one-tenth as much plutonium as those in the other groups, and the data for blood and urinary plutonium were not as reliable.

The set of four logarithmic curves shown in Figure C.1 was obtained from the combined data for 20 dogs using the Origin® graphics program; their equations are:

$$B_1 \ (1-10 \ \text{d}) = 5.2t^{-1.21} \text{ and } B_2 \ (10-185 \ \text{d}) = 0.85t^{-0.48}, \qquad \text{(C.1)}$$

where B_1 and B_2 are plutonium in the blood volume (% *ID*), and t is days after injection, and:

$$U_1 \ (1-10 \ \text{d}) = 1.2t^{-2.16} \text{ and } U_2 \ (10-185 \ \text{d}) = 0.039t^{-0.38}, \qquad \text{(C.2)}$$

where U_1 and U_2 are daily urinary plutonium excretion rates (percent of injected dosage excreted per day), and t is days after injection.

The percent of the blood volume cleared per day by urinary excretion is the quotient of the integrals of $B(t)$ and $U(t)$ and from Equations C.1 and C.2 are:

$$U_1 B_1^{-1} = 10 \text{ % and } U_2 B_2^{-1} = 8 \text{ %} \qquad \text{(C.3)}$$

of the blood volume plutonium cleared per day to urine.

The agreement between the estimated renal clearance of plutonium dogs s.c. injected with colloidal Pu^{4+} hydroxide and those i.v. injected with soluble Pu^{4+} citrate is evidence for the gradual solubilization and transfer to blood of some of the colloidal plutonium hydroxide deposited at the wound site.

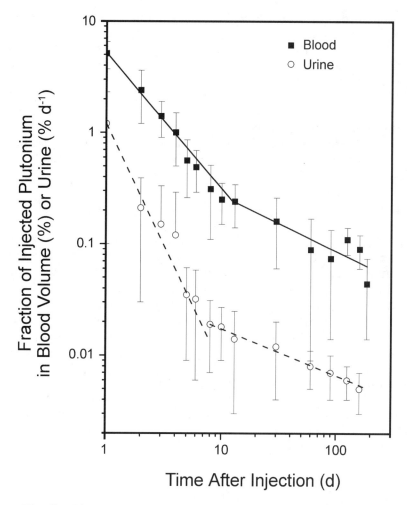

Fig. C.1. Plutonium in the blood volume and daily urinary excretion of dogs s.c. injected in a paw with 15 to 52 µg of colloidal ^{239}Pu hydroxide. Curves correspond to Equation C.1 for blood plutonium and Equation C.2 for urinary plutonium excretion rate (Bistline, 1973).

C.1.2 *Autoradiographic Studies*

C.1.2.1 *Radionuclide Penetration of Tissue Fluid.* Studies in mice demonstrate dispersion of Pu^{4+} locally in tissue fluid. Mice were s.c. injected on the back with 0.1 mL of a solution containing "monomeric" ^{239}Pu^{4+} citrate (at least partly in the form of 5 nm diameter particles) (Matsuoka *et al.*, 1972). Penetration into the tissue surrounding the injection site 1 to 3 d later was demonstrated in whole-body autoradiographs. An estimate of the volume of tissue penetrated was obtained from measurement of the length and thickness of the autoradiographic images. Assuming that the three-dimensional shape was a thin circular disc, the volume penetrated was estimated to be ~0.8 cm^3. That tissue mass contains ~0.25 mL of tissue fluid or more than twice the volume of fluid injected, demonstrating that small solutes initially flow with the tissue fluid. Transport of plutonium from the s.c. site was shown by the presence at 3 d of substantial amounts of plutonium demonstrated as single alpha tracks in liver and on endosteal bone surfaces.

C.1.2.2 $^{239}Pu(NO_3)_4$ *Injected Intramuscularly in Rats.* Studies in rats have shown the retention pattern of i.m.-injected Pu^{4+}. ^{239}Pu(NO$_3$)$_4$ (~0.1 μg in 50 μL, pH 1) was injected into the *exterior cruris* muscle of rats *via* an incision in the pelt, and the histopathology and microscopic distribution of the plutonium retained at the wound site were investigated (Harrison *et al.*, 1978a). At 1 d, local damage caused by passage of the injection needle and introduction of the small amount of excess H$^+$ had elicited an inflammatory reaction with in-migration of polymorphonuclear leukocytes. The plutonium was distributed rather uniformly throughout the connective tissue separating the muscle fiber bundles as single tracks and a few small aggregates of tracks. By 7 d, the plutonium was still limited to the intermuscular connective tissue, single alpha tracks were fewer in number, and most of the plutonium was present as aggregates (some quite large). Those results imply progressive polymerization and phagocytosis of Pu^{4+} hydroxide formed at the injection site.

C.1.2.3 $^{210}Po^{4+}$ *and* $^{241}Am^{3+}$ *Applied to Lacerations or Abraded Skin of Rats.* Studies of wounded skin of rats show local migration of radionuclides applied to the surface. Autoradiographs were prepared of lacerated skin contaminated with ^{210}Po and ^{241}Am. At 1 d, most of the alpha tracks from both radionuclides were seen as aggregates associated with the cut surface, but there was evidence of radionuclide migration, as shown by some smaller cluster and single tracks in the adjacent connective tissue and the connective tissue layers of the cut muscle. Autoradiographs of abraded rat skin cut perpendicularly to the surface showed that at 1 d nearly all of the applied ^{210}Po and ^{241}Am were present as large aggregates on the epidermal surface. There were spatially separated "stripes" of less dense clusters of tracks and single alpha tracks that penetrated deeply into the dermis and connective tissue of the underlying muscle. That pattern of radionuclide distribution provides evidence for radionuclide migration through the perforations in the abraded epidermis (Ilyin, 2001; Ilyin and Ivannikov, 1979; Ilyin *et al.*, 1977).

C.2 Status of Soluble Radionuclides Deposited in a Wound

C.2.1 *Initial Observations*

The restoration of tissue structural relationships, osmotic equilibrium, and acid-base balance begins immediately after injection of an aqueous solution *via* a puncture wound. Excess injected water and small mobile solutes, H^+, Na^+, Cl^-, NO_3^-, diffuse away from the site rapidly into the blood and lymph capillaries, reducing any edema and restoring osmotic equilibrium. Diffusion of H^+ and neutralization by the abundant HCO_3^- of extracellular fluid promptly reduce the local H^+ concentration in the tissue fluid at the wound site to reestablish physiological pH (Cronkite, 1973). All of those processes combine to increase the local concentration of the deposited contaminant.

C.2.1.1 *Elements That Do Not Hydrolyze at Physiological pH*. Radionuclides in stable oxidation states that do not react with water (hydrolyze) or form stable compounds or complexes with fixed tissue constituents at pH 7.4 are rapidly translocated from a wound site *via* the tissue fluid. The injected salts and water, for example, anions and most mono- and divalent cations are also cleared in this manner. However, some of those elements form sparingly soluble compounds with tissue fluid constituents, such as Cl^-, CO_3^{2-}, or SO_4^{2-}, which, depending on the mass of element deposited appear to dissolve gradually and translocate from the wound site within days to weeks.

C.2.1.2 *Elements That Hydrolyze at Physiological pH*. Many of the elements of Periodic Groups IIIB and IIIA (3, 13) have e/r ratios that are sufficiently large for them to be regarded as "hard" metal ions (Shannon, 1976). Their affinities for oxy anions range from moderate to strong, and they react with water (hydrolyze) at physiological pH to form hydroxide microcolloids at low concentrations and crystalline hydroxide precipitates at high concentrations. The trivalent metal ions form variably stable transportable soluble complexes with the organic acids and transferrin in plasma and tissue fluid and immobile complexes with the carboxyl side chains of fixed proteins. Trivalent $^{241}Am^{3+}$ is representative of elements with these properties. Variable fractions of the trivalent radionuclides (<5 μg deposited), ranging from 15 % of $^{241}Am^{3+}$ to 68 % of $^{67}Ga^{3+}$ with a mean of 34 ± 13 % of the amounts injected, were cleared from an i.m. wound site in rats in 1 d (Table A.5), presumably as soluble complexes.

Those metals for which 4+ is the stable oxidation state under physiological conditions and some very small trivalent metal ions like Sc^{3+} have large e/r ratios (Shannon, 1976), and these "hard" metal ions have such high affinities for oxy anions that they begin to hydrolyze at about pH 2 to form hydroxide microcolloids at very low concentrations. Even low concentrations of the tetravalent cations like Pu^{4+} tend to form hydroxide polymers. They all form stable complexes with the circulating organic acids and transferrin in plasma and tissue fluid and stable complexes with the immobile carboxyl and phenolic side chains of fixed tissue proteins (Section 2.2.2 and Appendix C.1.1). Most of the biological investigations of the tetravalent metal ions have been conducted with isotopes of plutonium. Only small fractions of these radionuclides (<5 μg deposited from solutions at pH <2), ranging from 10 % of $^{114}Sn^{4+}$ to 24 % of $^{239}Pu^{4+}$ of the amounts deposited, were cleared from an i.m. wound site in rats in 1 d (Table A.5). At physiological pH, the competition for the tetravalent metal ions among water (hydrolysis), complexation with soluble bioligands, and complexation with fixed tissue ligands greatly reduce the fraction of the amount deposited that can be cleared rapidly from a puncture wound as soluble complexes.

$^{239}Pu^{4+}$, which has been well studied as a wound contaminant, can be regarded as a worst case representative of multivalent cationic radionuclides that form insoluble, and in some cases, polymerized hydroxides at physiological pH.

During the brief initial interval between an i.m. or s.c. injection and neutralization of the excess H^+ at the wound site, Pu^{4+} may exist as a hydrated ion or an incomplete hydrolysis product that is amenable to complexation by bioligands in the circulating tissue fluid. For example, as late as 1 h after an i.m. injection in rats of 8 μg of $^{239}Pu(NO_3)_4$ in 3 mol L^{-1} HNO_3, local infiltration with sodium citrate or $CaNa_3$-DTPA significantly reduced retention of the plutonium at the wound site (Volf, 1975). During the first 1 to 2 h after colloidal $^{239}Pu(NO_3)_4$ was s.c. injected into a dog paw, important fractions (from 10 to 25 % of the injected amount depending inversely on the mass of plutonium deposited) were present in the lymph draining the wound site and in the blood (Appendices B.1.1.6.3 and C.1.1.1).

The ability of the tissue fluid bioligands to form soluble metal ion complexes is severely limited, because their concentrations are so low, no more than $\sim 10^{-4}$ mol L^{-1}. If, for example, 1 μg of Pu^{4+} initially in solution in a medium of pH 1 is deposited in a wound, and if it is rapidly distributed in 0.2 mL of tissue fluid, the initial local plutonium concentration will be $\sim 10^{-4}$ mol L^{-1}, nearly the same as the estimated concentration of circulating bioligands. Larger masses of plutonium and other elements with similar chemical properties, even if deposited in solution in a suitably acidic medium, overwhelm the carrying capacity of the bioligands immediately available in the slowly flowing tissue fluid and hydrolyze *in situ*.

By the end of the first day after injection, Pu^{4+} hydroxide precipitation is likely to be complete. The slower process of hydroxide polymerization, a mass dependent reaction in which oxo (-O-) bridges form between Pu^{4+} atoms, is in progress; it is possible that some very small hydroxide particles escape from the wound site.

Phagocytosis of the hydroxide particles is expected to begin as soon as they form, but the macrophage populations of connective tissue and dermis are not large, and time is needed to recruit additional phagocytic cells to the site. As the injected mass of radionuclide is increased from nanograms to tens of micrograms, the tendency of hydroxide self-aggregation is expected to increase, leading to formation of larger and more efficiently phagocytized particles, and to stimulation of a more intense inflammatory reaction with recruitment of additional macrophages. By 7 d, the number of macrophages appears to be sufficient to scavenge nearly all of the hydroxide particles, and in autoradiographs, those accumulated particles appear as ragged clusters of tracks.

With the passage of time, the hydroxide aggregates within the macrophages grow larger, as the individual macrophages accumulate more hydroxide particles and radionuclide-containing cell debris and/or remnants of remodeled structural protein. Formation of encapsulating or confining scar tissue (fibrosis) further immobilizes the residual radionuclide. Small amounts of radionuclides that, similarly to Pu^{4+}, form insoluble hydroxides in a wound appear to be slowly translocated from the wound in soluble form. For example, six months after s.c. injection of colloidal $^{239}Pu(NO_3)_4$ in the paws of dogs, plutonium was detectable in both blood and urine, and the renal clearance of the plutonium was that expected for soluble plutonium (Appendix C.1.1.2).

C.2.2 *Long-Term Observations*

Two autoradiographic studies provide general descriptions of the changing status at a wound site of $^{239}Pu^{4+}$ deposited in soluble or ultrafilterable form.

C.2.2.1 $^{239}Pu(NO_3)_4$ *in Strong Acid Injected Intradermally in Swine.* The sites of swine skin injected intradermally with >0.13 µg of plutonium in 0.2 mol L^{-1} HNO$_3$ were detectable visually at 3 y, with the higher dosage sites exhibiting varying degrees of depression, thickening, and hyperkeratinization (McClanahan *et al.*, 1964). At 4 y, the sites injected with >16 µg of plutonium contained plutonium associated with macrophages, collagen fibrils, hypereratotic areas, and connective tissue. At the lower dosage sites, which appeared normal except for hyperkeratosis, the residual plutonium was associated with macrophages and connective tissue cells of the dermis (McClanahan and Ragan, 1967).

C.2.2.2 *Colloidal* $^{239}Pu(NO_3)_4$ *Injected Subcutaneously in Dog Paws.* $^{239}Pu(NO_3)_4$ injected under the skin of the dog paw resulted in degenerative lesions at the site. Eight dogs were held for long-term study (5 y) of local and systemic biological effects of a s.c. injection in a forepaw of about the same amount of a colloidal suspension of $^{239}Pu^{4+}$ used in Bistline's (1973) study, that is, ~20 µg of $^{239,240}Pu(NO_3)_4$ at pH 2.4 (Dagle *et al.*, 1984). Small, gray, firm areas developed at the injection site of several dogs. Histologically, at 5 y after implant, focal atrophy and scarring of the subcubitis were observed at the wound site in all but one dog. Atrophy of adjacent adnexal tissues was seen in three dogs. Autoradiographs showed a few single tracks and pronounced accumulations of overlapping plutonium aggregates concentrated in the central area of the scar tissue. No gross or microscopic evidence suggestive of neoplastic changes were seen in the tissues in or around the injection sites.

The regional lymph node of one dog contained a marked amount of nodular scar tissue with sequestered pigment granules and alpha activity. The structure of the regional nodes of the other seven dogs was intact, except for occasional small foci of atrophy, scar tissue, and small amounts of hemosiderin. Alpha activity, both occasional single tracks and aggregates, was present in the nodes of three dogs with significant lymph-node scarring.

Autoradiographs showed a few randomly distributed aggregates of alpha tracks and rare single tracks in the liver (six dogs), spleen (two dogs), and kidney (one dog). The amounts of plutonium translocated to the liver were sufficient to induce adenomatous hyperplasia in two dogs, and the amount translocated to the skeleton may have induced a rare osteoma in one dog.

C.3 Radioactive Solids Deposited in Wounds

The fate of solids deposited in wounds depends on their solubilities in tissue fluid at pH 7.4 and within macrophage lysosomes at pH 4.5 to 5.5 (Appendix A.5; Section 2.2.3), their affinities for specific tissue fluid bioligands [for example, the affinity of uranyl ion for carbonate (Appendix A.5.1.1)], their stability to oxidation-reduction [for example, oxidation of UO_2 to uranyl ion (Appendices B.3.1 and B.3.2) and probable reduction of AmO_2 to Am^{3+} and $CmO_{1.7}$ to Cm^{3+} (Stradling *et al.*, 1978; Thomas *et al.*, 1972)], how finely the solid is divided [particle size (Smith *et al.*, 1977)], and at least for the alpha-emitting radionuclides, specific activity (Stradling *et al.*, 1978). The chemical composition of the solid and its particle size combined with the local tissue response determine the amounts and rates at which deposited solids will be dissolved and/or translocated away from the wound site in solid form.

Very small particles of $^{239}PuO_2$, on the order of 1 nm diameter, can dissolve *in vivo* and also be filtered by the kidneys into the urine (Harrison *et al.*, 1978a; Smith *et al.*, 1977). Particles smaller than ~0.2 μm diameter can penetrate the connective tissue gel (Section 2.2.1). Particles with diameters ranging from ~0.01 to 20 μm diameter can be ingested and transported by macrophages in lymph and deposited in lymph nodes (Matsuoka *et al.*, 1972; Schallberger, 1974). The local foreign-body reaction stimulated by larger particles and fragments that eventually results in their entrapment in scar tissue or encapsulation by fibrous connective tissue and a great reduction in radionuclide transport away from the deposition site.

C.3.1 *Dispersion of Subcutaneously Deposited Particles into Tissue Fluid*

Studies in mice show that the volume of tissue fluid penetrated by deposited particles depends inversely on particle size. Mice were s.c. injected on the back with aqueous suspensions containing 16 μg of "monomeric plutonium" in 2 % sodium citrate or "polymeric plutonium" in 0.02 % sodium citrate, pH 4 to 5. Particle diameters, measured in a diffusion chamber, were 2.5 to 25 nm and 450 to 1,200 nm, respectively. These were compared to three reference particles: large, ^{32}P-labelled $Cr(OH)_3$ 500 nm diameter; medium,

[198]Au colloid 300 nm diameter; and small, [198]Au colloid 5 nm diameter (Matsuoka *et al.*, 1972). The injected volumes of fluid containing the particles were not reported, but because of the small body size of the mouse, they probably were on the order of 0.1 mL.

Penetration of the particles into the tissue around the injection site at 1 to 3 d after injection was shown in whole-body autoradiographs. The tissue volumes penetrated were estimated from measurements of the autoradiographic images, assuming that their three-dimensional shapes were thin circular discs. The penetrated tissue volumes were 0.9 cm^3 for the "monomeric plutonium" particles and 0.05 cm^3 for the "polymeric plutonium" particles and 0.20, 1.3, and 1.3 cm^3 for the large, medium and small diameter reference particles, respectively. The two larger particles penetrated tissue volumes containing only ~0.013 to 0.05 mL of tissue fluid, much smaller volumes than that estimated to have been injected. The connective tissue gel, acting as a filter, allowed the smaller particles (<30 nm) to flow into larger tissue volumes, while the largest particles were retained close to the point of entry. In 1 to 3 d no detectable amounts of the two larger particles had been translocated away from the injected site. In contrast, large fractions of the "monomeric plutonium" had been transported *via* the blood to bone and liver, and large fractions of the two smaller [198]Au particles had been translocated to lymph nodes, liver, and spleen, and in the case of the smallest [198]Au particles (5 nm), also to the bone marrow.

C.3.2 *Very Small Particles of PuO₂ Implanted Intramuscularly in Rats*

The clearance pattern of minute particles of $^{239}PuO_2$ from an i.m.-implant site in rats was similar to that of dissolved $^{239}Pu(NO_3)_4$. Very small particles of $^{239}PuO_2$ (1 nm diameter) were i.m. injected in rats (0.01 μg of plutonium in <0.05 mL of water) (Harrison *et al.*, 1978a). Retention of the plutonium at the wound site was about the same as that of 0.011 μg of $^{239}Pu(NO_3)_4$ in solution at pH 1 (Table A.2). A significant and unusually large fraction of the plutonium cleared from the injection site was excreted in the urine, presumably as intact particles small enough to be filtered through the glomeruli, which are estimated to retain particles larger than 0.01 μm diameter (Berliner, 1973). The tissue distribution of the translocated $^{239}PuO_2$ was similar to that of i.m.-injected $^{239}Pu(NO_3)_4$, with very little accumulation of plutonium in the local lymph nodes. These very small particles, which are estimated to contain only ~50 plutonium atoms, are amenable to dissolution by citrate ion and complexation with $CaNa_3$-DTPA (Smith *et al.*, 1977).

C.3.3 *Transport of Small High-Fired PuO$_2$ Particles in Lymph*

Pairs of dogs were s.c. injected above the metatarsals of a hind paw with one of four suspensions of high-fired PuO$_2$ particles: polydisperse particles 0.7 μm GMD in 0.1 mL of water in a preparation similar to that reported by Bistline (1973), or monodisperse particles 0.16, 0.54, or 1.05 μm in diameter suspended in 1 mL of water (Schallberger, 1974; Schallberger *et al.*, 1976). The amounts of plutonium implanted were not reported. The methods used were described briefly in Appendix C.1.1. The distributions of the injected plutonium between the acellular (fluid) and cellular fractions of the afferent and efferent lymph in the dogs implanted with the PuO$_2$ particles are summarized in Table C.1. For all four particle sizes, the fraction of plutonium migrating from the s.c. site in the afferent lymph were small during the 4 h study period, <0.2 % of the amounts assumed to have been implanted. These results support other findings (Appendix B.1.4) that the outflow from the wound site of plutonium implanted as small particles of high-fired PuO$_2$ is severely inhibited. Initial transport of plutonium in lymph was least for the polydisperse 0.7 μm particles and greatest for the

TABLE C.1—*Plutonium in afferent and efferent popliteal lymph of dogs s.c. injected in a hind paw with ^{239}PuO$_2$ particles.*[a,b]

^{239}PuO$_2$ Particles (μm)	Total ^{239}Pu Collected in 0 to 4 h (percent of injected amount)[c]			
	Afferent Lymph		Efferent Lymph	
	Acellular	Cellular	Acellular	Cellular
Polydisperse				
0.7 GMD	0.028	0.011	0.0022	0.001
Monodisperse				
0.16	0.044	0.13	0.0053	0.003
0.54	0.046	0.066	0.00035	5.2×10^{-5}
1.05	0.032	0.037	< detection limit	0.0009

[a]PuO$_2$ particles dispersed in water.

[b]Main lymph ducts cannulated with continuous collection of lymph from pairs of dogs; afferent lymph collected from one dog, efferent lymph collected from the other.

[c]Summed from data for 30 min intervals (Table 13 of Schallberger, 1974).

smallest (0.16 μm) monodisperse particles. The association of plutonium with the cellular fraction of the afferent lymph appeared to be inversely proportional to particle size for the monodisperse particles, that is, 75, 59 and 54 % of the total afferent lymph from 0.16, 0.54, and 1.05 μm particles, respectively. For the polydisperse particles only 28 % of total afferent lymph plutonium was in the cellular fraction, suggesting the presence of some very small filterable particles.

The amount of plutonium in the efferent lymph was much less than that in the afferent lymph, ranging from 0.36 % (0.54 μm monodisperse particles) to 7.7 % (0.7 μm polydisperse particles). For three of the four particle sizes, the fraction of total lymph plutonium exiting the nodes in association with cells was 15 to 36 %. The major fraction of the plutonium transported away from the wound site to the lymph nodes is presumed to have been retained there. On average, about one-half of the plutonium initially migrating from the wound site in the lymph was associated with cells, and dense particles, presumably PuO_2, were seen in phagocytes in the afferent lymph.

As had been found in the case of similarly injected $^{239}Pu(NO_3)_4$ at pH 2.4, transferrin, and to a lesser degree, albumin, were the major protein carriers of plutonium in the acellular fractions of both afferent and efferent lymph.

C.3.4 $^{239}PuO_2$ and $^{232}ThO_2$ Particles Injected Intramuscularly in Rats

Retention at an i.m. wound site in rats was determined for $^{239}PuO_2$ particles 0.22 to 1.2 μm in diameter (Harrison *et al.*, 1978a). At 7 and 28 d after the injection, respectively, retention in the injected leg was 99 and 96.5 %, and translocation was mainly to the local lymph nodes.

Thorotrast® (colloidal $^{232}ThO_2$, particle size ~0.01 μm) was i.m. injected in the legs of rats that were followed for lifespan (Hahn *et al.*, 2002). Retention of the ^{232}Th at the injection site was not measured. Nearly all of the organs and tissues were examined histopathologically, and the regional lymph nodes (lumbar and popliteal) were the only tissues other than the i.m.-injection site reported to contain identifiable $^{232}ThO_2$ particles.[9]

[9]Hahn, F.F. (2003). Personal communication (Lovelace Respiratory Research Institute, Albuquerque, New Mexico).

C.3.5 *$^{239}PuO_2$ Particles Implanted Subcutaneously in Dog Paws*

Particles of air-oxidized $^{239}PuO_2$ [7 μm GMD (Johnson, 1969; Appendix B.1.3)] or high-fired $^{239}PuO_2$ [0.7 μm GMD (Appendix B.1.4; Bistline, 1973)] were implanted as aqueous s.c. suspensions in the forepaws of dogs to determine transport from the wound site. Accumulation of plutonium in the regional lymph nodes (LSCLN) began almost immediately after the PuO_2 particles were implanted and continued through the year of observation (Figures B.5 and B.6).

The equations derived from the combined data for plutonium in the paw and plutonium accumulation in the regional lymph nodes and tissues plus excretion in the dogs implanted with the larger (7 μm GMD) air-oxidized PuO_2 particles provide estimates at 365 d of 16.6 % in the lymph nodes (Equation B.11) and 1.8 % in the combined tissues and excretion (Equation B.12). Estimates could also be made of tissue plutonium and plutonium excretion for three dogs killed at 365 d, based on material recovery; the total amounts of plutonium in the tissues plus estimated excretion ranged from 0.95 to 1.8 % of that implanted. About 90 % of the plutonium translocated from the wound could be accounted for by accumulation and retention in the lymph nodes.

For the dogs implanted with the smaller (0.7 μm GMD) particles of high-fired PuO_2, the modified equation for wound plutonium retention, Equations B.14 and B.15, derived for accumulation of plutonium in the lymph nodes, predict that at 365 d after the implant the lymph nodes will contain 20.4 % and the tissues plus estimated excretion will account for only ~0.6 % of the implanted plutonium. About 97 % of the plutonium translocated from the wound site could be accounted for by accumulation and retention in the regional lymph nodes. These estimates suggest that plutonium in the form of smaller more refractory particles of high-fired PuO_2 was less soluble and less transportable than plutonium in the form of the larger air-oxidized particles of PuO_2.

C.3.5.1 *Renal Clearance of Plutonium Implanted in Dog Paws as Air-Oxidized $^{239}PuO_2$ Particles.* The method of Stover *et al.* (1959) was used to analyze the blood and urine data from eight untreated dogs that were s.c. implanted with air-oxidized 7 μm GMD particles of $^{239}PuO_2$ (Johnson, 1969). The recalculated blood and urine data are summarized in Table C.2 and plotted logarithmically in Figure C.2. The equations of the curves, obtained using the Origin® graphics program for the interval 1 to 365 d, where *t* is days after injection, are:

TABLE C.2—*Kinetics of ^{239}Pu in blood and urine of eight untreated dogs s.c. implanted in a paw with air-oxidized ^{239}PuO$_2$ particles (7 μm GMD).*[a]

Days	Fraction of Recovered Plutonium (% ± SD)			
	Blood Volume (% × 10^{-2})[b]		Urinary Excretion Rate (% d^{-1} × 10^{-3})[c]	
	Number of Samples[d]	Mean ± SD	Number of Samples[d]	Mean ± SD
1	8	2.4 ± 1.9	8	2.4 ± 2.1
2	8	1.9 ± 1.1	8	2.2 ± 2.4
3	8	1.9 ± 0.9	8	3.8 ± 3.3
4	8	2.1 ± 2.1	8	3.8 ± 2.7
5	8	1.5 ± 0.9	8	2.4 ± 1.9
6	8	1.8 ± 1.3	8	2.4 ± 2.1
7	8	1.4 ± 0.7	8	1.7 ± 1.4
9	8	1.6 ± 1.1	8	1.3 ± 0.8
11	8	1.4 ± 1.3	8	2.4 ± 1.4
14	8	1.5 ± 0.7	8	3.2 ± 3.2
32 – 34	7	1.8 ± 1.6	7	1.0 ± 0.4
60 – 62	7	1.7 ± 0.8	7	1.1 ± 0.9
88 – 90	7	1.5 ± 1.1	7	0.72 ± 0.5
123 – 125	7	1.7 ± 1.5	6	0.75 ± 0.49
160 – 161	5	1.2 ± 0.9	5	0.44 ± 0.24
188 – 190	4	1.1 ± 0.7	4	1.05 ± 0.57
223 – 225	4	0.86 ± 0.4	4	0.94 ± 0.45
250 – 252	4	0.84 ± 0.2	4	0.68 ± 0.19
285 – 286	2	0.65	2	0.64
334 – 335	2	1.1	2	0.46
362 – 364	2	0.83	4	0.46 ± 0.24

[a]Calculated from the data of Johnson (1969). The injected paws of the eight dogs not treated with CaNa$_3$-DTPA were radiochemically analyzed. Material recovery, an approximation of the amount of plutonium implanted, was estimated as described in Appendix B.1.3 and Table B.5

[b]The mean body weight of male beagles from this study was 15 ± 1.9 kg, and their average measured blood volume was 93 ± 10 mL kg^{-1} (Table 4 of Johnson, 1969). Blood plutonium concentration was reported as dpm mL^{-1} for each dog at each sampling time, and plutonium in the whole blood volume was calculated as:

$$100 \times 1,395 \ (mL) \times [\text{plutonium concentration (dpm mL}^{-1})]$$
$$\times [\text{recovered plutonium (dpm)}]^{-1} \% \text{ of recovered amount.}$$

[c]Urinary plutonium was reported as dpm per 24 h sample. The daily urinary plutonium excretion rate (% d^{-1}) was calculated for each dog at each sampling time as:

$$100 \times [\text{daily urinary plutonium (dpm d}^{-1})]$$
$$\times [\text{recovered plutonium (dpm)}]^{-1} \% \text{ recovered amount per day.}$$

[d]Number of samples in interval.

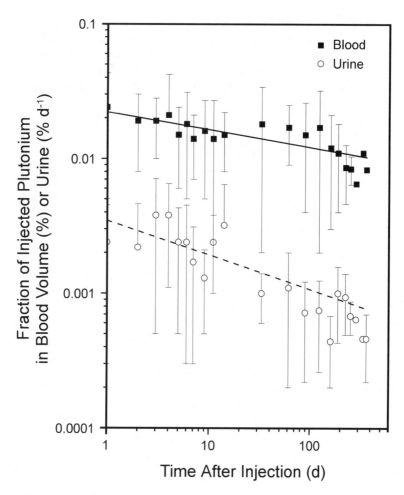

Fig. C.2. Plutonium in the blood volume and daily urinary plutonium excretion of eight dogs that received 13 to 139 µg of air-oxidized PuO_2 particles (7 µm GMD) by s.c. implantation in a paw. Curves correspond to Equations C.4 and C.5, respectively (recalculated from the data of Johnson, 1969).

$$\text{Pu in blood volume} = 0.022t^{-0.13}\% \qquad (C.4)$$

of recovered amount, and

$$\text{Pu urinary excretion rate} = 0.0035t^{-0.26}\% \qquad (C.5)$$

of recovered amount per day.

The ratio of the integrals of those equations over the entire observation interval, 1 to 365 d, is 8.6 % of the plutonium in one blood volume cleared to urine per day. That renal plutonium clearance is nearly the same as was obtained for colloidal Pu^{4+} hydroxide [$^{239}Pu(NO_3)_4$, pH 2.4] s.c. injected in the paws of dogs (Appendix C.1.1.2), and it agrees with the renal clearance of Pu^{4+} i.v. injected in dogs in soluble form as plutonium citrate (Stover *et al.*, 1959).

After s.c. implantation of the air-oxidized PuO_2 particles, neither the blood plutonium nor the urinary plutonium excretion rate displayed a prominent initial, rapidly diminishing component like those observed after a similar implant of colloidal plutonium nitrate (Figure C.1). The fraction of plutonium implanted as 7 μm GMD particles of PuO_2 that could be transported immediately to blood and filtered by the kidneys is small, only ~1 % of the initially transportable fraction of plutonium that was found after s.c. injection of $Pu(NO_3)_4$ in the dog paws. After ~10 d, the amounts of plutonium in the blood and daily urine are about one-tenth of those found after implantation of the colloidal plutonium hydroxide (compare Figures C.1 and C.2). Both blood and urinary plutonium declined slowly with half-times of 250 and 400 d, respectively. The presence of plutonium in blood and urine at 1 y after the PuO_2 implant suggests a slow, but apparently diminishing, solubilization of a small fraction of the implanted air-oxidized PuO_2 particles at the wound site or in the lymph nodes.

C.3.5.2 *Renal Clearance of Plutonium Implanted in Dog Paws as High-Fired $^{239}PuO_2$ Particles.* The method of Stover *et al.* (1959) was used to analyze the blood and urine plutonium data from four dogs not treated with $CaNa_3$-DTPA that were followed for 360 d after implantation of 0.7 μm GMD particles of high-fired $^{239}PuO_2$. Although the radiochemical analyses of most of the biological samples from this study are considered to be unreliable (discussed in Appendix B.1.4), those of blood and urine may be less problematic. Urinary plutonium would have been filtered from the blood through the renal glomeruli, which, with a pore size of ~0.01 μm, allows passage only of molecules of <60,000 molecular weight and very small particles (0.001 μm diameter) of $^{238}PuO_2$ or $^{239}PuO_2$ (Brobeck, 1973; Harrison *et al.*, 1978a; Smith *et al.*, 1977; Stradling *et al.*, 1978). Even if they had penetrated the central circulation, particles large enough to be phagocytized would be rapidly recognized by and accumulated in reticuloendothelial cells in the liver, spleen, and bone marrow (Matsuoka *et al.*, 1972). Consequently, plutonium in the blood of these dogs would be expected to be protein-bound as the nonfilterable transferrin complex or as filterable complexes with small ligands like citrate ion or minute PuO_2 particles. The wet digestion step in the analytical procedure for plutonium should have dissolved all of those forms of plutonium in the blood and urine samples.

Blood samples and 24 h collections of urine were taken from most of the dogs on nine of the first 13 d after the PuO_2 implant and on three consecutive days every 30 d thereafter. The radiochemical results for plutonium in the blood volume (dpm) and daily urinary excretion (dpm d^{-1}) are collected in Table C.3 for the four dogs of Group 1 that were not treated with $CaNa_3$-DTPA and followed for 1 y. Plutonium was detected in all of the urine and blood samples collected for 357 d after the implant. Blood and urine sampled at the same post-implant times varied widely among the dogs of the group, at least in part, reflecting the variability of the amounts of plutonium implanted. Blood and urine plutonium were only weakly correlated with $w(0)$, which was assumed to be a surrogate for, and proportional to, the quantity of plutonium implanted in each dog (Appendix B.1.4). The amounts of plutonium in the blood and filtered into the urine were very small, indicating that the fractions of the implanted particles undergoing solubilization and/or mobilization as minute particles were also very small.

The following set of logarithmic equations was obtained using the Origin® graphics program:

$$B_1 \ (0.5 - 8 \ \mathrm{d}) \ = \ 77t^{-0.60} \ \text{and} \ B_2 \ (8 - 357 \ \mathrm{d}) = 24.5t^{-0.054}, \quad \text{(C.6)}$$

where B_1 and B_2 are plutonium in the blood volume (dpm), and t is days after injection, and:

$$U_1 \ (1 - 8 \ \mathrm{d}) \ = \ 26.8t^{-0.59} \ \text{and} \ U_2 \ (8 - 357 \ \mathrm{d}) = 10.3t^{-0.14}, \quad \text{(C.7)}$$

where U_1 and U_2 are the daily plutonium urinary excretion (dpm d^{-1}), and t is days after injection. The curves represented by those equations are shown in Figure C.3.

The ratios of the integrals of daily urinary plutonium excretion rate to plutonium in the blood volume, calculated from the four equations are:

$$U_1 B_1^{-1} \ = 27 \ \% \ \text{and} \ U_2 B_2^{-1} \ = 35 \ \% \quad \text{(C.8)}$$

of blood plutonium cleared daily to urine.

TABLE C.3—*Plutonium in the blood volume (dpm) and daily urinary excretion (dpm d⁻¹) of four dogs during 1 y after s.c. implantation in a paw of small (0.7 μm GMD) particles of high-fired PuO₂.*[a]

Time (d)	Plutonium Content	
	Blood Volume[b] (dpm) [c,d]	Daily Urinary Excretion (dpm d⁻¹) [c,d]
0.5	125 ± 110	—
1	59 ± 27	26 ± 27
2	45 ± 16	18 ± 15
3	51 ± 20	20 ± 12
4	48 ± 18	9.5 ± 2.4
5	33 ± 18	3.0 ± 1.6
6	15 ± 8.3	13 ± 12
8	19 ± 5.5	5.2 ± 3.6
10	24 ± 15	11 ± 7.2
13	19 ± 14	5.0 ± 3.7
49	—	8.6 ± 7.9
64 – 69	28 ± 17	2.9 ± 3.2
101 – 104	54 ± 30	8.9 ± 3.7
134 – 139	22 ± 80	5.5 ± 2.4
182	10 ± 4.7	7.4 ± 2.2
216	39 ± 24	3.8 ± 0.4
257	20 ± 13	3.2 ± 1.7
286	23 ± 13	4.3 ± 2.4
328	—	1.8 ± 0.5
357	—	3.5 ± 3.3

[a]Original data for individual dogs were obtained from the project records supplied by Bistline, R.W. (2000) personal communication (Abilene, Kansas).

[b]Plutonium in the blood volume was calculated by using Equation B.5 and the recorded initial body weights of the individual dogs.

[c]Data are expressed as mean ± SD (Mack, 1967).

[d]From 0.5 to 13 d, means are for daily blood and urine samples from the four dogs of Group 1 not treated with CaNa₃-DTPA. After 30 d, blood and urine were collected on three consecutive days about every 30 d; the collection times shown are the mid-points of the collection times, and the mean activities are the 3 d averages for the four dogs.

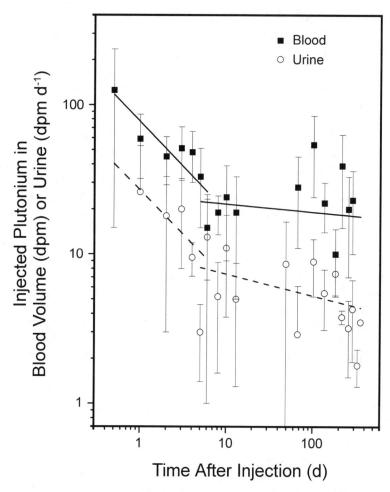

Fig. C.3. Plutonium in the blood volume and daily urinary excretion from 0.5 to 357 d of the four dogs of Group 1 that were implanted s.c. in a paw with small (0.7 μm GMD) particles of high-fired PuO_2 and not treated with $CaNa_3$-DTPA (recalculated data of Bistline, 1973). The curves correspond to Equation C.6 for blood plutonium and Equation C.7 for urinary plutonium excretion rate.

Daily renal clearance of 27 to 35 % of the plutonium in the blood volume is three to four times the renal clearances calculated for plutonium injected into the dog paw as colloidal $Pu(NO_3)_4$ (Appendix C.1.1.2) or as larger air-oxidized PuO_2 particles (Appendix C.3.5.1). This result suggests that, assuming the radiochemical analyses were accurate, in addition to a small fraction of the implanted high-fired PuO_2 that may be solubilized, the circulating blood may also contain a small fraction of the PuO_2 in the form of filterable minute particles.

C.3.6 Plutonium Metal Wire Implanted Subcutaneously in Rats and Rabbits

The plutonium wire implanted in the rabbit that died at 2 d had already disintegrated into numerous small fragments coated with green-black granules of hydrous plutonium oxides, and these were confined within the original volume of the implant site (Lisco and Kisieleski, 1953; Appendix B.1.5). Fragmentation and corrosion and dispersion of the fragments and corrosion products locally within the slowly expanding volume of affected tissue continued until death. Measurable levels of plutonium in bone and liver, the target tissues for soluble Pu^{4+}, and in the excreta of rats similarly implanted with plutonium wire demonstrated the dissolution of small amounts of plutonium oxide corrosion products (Appendix B.1.5). Excretion of plutonium by the rats declined early, and plutonium absorption did not depend on time elapsed after the plutonium implants. Fibrosis and mineralization of the tissue surrounding the implant sites created a barrier that efficiently impeded long-term plutonium transport.

C.3.7 Dry UO_2 Powder Implanted Subcutaneously in Rats

At times <6 h after s.c. deposition of 1.6 to 160 mg per rat of heat-treated UO_2 powder (4 to 40 μm diameter), the uranium at the implant sites was randomly scattered in the intercellular spaces among large numbers of polymorphonuclear leukocytes (De Rey et al., 1984). After 24 h, there were few polymorphonuclear leukocytes present, and the spaces had been invaded by large numbers of macrophages. The macrophages contained electron-dense uranium granules within phagosomes, and some granules were also seen in cytoplasmic vesicles in fibroblast-like cells. Dense trails of uranium were seen between endothelial cells in blood capillaries in organized granular tissue and deep within muscle bundles.

C.3.8 Depleted Uranium Metal Fragments Implanted Intramuscularly in Rats

Within three weeks the edges of the DU metal wafers implanted in rat leg muscle began to corrode and shed particles of UO_2 (Hahn *et al.*, 2002). In addition to the small fraction of the implanted uranium that dissolved and was excreted in urine (Appendix B.3.4.1), there was evidence for the migration of a small fraction of the UO_2 corrosion products from the wound site to the regional lymph nodes (Appendix B.3.4.2).[10]

[10]Hahn, F.F. (2003). Personal communication (Lovelace Respiratory Research Institute, Albuquerque, New Mexico).

Appendix D

Worked Examples of the Application of the NCRP Wound Model to Bioassay and Dose Assessment for Uranium

One of the important uses of the NCRP wound model is to aid in the interpretation of bioassay data, for example, for supplementing data from *in situ* measurements of the radioactive contaminant. Such application allows for both prospective dose assessment, which may be useful in planning medical management, and retrospective dose assessment in cases of actual wound contamination in which doses need to be assessed by interpreting *in vivo* or *in vitro* bioassay data.

In this example, the NCRP wound model is coupled with the uranium systemic biokinetic model of ICRP Publication 69 (ICRP, 1995a; Figure D.1) and is used to calculate the uranium urinary excretion patterns as well as tissue retention patterns for the wound site and an important target organ, the kidney. To do this, the blood compartment of the NCRP model is made identical to the plasma or blood compartment of the uranium systemic biokinetic model. Accordingly, clearance of uranium from the wound to blood is equivalent to clearance directly to the plasma compartment. Similarly, clearance from lymph node in the NCRP model goes to plasma in the ICRP (1995a) model. All default systemic transfer rates from ICRP were used in these calculations, which were performed for three default categories that could be reasonably expected for uranium materials (*i.e.*, weak, particle and fragment). The calculated retention functions are given for the wound site

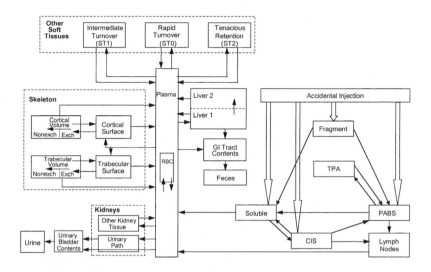

Fig. D.1. Schematic diagram of the NCRP wound model coupled with ICRP (1995a) uranium systemic biokinetic model.

(Figure D.2) and kidneys (Figure D.3) as well as for 24 h excretion of uranium in urine (Figure D.4).

The dose coefficients (Table D.1) were calculated for the set of organs that are typically shown in ICRP publications using the radiation weighting factors and tissue weighting factors from ICRP Publication 60 (ICRP, 1991a). The coefficients in Table D.1 include the dose contributions from the radioactive progeny of ^{238}U, assuming ingrowth *in vivo* and independent biokinetics, as described in ICRP Publications 69 (ICRP, 1995a) and 71 (ICRP, 1995b). The intake retention fractions [$m(t)$; Section 5.3.4], which are shown for the wound site, kidneys and 24 h urine excretion for weak (Table D.2) particle (Table D.3), and fragment (Table D.4) categories, were calculated for ^{238}U only but are applicable to other isotopic mixtures of uranium, as they are element-specific, and differences in radioactive decay rates are negligible. All calculations shown in Tables D.1 through D.4 were done by two scientists[11] at the Los Alamos National Laboratory using different computational approaches, both of which have been previously benchmarked for accuracy against published ICRP dose coefficients. The calculated results agreed to better than 1 %.

[11]NCRP expresses its appreciation to Drs. Luiz Bertelli and Guthrie Miller for their derivation of the values provided in this Appendix.

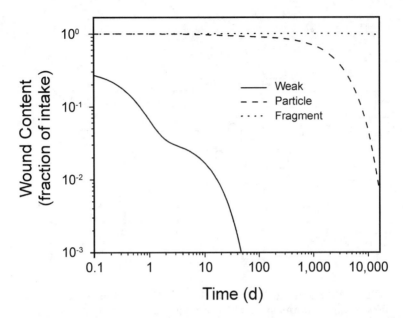

Fig. D.2. Predicted retention of uranium at the wound site for weak, particle and fragment categories.

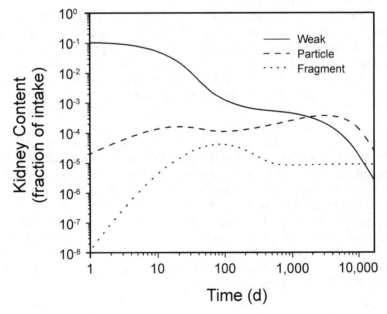

Fig. D.3. Predicted retention of uranium in kidneys for weak, particle and fragment categories.

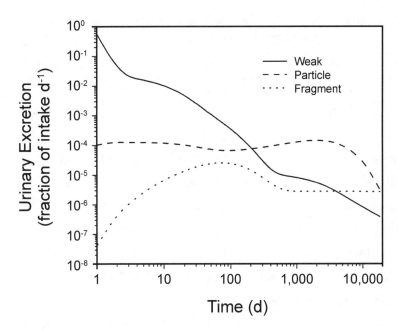

Fig. D.4. Predicted uranium urinary excretion for weak, particle and fragment categories.

TABLE D.1—*Fifty-year dose coefficients (h_T Sv Bq^{-1}) for ^{238}U and progeny for three wound retention categories.*

Organ	Weak	Particle	Fragment
Adrenals	1.21E–06	9.35E–07	3.96E–08
Bladder wall	1.21E–06	9.39E–07	3.99E–08
Bone surface	3.50E–05	3.18E–05	1.54E–06
Brain	1.21E–06	9.34E–07	3.96E–08
Breasts	1.21E–06	9.34E–07	3.96E–08
Esophagus	1.21E–06	9.34E–07	3.96E–08
Stomach wall	1.21E–06	9.34E–07	3.96E–08
Small-intestine wall	1.21E–06	9.34E–07	3.96E–08
Upper large-intestine wall	1.21E–06	9.34E–07	3.96E–08
Lower large-intestine wall	1.21E–06	9.35E–07	3.97E–08
Colon	1.21E–06	9.35E–07	3.97E–08
Kidneys	1.23E–05	1.22E–05	6.43E–07
Liver	4.70E–06	4.33E–06	2.02E–07
Muscle	1.21E–06	9.34E–07	3.96E–08
Ovaries	1.19E–06	9.27E–07	3.94E–08
Pancreas	1.21E–06	9.34E–07	3.96E–08
Red marrow	3.80E–06	3.50E–06	1.72E–07
Extrathoracic airways	1.21E–06	9.34E–07	3.96E–08
Lungs	1.21E–06	9.34E–07	3.96E–08
Skin	1.21E–06	9.34E–07	3.96E–08
Spleen	1.21E–06	9.34E–07	3.96E–08
Testes	1.19E–06	9.27E–07	3.94E–08
Thymus	1.21E–06	9.34E–07	3.96E–08
Thyroid	1.21E–06	9.34E–07	3.96E–08
Uterus	1.21E–06	9.34E–07	3.96E–08
Remainder	3.20E–05	1.05E–06	4.57E–08
Effective dose	2.03E–06	1.73E–06	7.89E–08

TABLE D.2—*Intake retention fractions [m(t)] for the wound site and kidney and daily urine excretion fractions (d⁻¹) for* ^{238}U — *weakly-retained category.*

Time (d)	Wound	Kidneys	24 h Urine
1	6.76E–02	1.04E–01	5.87E–01
2	3.55E–02	1.00E–01	5.16E–02
3	2.98E–02	9.32E–02	2.26E–02
4	2.72E–02	8.61E–02	1.78E–02
5	2.51E–02	7.94E–02	1.60E–02
6	2.32E–02	7.32E–02	1.45E–02
7	2.15E–02	6.75E–02	1.33E–02
8	2.00E–02	6.22E–02	1.22E–02
9	1.84E–02	5.74E–02	1.12E–02
10	1.71E–02	5.29E–02	1.03E–02
11	1.58E–02	4.88E–02	9.54E–03
12	1.46E–02	4.50E–02	8.81E–03
13	1.36E–02	4.15E–02	8.15E–03
14	1.26E–02	3.83E–02	7.56E–03
15	1.17E–02	3.54E–02	7.01E–03
16	1.07E–02	3.27E–02	6.52E–03
17	9.96E–03	3.02E–02	6.06E–03
18	9.22E–03	2.79E–02	5.65E–03
19	8.53E–03	2.58E–02	5.27E–03
20	7.90E–03	2.39E–02	4.92E–03
21	7.32E–03	2.21E–02	4.60E–03
22	6.77E–03	2.05E–02	4.31E–03
23	6.27E–03	1.90E–02	4.05E–03
24	5.81E–03	1.76E–02	3.80E–03
25	5.37E–03	1.64E–02	3.57E–03
26	4.98E–03	1.52E–02	3.37E–03
27	4.60E–03	1.42E–02	3.17E–03
28	4.27E–03	1.32E–02	3.00E–03
29	3.95E–03	1.23E–02	2.83E–03
30	3.66E–03	1.15E–02	2.68E–03

TABLE D.2—(*continued*)

Time (d)	Wound	Kidneys	24 h Urine
35	2.48E–03	8.25E–03	2.08E–03
40	1.69E–03	6.12E–03	1.66E–03
45	1.15E–03	4.70E–03	1.36E–03
50	7.82E–04	3.74E–03	1.14E–03
55	5.32E–04	3.07E–03	9.71E–04
60	3.62E–04	2.60E–03	8.42E–04
65	2.46E–04	2.26E–03	7.38E–04
70	1.67E–04	2.01E–03	6.54E–04
75	1.14E–04	1.82E–03	5.84E–04
80	7.74E–05	1.66E–03	5.25E–04
85	5.26E–05	1.54E–03	4.74E–04
90	3.58E–05	1.44E–03	4.30E–04
95	2.43E–05	1.35E–03	3.92E–04
100	1.65E–05	1.28E–03	3.58E–04
105	1.12E–05	1.22E–03	3.28E–04
110	7.66E–06	1.16E–03	3.02E–04
115	5.21E–06	1.12E–03	2.78E–04
120	3.55E–06	1.07E–03	2.56E–04
125	2.41E–06	1.03E–03	2.37E–04
130	1.64E–06	1.00E–03	2.20E–04
135	1.11E–06	9.69E–04	2.04E–04
140	7.58E–07	9.40E–04	1.89E–04
145	5.16E–07	9.15E–04	1.76E–04
150	3.51E–07	8.91E–04	1.64E–04
155	2.38E–07	8.70E–04	1.53E–04
160	1.62E–07	8.50E–04	1.43E–04
165	1.10E–07	8.32E–04	1.34E–04
170	7.50E–08	8.16E–04	1.26E–04
180	3.47E–08	7.86E–04	1.10E–04
195	1.09E–08	7.49E–04	9.19E–05
210	3.44E–09	7.19E–04	7.70E–05

TABLE D.2—(*continued*)

Time (d)	Wound	Kidneys	24 h Urine
225	1.08E–09	6.95E–04	6.51E–05
240	3.39E–10	6.75E–04	5.54E–05
255	1.06E–10	6.58E–04	4.75E–05
270	3.36E–11	6.43E–04	4.10E–05
285	1.05E–11	6.30E–04	3.57E–05
300	3.32E–12	6.20E–04	3.13E–05
315	1.04E–12	6.10E–04	2.77E–05
330	3.29E–13	6.02E–04	2.47E–05
345	1.03E–13	5.94E–04	2.22E–05
360	3.25E–14	5.88E–04	2.01E–05
400	1.49E–15	5.73E–04	1.61E–05
500	3.35E–19	5.45E–04	1.16E–05
600	3.20E–19	5.24E–04	9.99E–06
720	3.05E–19	5.00E–04	9.17E–06
900	2.83E–19	4.68E–04	8.43E–06
1,000	2.72E–19	4.51E–04	8.09E–06
1,500	2.22E–19	3.75E–04	6.63E–06
2,000	1.82E–19	3.12E–04	5.47E–06
2,500	6.08E–19	2.60E–04	4.55E–06
3,000	1.04E–18	2.16E–04	3.81E–06
3,500	1.36E–18	1.80E–04	3.22E–06
4,000	1.58E–18	1.50E–04	2.75E–06
4,500	1.73E–18	1.25E–04	2.37E–06
5,000	1.83E–18	1.04E–04	2.06E–06
6,000	1.90E–18	7.24E–05	1.61E–06
7,000	1.88E–18	5.06E–05	1.30E–06
8,000	1.79E–18	3.56E–05	1.09E–06
9,000	1.69E–18	2.52E–05	9.31E–07
10,000	1.57E–18	1.80E–05	8.15E–07

TABLE D.3—*Intake retention fractions [m(t)] for the wound site and kidneys and daily urine excretion fraction (d^{-1}) for ^{238}U — particle category.*

Time (d)	Wound	Kidneys	24 h Urine
1	9.96E–01	2.05E–05	1.03E–04
2	9.92E–01	4.10E–05	1.26E–04
3	9.89E–01	5.91E–05	1.26E–04
4	9.86E–01	7.52E–05	1.25E–04
5	9.83E–01	8.93E–05	1.24E–04
6	9.80E–01	1.02E–04	1.23E–04
7	9.77E–01	1.13E–04	1.22E–04
8	9.74E–01	1.22E–04	1.21E–04
9	9.72E–01	1.30E–04	1.20E–04
10	9.69E–01	1.37E–04	1.18E–04
11	9.67E–01	1.43E–04	1.17E–04
12	9.64E–01	1.48E–04	1.15E–04
13	9.62E–01	1.52E–04	1.14E–04
14	9.60E–01	1.55E–04	1.12E–04
15	9.58E–01	1.58E–04	1.10E–04
16	9.56E–01	1.60E–04	1.09E–04
17	9.55E–01	1.62E–04	1.07E–04
18	9.52E–01	1.63E–04	1.06E–04
19	9.51E–01	1.64E–04	1.04E–04
20	9.49E–01	1.64E–04	1.03E–04
21	9.47E–01	1.64E–04	1.01E–04
22	9.46E–01	1.64E–04	9.96E–05
23	9.45E–01	1.64E–04	9.81E–05
24	9.43E–01	1.63E–04	9.67E–05
25	9.41E–01	1.63E–04	9.54E–05
26	9.40E–01	1.62E–04	9.40E–05
27	9.39E–01	1.61E–04	9.27E–05
28	9.38E–01	1.59E–04	9.15E–05
29	9.36E–01	1.58E–04	9.03E–05

TABLE D.3—(*continued*)

Time (d)	Wound	Kidneys	24 h Urine
30	9.35E–01	1.57E–04	8.91E–05
35	9.30E–01	1.50E–04	8.39E–05
40	9.26E–01	1.43E–04	7.96E–05
45	9.22E–01	1.36E–04	7.61E–05
50	9.19E–01	1.31E–04	7.33E–05
55	9.16E–01	1.26E–04	7.12E–05
60	9.13E–01	1.22E–04	6.95E–05
65	9.11E–01	1.19E–04	6.83E–05
70	9.10E–01	1.17E–04	6.74E–05
75	9.07E–01	1.15E–04	6.68E–05
80	9.06E–01	1.14E–04	6.64E–05
85	9.04E–01	1.13E–04	6.62E–05
90	9.02E–01	1.13E–04	6.61E–05
95	9.00E–01	1.12E–04	6.61E–05
100	8.99E–01	1.13E–04	6.63E–05
105	8.98E–01	1.13E–04	6.65E–05
110	8.97E–01	1.13E–04	6.67E–05
115	8.95E–01	1.14E–04	6.70E–05
120	8.94E–01	1.14E–04	6.74E–05
125	8.93E–01	1.15E–04	6.78E–05
130	8.91E–01	1.16E–04	6.82E–05
135	8.90E–01	1.17E–04	6.86E–05
140	8.88E–01	1.18E–04	6.90E–05
145	8.87E–01	1.19E–04	6.95E–05
150	8.86E–01	1.19E–04	6.99E–05
155	8.84E–01	1.20E–04	7.04E–05
160	8.83E–01	1.21E–04	7.09E–05
165	8.82E–01	1.22E–04	7.13E–05
170	8.81E–01	1.23E–04	7.18E–05
180	8.78E–01	1.25E–04	7.28E–05
195	8.74E–01	1.28E–04	7.42E–05

TABLE D.3—(*continued*)

Time (d)	Wound	Kidneys	24 h Urine
210	8.71E–01	1.31E–04	7.56E–05
225	8.66E–01	1.34E–04	7.71E–05
240	8.63E–01	1.37E–04	7.85E–05
255	8.59E–01	1.40E–04	7.98E–05
270	8.55E–01	1.43E–04	8.12E–05
285	8.51E–01	1.46E–04	8.26E–05
300	8.48E–01	1.49E–04	8.39E–05
315	8.45E–01	1.52E–04	8.52E–05
330	8.40E–01	1.55E–04	8.65E–05
345	8.37E–01	1.58E–04	8.77E–05
360	8.34E–01	1.60E–04	8.90E–05
400	8.24E–01	1.68E–04	9.22E–05
500	8.00E–01	1.86E–04	9.97E–05
600	7.77E–01	2.02E–04	1.06E–04
720	7.50E–01	2.21E–04	1.13E–04
900	7.12E–01	2.47E–04	1.22E–04
1,000	6.92E–01	2.59E–04	1.26E–04
1,500	5.99E–01	3.12E–04	1.39E–04
2,000	5.18E–01	3.45E–04	1.43E–04
2,500	4.47E–01	3.65E–04	1.40E–04
3,000	3.88E–01	3.72E–04	1.34E–04
3,500	3.35E–01	3.70E–04	1.25E–04
4,000	2.89E–01	3.62E–04	1.15E–04
4,500	2.50E–01	3.48E–04	1.05E–04
5,000	2.17E–01	3.31E–04	9.49E–05
6,000	1.62E–01	2.91E–04	7.60E–05
7,000	1.21E–01	2.49E–04	5.97E–05
8,000	9.06E–02	2.08E–04	4.64E–05
9,000	6.78E–02	1.71E–04	3.57E–05
10,000	5.07E–02	1.39E–04	2.74E–05

TABLE D.4—*Intake retention fractions [m(t)] for the wound site and kidneys and daily urine excretion fraction (d⁻¹) for ^{238}U — fragment category.*

Time (d)	Wound	Kidneys	24 h Urine
1	1.00E+00	1.27E–08	4.39E–08
2	1.00E+00	9.40E–08	4.10E–07
3	1.00E+00	2.78E–07	1.02E–06
4	1.00E+00	5.75E–07	1.74E–06
5	1.00E+00	9.81E–07	2.53E–06
6	1.00E+00	1.49E–06	3.33E–06
7	1.00E+00	2.08E–06	4.14E–06
8	1.00E+00	2.76E–06	4.94E–06
9	1.00E+00	3.50E–06	5.74E–06
10	1.00E+00	4.30E–06	6.52E–06
11	1.00E+00	5.16E–06	7.29E–06
12	9.99E–01	6.05E–06	8.04E–06
13	9.99E–01	6.98E–06	8.77E–06
14	9.99E–01	7.93E–06	9.49E–06
15	9.99E–01	8.90E–06	1.02E–05
16	9.99E–01	9.89E–06	1.09E–05
17	9.99E–01	1.09E–05	1.15E–05
18	9.99E–01	1.19E–05	1.22E–05
19	9.99E–01	1.29E–05	1.28E–05
20	9.99E–01	1.39E–05	1.34E–05
21	9.99E–01	1.49E–05	1.40E–05
22	9.99E–01	1.59E–05	1.45E–05
23	9.99E–01	1.69E–05	1.51E–05
24	9.99E–01	1.78E–05	1.56E–05
25	9.99E–01	1.88E–05	1.61E–05
26	9.99E–01	1.97E–05	1.66E–05
27	9.99E–01	2.06E–05	1.71E–05
28	9.99E–01	2.15E–05	1.76E–05
29	9.99E–01	2.24E–05	1.80E–05
30	9.99E–01	2.33E–05	1.84E–05

TABLE D.4—(*continued*)

Time (d)	Wound	Kidneys	24 h Urine
35	9.99E–01	2.73E–05	2.03E–05
40	9.99E–01	3.07E–05	2.19E–05
45	9.98E–01	3.36E–05	2.31E–05
50	9.98E–01	3.60E–05	2.40E–05
55	9.98E–01	3.79E–05	2.47E–05
60	9.98E–01	3.94E–05	2.52E–05
65	9.98E–01	4.05E–05	2.55E–05
70	9.97E–01	4.13E–05	2.56E–05
75	9.97E–01	4.18E–05	2.56E–05
80	9.97E–01	4.21E–05	2.55E–05
85	9.97E–01	4.22E–05	2.54E–05
90	9.97E–01	4.21E–05	2.51E–05
95	9.97E–01	4.19E–05	2.48E–05
100	9.97E–01	4.15E–05	2.44E–05
105	9.97E–01	4.10E–05	2.40E–05
110	9.97E–01	4.05E–05	2.35E–05
115	9.97E–01	3.99E–05	2.30E–05
120	9.97E–01	3.92E–05	2.25E–05
125	9.97E–01	3.85E–05	2.20E–05
130	9.96E–01	3.78E–05	2.15E–05
135	9.96E–01	3.70E–05	2.09E–05
140	9.96E–01	3.62E–05	2.04E–05
145	9.96E–01	3.54E–05	1.99E–05
150	9.96E–01	3.46E–05	1.94E–05
155	9.96E–01	3.39E–05	1.88E–05
160	9.96E–01	3.31E–05	1.83E–05
165	9.96E–01	3.23E–05	1.78E–05
170	9.95E–01	3.15E–05	1.73E–05
180	9.95E–01	3.00E–05	1.63E–05
195	9.95E–01	2.79E–05	1.50E–05
210	9.95E–01	2.59E–05	1.37E–05

TABLE D.4—(*continued*)

Time (d)	Wound	Kidneys	24 h Urine
225	9.95E–01	2.40E–05	1.26E–05
240	9.95E–01	2.24E–05	1.15E–05
255	9.95E–01	2.09E–05	1.06E–05
270	9.94E–01	1.95E–05	9.76E–06
285	9.94E–01	1.83E–05	9.01E–06
300	9.94E–01	1.72E–05	8.33E–06
315	9.94E–01	1.62E–05	7.72E–06
330	9.94E–01	1.53E–05	7.17E–06
345	9.94E–01	1.45E–05	6.69E–06
360	9.94E–01	1.38E–05	6.25E–06
400	9.94E–01	1.23E–05	5.31E–06
500	9.93E–01	1.01E–05	3.92E–06
600	9.93E–01	9.07E–06	3.28E–06
720	9.93E–01	8.58E–06	2.95E–06
900	9.92E–01	8.39E–06	2.79E–06
1,000	9.92E–01	8.38E–06	2.77E–06
1,500	9.91E–01	8.50E–06	2.74E–06
2,000	9.89E–01	8.62E–06	2.74E–06
2,500	9.88E–01	8.72E–06	2.74E–06
3,000	9.87E–01	8.80E–06	2.74E–06
3,500	9.85E–01	8.87E–06	2.74E–06
4,000	9.84E–01	8.92E–06	2.73E–06
4,500	9.82E–01	8.97E–06	2.73E–06
5,000	9.81E–01	9.00E–06	2.73E–06
6,000	9.78E–01	9.05E–06	2.72E–06
7,000	9.75E–01	9.07E–06	2.72E–06
8,000	9.73E–01	9.08E–06	2.71E–06
9,000	9.70E–01	9.09E–06	2.71E–06
10,000	9.67E–01	9.08E–06	2.70E–06

Appendix E

Radiation Detectors and Calibration

Frequently the assessment of the radiological consequences of a contaminated wound is based on direct measurements of radioactive material at the wound site with an external detector. This Appendix describes the detectors normally used for wound monitoring, associated apparatus, and calibration.

E.1 Solid-State Detectors

Because of their high resolution and small sizes, solid-state detectors offer advantages in both identifying and localizing contamination in a wound. The following types of detectors are commonly used for wound monitoring.

E.1.1 *Germanium Diodes*

The most common type of wound monitor in use for photon emitters is a high-purity, or intrinsic germanium diode. These detectors offer superior resolution, ~700 eV at the x-ray energy of 5.9 keV; thus, multiple radionuclides can be identified by their different photon emissions. In addition, germanium diodes have a relatively high intrinsic efficiency, but are necessarily limited in size, and so cannot provide high geometric efficiency. However, for wound monitoring, small detector size is an advantage, because it is easier to shield the detector from interferences, and a small detector can more easily determine the distribution of activity in a larger-area wound. Germanium detectors are operated at liquid nitrogen temperature, and it is recommended that intrinsic germanium detectors used for wound monitoring be maintained at liquid nitrogen temperature because it takes hours for the detector to cool down to operating temperature, and time may be of the essence when responding to a contaminated wound situation. Some manufacturers now offer electric refrigeration systems to cool germanium detectors to operating temperature without the use of liquid nitrogen; this technology would offer an advantage in a field location.

The high resolution of germanium detectors frequently enables direct measurements to be made of the depth of contamination in a wound. For example, the principal photon emissions of ^{239}Pu are uranium L-shell x rays with energies of 13.6, 17.2, and 20.2 keV. Because the attenuation coefficient of soft tissues changes by a factor of two over this energy range, the depth of activity in the wound can be determined by comparing the relative counts observed in each peak with those observed from a bare source (Berger and Lane, 1984). When ^{241}Am is present a similar technique compares the x-ray counts with those from the 59.6 keV gamma ray. This method is applicable to any radionuclide that emits low-energy photons of at least two different energies. Sequential measurements of these ratios over time may also provide information on changes in the size or shape of the embedded fragments or particles, changes in depth, or encapsulation.

E.1.2 *Lithium-Drifted Silicon Diodes*

Although not in common use, small lithium-drifted silicon [Si(Li)] detectors may be used for wound monitoring. These detectors are operated at liquid nitrogen temperature, and have superior resolution to germanium diodes. In trying to determine the depth of burial of a transuranic radionuclide in a wound by comparing the relative attenuation of the L-shell x rays, a Si(Li) detector has an advantage over an intrinsic germanium detector because its greater resolution makes it possible to separate out the subpeaks within the three groups of x rays, and so more detailed information on the relative attenuation is available. This methodology has been thoroughly described by Sherman *et al.* (1984) in an application of Si(Li) detectors to detection of transuranics in lung.

E.1.3 *Cadmium Telluride Detectors*

Another type of diode is the cadmium telluride (CdTe) detector, which has one major advantage over germanium and silicon; it can be operated at room temperature. However, its resolution is much poorer, ~3 keV at 30 keV, and so it cannot, for example, separate the L-shell x-ray complex of plutonium at 13.6, 17.2, and 20.2 keV. It has excellent efficiency; a detector only 2 mm thick will absorb 85 % of incident 100 keV photons (Entine, 1976). It may well be the detector of choice for detection of ^{241}Am and other radionuclides with primary photon emissions in the range of 30 to 200 keV, and because it need not be cooled, it is preferable for field operations where immediate screening of a wound is desired before transporting the injured worker to a central facility.

E.2 Scintillation Detectors

Scintillation detectors operate by a fundamentally different mechanism from solid-state detectors. Although electrons are initially liberated in both types of crystal by incoming photons, in solid-state detectors those electrons themselves are collected to produce a signal, whereas in scintillation detectors, the signal is produced by light emitted by outer shell electrons filling vacancies created in the lower shells by photon ionization. The emitted light, usually in the ultraviolet region of the spectrum, is collected, converted to an electrical output, and amplified by a photomultiplier tube optically coupled to the scintillator crystal. The advantages of scintillators over solid-state detectors include the facts that they are operated at room temperature and can be made quite large and, therefore have high geometric and intrinsic efficiencies. The disadvantages include poorer resolution and generally higher backgrounds than germanium detectors.

E.2.1 *Thallium-Activated Sodium-Iodide Scintillators*

Small NaI(Tl) detectors may be used for wound monitoring if the radionuclides of interest emit energetic gamma rays (*i.e.*, photon energies greater than ~100 keV) and the mixture of radionuclides is well known. However, the limited resolution of these detectors limits their usefulness if the composition of radioactive material is variable or unknown. Thin crystals (*i.e.*, 1 to 3 mm thick) may be used for detection of low-energy photons, but the high background counting rates in these crystals generally result in their being less useful than other detectors. It should be noted, however, that some survey meters use NaI(Tl) crystals as the detector element.

E.2.2 *Dual-Crystal Scintillators*

Perhaps the most commonly used scintillation detectors for low-energy photons are the dual-crystal or so-called "phoswich" (phosphor sandwich) detectors developed by Laurer at New York University (Laurer and Eisenbud, 1968). These detectors consist of two scintillators optically coupled and viewed by the same photomultiplier tube(s). The front scintillator is a thin (~3 mm thick) NaI(Tl) crystal, backed by a thick (~50 mm) thallium-doped cesium iodide [CsI(Tl)] or other crystal, which has a different fluorescent decay time from the front crystal. Thus, the electronic outputs from the two scintillators will have different rise times, and so can be distinguished by pulse-shape analysis techniques. The thicker (backing) crystal is then used as an anti-coincidence shield, and any photon interactions that occur in the front crystal are rejected if the photon also interacts in the thick crystal. Thus, the detector will record only low-energy photon interactions, that is, only photons that are completely absorbed in the front crystal. Typical phoswich detectors are ~650 mm in diameter, and so are frequently collimated or partially covered with shielding when used as wound monitors, in order to reduce the background and provide better spatial resolution to locate the buried contamination. If the type of contamination is known, and if higher-energy photons, such as the 59.6 keV gamma ray from ^{241}Am are to be measured, the higher efficiency of the phoswich may offer some advantage. Depth measurements can still be performed by comparing x-ray counting rates or scattered photon counting rates to peak gamma-ray counts, but are not as sensitive as those made with a high-resolution detector by comparing the counting rates in the various x-ray groups. However, due to its high efficiency and low background, a phoswich detector may be better able to quantify the amount of activity at a wound site than other scintillators.

E.3 Proportional Counters

Some facilities still use gas-filled proportional counters for measurements of low-energy photon emitters *in vivo* and such detectors may also be used for wound monitoring. Typically such detectors will be argon-methane gas-flow counters or sealed xenon-methane counters, frequently with separate anodes or chambers serving as anti-coincidence shields. Proportional counters offer the high resolution of solid-state detectors combined with low backgrounds, but also with low efficiencies, since the absorbing medium is a gas rather than a solid. Such detectors are normally used only for detection of photons with energies below ~30 keV, because detection efficiencies fall off rapidly above that energy, and become essentially nil at ~100 keV. The high resolution offers the ability to make fine distinctions in burial depth of the contamination. Although proportional counters can be made quite large, such as to cover the entire chest area, this does not offer an advantage for wound monitoring.

E.4 Other Apparatus

Although a full description of other apparatuses used in wound monitoring is beyond the scope of this Report, a brief description is included here for completeness.

E.4.1 *Electronic Modules*

Typical electronic modules used in photon spectrometry include pre-amplifiers, amplifiers, discriminators, pulse-shape analyzers, amplitude to digital converters, and multi-channel analyzers. Almost all current multi-channel analyzers are computer-based, usually consisting of a plug-in board and accompanying software. The analog to digital converter circuit is usually intrinsic to the board, so that the amplified signal from the detector is fed directly into the computer. Personal computers are frequently used in a stand-alone configuration for spectroscopy, and laptops may be used for field locations.

E.4.2 *Positioning Apparatus*

Frequently some sort of positioning apparatus will be employed to provide a constant and reproducible geometry for wound monitoring. This is especially important if a series of wound counts is made before and after surgical excision of contaminated tissue. Some facilities, if time permits, will make a plaster-of-paris mold to hold the subject's extremity in the initial counting position, so that the limb can later be placed in the exact same orientation. Other devices may include such simple apparatus as an armrest, or merely using foam pillows to cushion and position the extremity. A careful record should always be made of the counting geometry, and documented with photographs. Digital or instant-developing photographs are preferred, so as to ensure that an adequate visual record of the counting geometry has been made. Photos should be supplemented with detailed measurements of the distance from the detector window to the wound, and from various landmarks on the detector or its mounting apparatus to landmarks on the subject. These measurements should be recorded in a logbook and cross-referenced to the photographs.

E.5 Detector Calibration

Calibration of a wound monitor is no different in principle from calibration of any other radiation detector. A source of known activity is counted in a configuration that approximates as closely as possible that of the unknown to be assayed. For wound monitoring, a point source of the radionuclide of interest usually a planchet with electrodeposited activity or a sealed drop of solution encased in plastic (*i.e.*, a "button" source) is used. The source is placed in the positioning apparatus and covered with an appropriate thickness of tissue-equivalent absorber, such as sugar, wax or water. As the photon energy increases above 200 keV, the exact tissue equivalence of the absorber becomes less important. The detector efficiency (*i.e.*, counts per minute in a designated region of interest per radioactive transformation) is measured and then applied to the net counting rate observed from the wound. Some facilities prefer to use the inverse of the efficiency, known as the calibration factor (*i.e.*, disintegrations per count per minute) to relate the observed counting rate to the activity in the wound. Actual samples of the contaminating material should also be examined if available, in order to obtain data on self-absorption, dissolution rates, and other parameters that could affect dose calculations.

Appendix F

Wound Pathobiology

The skin is the largest organ in the body and its primary function is to serve as a protective barrier against the environment. Other important functions include fluid homeostasis, thermoregulation, immune surveillance, sensory detection, and self-healing (Holbrook and Wolff, 1993). Loss of the integrity of large portions of the skin due to injury may result in significant disability or even death. The most common cause of significant skin loss is thermal injury with an estimated 2.5 million burns each year in the United States alone (CDC, 1982).

Wound repair is an integration of dynamic interactive processes involving soluble mediators, formed blood elements, extracellular matrix, and parenchymal cells. Unencumbered, these wound repair processes follow a specific time sequence and can be temporally categorized into three major groups: inflammation, tissue formation, and tissue remodeling. The three phases of wound repair, however, are not mutually exclusive but rather overlap in time [see Clark (1996) for a detailed discussion].

F.1 Inflammation

Severe tissue injury causes blood vessel disruption with concomitant extravasation of blood constituents. Blood coagulation and platelet aggregation generate a fibrin-rich clot that plugs severed vessels and fills discontinuities in the wounded tissue. While the blood clot within vessel lumen reestablishes hemostasis, the clot within wound space provides a provisional matrix for cell migration. Proper clearance of the clot provisional matrix appears just as important as its deposition. Inadequate removal of the fibrin-rich provisional matrix or continual deposition of clot, as in chronic inflammation, may lead to fibrosis (Olman *et al.*, 1995).

F.1.1 *Neutrophils*

The coagulation pathways activate complement pathways and injured parenchymal cells generate numerous vasoactive mediators and chemotactic factors which together recruit inflammatory leukocytes to the wound site (Baggiolini *et al.*, 1994; Williams, 1988). Infiltrating neutrophils cleanse the wounded area of foreign particles, including bacteria. If excessive microorganisms or indigestible foreign particles have lodged in the wound site, neutrophils will continue to be recruited causing further tissue damage as they attempt to clear these contaminants through the release of enzymes and toxic oxygen products. When particle clearance has been completed, generation of granulocyte chemoattractants ceases and the remaining neutrophils become effete.

F.1.2 *Monocytes*

In unhampered wound repair monocyte accumulation persists for several days after the neutrophil influx has ceased. Although many of the same general chemoattractants that draw neutrophils into the wound also attract monocytes, specific monocyte chemoattractants are responsible for the prolonged recruitment of these cells. Outside of the circulation, probably through interaction with the connective tissue, monocytes undergo a metamorphosis to activated macrophages with increased capacity for phagocytosis of degraded extracellular matrix components, bacteria, and foreign particles. Besides promoting phagocytosis and debridement, interaction with the connective tissue also stimulates monocytes to induce platelet-derived growth factor (PDGF) (Juliano and Haskill, 1993; Shaw *et al.*, 1990), a potent chemoattractant and mitogen for fibroblasts (Heldin and Westermark, 1996). PDGF, along with other growth factors emanating from macrophages, such as transforming growth factor-β (TGF-β) (Roberts and Sporn, 1996), or from the blood, such as insulin-like growth factor, initiate tissue repair. Thus, macrophages appear to play a pivotal role in the transition between wound inflammation and repair (Riches, 1996).

F.2 Reepithelialization

Reepithelialization of a wound begins within hours after injury. It is clear that rapid reestablishment of any epithelial barrier decreases victim morbidity and mortality. Epithelial cells from residual epithelial structures move quickly to dissect clot and damaged stroma from the wound space and repave the surface of viable tissue. Extracellular matrix degradation is clearly required for the dissection of migrating wound epidermis between the collagenous dermis and the fibrin eschar (Bugge *et al.*, 1996) and probably depends on epidermal cell production of both collagenase (Pilcher *et al.*, 1997; Woodley *et al.*, 1986) and plasminogen activator (Grondahl-Hansen *et al.*, 1988). These proteases enzymatically digest the extracellular matrix in the plane of epidermal migration. Epidermal migration and dissection between viable and nonviable tissue ultimately results in sloughing the eschar.

One to two days after injury, epithelial cells at the wound margin begin to proliferate (Krawczyk, 1971). Many growth factors have been shown to stimulate reepithelialization in animal models (Brown *et al.*, 1989; Hebda *et al.*, 1990; Lynch *et al.*, 1989; Staino-Coico *et al.*, 1993) and lack of their receptors in transgenic animals leads to deficient reepithelialization (Werner, 1998). Together these data are compelling support for the hypothesis that growth factors are required for reepithelialization. As reepithelialization ensues, basement membrane proteins reappear in a very ordered sequence from the margin of the wound inward in a zipper-like fashion (Clark *et al.*, 1982). Epidermal cells revert to their normal phenotype, once again firmly attaching to reestablished basement membrane.

F.3 Granulation Tissue

New stroma, often called granulation tissue, begins to invade the wound space ~4 d after injury. The name granulation tissue derives from the granular appearance of newly forming tissue when it is incised and visually examined. Numerous new capillaries endow the neostroma with its granular appearance. Macrophages, fibroblasts and blood vessels move into the wound space as a unit (Hunt, 1980) that correlates well with the proposed biologic interdependence of these cells during tissue repair. The macrophages provide a continuing source of growth factors necessary to stimulate fibroplasia and angiogenesis, fibroblasts construct new extracellular matrix necessary to support cell ingrowth, and blood vessels carry oxygen and nutrients necessary to sustain cell metabolism.

F.3.1 *Fibroplasia*

Fibroblasts and the extracellular matrix that they synthesize are collectively known as fibroplasia. Growth factors, particularly

PDGF (Heldin and Westermark, 1996) and TGF-β (Roberts and Sporn, 1996), in concert with the clot matrix proteins fibrin and fibronectin (Gray *et al.*, 1993; Postlethwaite *et al.*, 1981; Xu and Clark, 1996), presumably stimulate fibroblasts of the peri-wound tissue to proliferate and migrate into the wound space.

The early wound extracellular matrix was designated provisional matrix (Clark *et al.*, 1982). It is initially composed of plasma-derived fibrin, fibronectin and vitronectin and later composed of *in situ*-produced hyaluronan and fibronectin. These provisional matrix constituents contribute to tissue formation by providing a scaffold or conduit for cell migration (fibronectin) (Greiling and Clark, 1997), low impedance for cell invasion (hyaluronic acid) (Toole, 1991), a reservoir for cytokines including growth and chemotactic factors (fibrinogen) (Sahni *et al.*, 1998) and direct signals to the cells through integrin receptors (Schwartz *et al.*, 1995). Once the fibroblasts have migrated into the wound they gradually switch their major function to collagen production (Welch *et al.*, 1990). After an abundant collagen matrix is deposited in the wound, fibroblasts cease collagen production.

F.3.2   *Neovascularization*

Fibroplasia would halt if neovascularization failed to accompany the newly forming complex of fibroblasts and extracellular matrix. The process of new blood vessel formation is called angiogenesis (Madri *et al.*, 1996). Angiogenesis is a complex process that relies on an appropriate extracellular matrix in the wound bed as well as endothelial cell phenotype alteration, stimulated migration, and mitogenic stimulation of endothelial cells (Madri *et al.*, 1996). Soluble factors that may be responsible for wound angiogenesis include basic fibroblast growth factor (Folkman and Klagsbrun, 1987), vascular endothelial growth factor (Keck *et al.*, 1989), angiopoietin (Suri *et al.*, 1996), PDGF (Battegay *et al.*, 1994), and many others (Clark and Singer, 2000). Several isoforms of vascular endothelial growth factor (Veikkola and Alitalo, 1999) and angiopoietins (Davis and Yancopoulos, 1999) have been identified that affect endothelial cell growth and angiogenesis differentially. Within a day or two after removal of angiogenic stimuli, capillaries undergo regression as characterized by mitochondria swelling in endothelial cells, platelet adherence to the blood vessel wall, vascular stasis, and endothelial cell apoptosis and ingestion of debris by macrophages.

F.4 Wound Contraction and Extracellular Matrix Reorganization

During the second and third week of healing, fibroblasts begin to assume a myofibroblast phenotype (Welch *et al.*, 1990). The appearance of the myofibroblasts corresponds to the commencement of connective tissue compaction and the contraction of the wound. Fibroblasts link to the extracellular matrix molecules and to each other. New collagen bundles in turn have the capacity to join end-to-end with collagen bundles at the wound edge and ultimately to form covalent crosslinks among themselves and with the collagen bundles of the adjacent dermis. These cell-cell, cell-matrix, and matrix-matrix links provide a network across the wound whereby the traction of fibroblasts on their pericellular matrix can be transmitted across the wound (Singer *et al.*, 1984).

PDGF, the major fibroblast mitogen in serum, stimulates fibroblast contraction of collagen gels *in vitro* (Clark *et al.*, 1989). Since PDGF is abundant in wounds (Ansel *et al.*, 1993), it may also provide the signal for wound contraction. TGF-β has also been shown to stimulate fibroblast-driven collagen gel contraction (Reed *et al.*, 1994) and persists in wound fibroblasts during the time of tissue contraction (Clark *et al.*, 1995). Perhaps both PDGF and TGF-β signal wound contraction; one more example of the many redundancies observed in the critical processes of wound healing. In summary, wound contraction represents a complex and masterfully orchestrated interaction of cells, extracellular matrix and cytokines.

Collagen remodeling during the transition from granulation tissue to scar is dependent on continued collagen synthesis and collagen catabolism. The degradation of wound collagen is controlled by a variety of collagenase enzymes from macrophages, epidermal cells, and fibroblasts. These collagenases are specific for particular types of collagens but most cells probably contain two or more different types of these enzymes (Hasty *et al.*, 1986). Wounds gain only ~20 % of their final strength by the third week, during which time fibrillar collagen has accumulated relatively rapidly and has been remodeled by myofibroblast contraction of the wound. Thereafter the rate at which wounds gain tensile strength is slow, reflecting a much slower rate of collagen accumulation. In fact, the gradual gain in tensile strength has less to do with new collagen deposition than further collagen remodeling with formation of larger collagen bundles and an accumulation of intermolecular crosslinks (Bailey *et al.*, 1975). Nevertheless, wounds fail to attain the same breaking strength as uninjured skin. At maximum strength, a scar is only 70 % as strong as intact skin (Levenson *et al.*, 1965).

F.5 Burns

F.5.1 *Zones of Injury*

Although burn etiologies are diverse and burn wounds may be nonuniform, there are common problems and healing characteristics encountered in the understanding of burns. No matter how diverse the mode of burn trauma, the determination of burn depth during the immediate post-burn period is frequently difficult and imprecise. Burn care specialists typically have little or no difficulty in diagnosing a full-thickness third-degree burn where immediate coagulation is evident. This "zone of coagulation" exhibits no blood flow, is insensitive to pinprick due to the destruction of cutaneous nerve endings, and must eventually be excised and replaced. By definition, two additional zones of injury are commonly present in burn injuries (Zawacki, 1974). Peripherally, a "zone of hyperemia" is present and exhibits increased blood flow in the early hours after burn trauma. The area of greatest importance is the "zone of stasis." This region is sandwiched between the zones of hyperemia and coagulation. This tissue zone is severely compromised with progressingly diminished blood flow in the immediate post-burn period and will ultimately lose viability as the microcirculation becomes nonfunctional. The dynamic nature of this zone renders it a most difficult region to make an immediate clinical or histologic determination as to whether it is a partial-thickness second-degree or full-thickness third-degree injury. Assessments of burn depth become easier on subsequent days after injury when the overlying dead eschar demarcates from the underlying viable tissue.

F.5.2 *Healing of Burn Wounds*

F.5.2.1 *Inflammation.* The most important pathophysiologic characteristic of a burn that determines the course of its healing is burn depth. Necrosis of the epidermis and varying degrees of dermal necrosis, depending on the initial depth of the burn, is exhibited within the zone of coagulation. Blood vessels are coagulated and blood flow ceases. Cellular debris is mixed with collagen fibers, and there is an absence of intact hair follicles and glandular structures. Viable epidermal cells within follicles and glandular structures are found only at the deeper levels. The epidermis itself will be separated from the dermis. It is this dead tissue that forms the burn eschar, which can serve as an excellent medium for microorganisms if it is not removed. Capillaries in the zone of stasis closest to the zone of coagulation are completely occluded, with decreasing degrees of partial occlusion moving further from that zone (Boykin *et al.*, 1980). Although leukocyte sticking and erythrocyte aggregation in these capillaries are characteristic of the zone of stasis, platelet microthrombi are indicative of permanent vessel occlusion (Boykin *et al.*, 1980).

The occurrence of edema is gradual, and is related to the progression of stasis. Early edema results from heat injury that causes increased vascular permeability and exudation of fluid into the tissue interstitium. Some of this fluid is reabsorbed *via* lymphatics and some may be expressed as blister fluid. Edema associated with delayed stasis occurs between 4 and 16 h post-burn, mainly in the lower two-thirds of the zone of stasis. As stasis and complete capillary occlusion progress, the area of skin necrosis expands. The zone of hyperemia at the outer margin of affected tissue is characterized by vasodilation secondary to the effects of heat and inflammatory mediators. Aside from the capillary stasis and occlusion described above, the recruitment and function of platelets, neutrophils and monocytes at sites of burn injury are similar to those mechanisms in play during excisional wound repair.

F.5.2.2 *Epidermis.* Once the destructive phase has waned, surviving keratinocytes that are either at the epidermal wound margin or in deeply positioned epithelial appendages, such as dermal sweat ducts, hair follicles, or sebaceous glands, exhibit the first morphologic evidence of healing. Reepithelialization proceeds from these sites as described in the section on excisional wound repair. However, large areas of full-thickness burn injury have no surviving epithelial cells to initiate the process of epithelialization. Deep partial-thickness injuries exhibiting destruction of the source of stem cells (deep to the bulge region of hair follicles) will be extremely slow to resurface. For these reasons the dead tissue (eschar) is routinely excised and a partial thickness meshed skin autograft is placed over this wound bed. In these cases, reepithelialization is extremely rapid. The patient's own grafted epidermis serves as a ready source of migrating, proliferating keratinocytes that quickly grow across the interstices of the graft. Resurfacing is also rather rapid if the movements of new epithelium are not impeded by the presence of an eschar. If the burn eschar is left in place, the granulation tissue will develop under the eschar. Separation of the eschar can take 10 to 14 d if there is no infection or if surgical debridement is not performed; if infection occurs, the eschar separates sooner due to the action of proteinases produced by inflammatory cells and bacteria, but with a resultant increase in the depth of tissue necrosis.

F.5.2.3 *Blood Vessels.* Endothelium responds to vasoactive amines (such as histamine and serotonin) and end products of the kinin system in two phases as described earlier. An immediate period of vasoconstriction, followed by a longer period of vasodilatation and increased microvascular permeability, which is mediated largely by the vasoactive amines. Extravasation of fluid into the interstitium and edema formation is the outcome. Endothelial cells and platelets produce the arachidonic acid metabolites, prostacyclins and thromboxanes, respectively. These mediators are released in response to burn injury (Arturson, 1983; Heggers *et al.*, 1980) and appear to work antagonistically to one another, having somewhat opposing effects on vessel contraction and relaxation. They also affect the ability of other cells to stick to vessel walls causing occlusion. Regeneration of new blood vessels takes place by the process of angiogenesis as discussed in Section F.2 on excisional wound healing.

F.6 Foreign-Body Reactions

If substantial wound contamination has not occurred, neutrophil infiltration usually ceases within a few days. Most invading neutrophils become entrapped within the wound clot and desiccated tissue. This eschar sloughs during tissue regeneration. Neutrophils within viable tissue become senescent within a few days and are phagocytosed by tissue macrophages (Newman *et al.*, 1982). These processes mark the end to neutrophil-rich inflammation. However, substantial wound contamination will provoke a persistent neutrophil-rich inflammatory response. Foreign objects that can precipitate chronic inflammatory events that lead to foreign-body granuloma formation include metal suspensions, colloids and fragments as documented by foreign-body granuloma formation from elemental mercury (Bradberry *et al.*, 1996), thorium dioxide (Thorotrast®) (Plent *et al.*, 1990) (Section F.7.1.4), and bomb fragments (Wijekoon *et al.*, 1995), respectively. The granulomas formed in reaction to inert metals are fundamentally different from those generated from microorganisms as exemplified by the stimulation of nitric oxide by the latter (Kreuger *et al.*, 1998). Nevertheless, granulomas generated from inert material have biochemical evidence of ongoing inflammation (Lukacs *et al.*, 1994). As with burns, TNF-α generated from widespread granulomas can have adverse systemic effects such as the generation of an acute phase response and bone loss (Vukicevic *et al.*, 1994). Once granulomas begin to resolve they do so by apoptosis (Honma and Hamasaki, 1996).

F.6.1 *Foreign-Body Carcinogenesis in Humans*

The reaction of human tissues to foreign materials is important because of the paucity of information on radioactive materials and the view that radioactive solids may be handled in the body just like any other foreign body (Lushbaugh *et al.*, 1967). The risk of cancers associated with implanted prostheses has been stated to be small because the incidence of these cancers was low in the face of an increasing usage of such prostheses (Brand, 1994). The sole epidemiological study of artificial implants and soft-tissue sarcomas used a case-control approach with a population of 217 Vietnam War veterans with soft-tissue sarcomas (Morgan and Elcock, 1995). No association was found between having an implant of a pin, plate, staple or screw and presence of a soft-tissue sarcoma. Although the incidence is low, case reports of sarcomas associated with implanted materials continue (Lindeman *et al.*, 1990). A literature review (Jennings *et al.*, 1988) revealed 39 cases of sarcoma intimately associated with metallic foreign bodies such as shrapnel, or metallic implants such as plates. Of these 39 cases, 23 arose from soft tissues. The latency period ranged from four months to 63 y with a median of 15 y. A wide range of tumor types was reported. Five were malignant fibrous histiocytomas, three were fibrosarcomas, and two each were angiosarcomas, spindle-cell sarcomas, or polymorphic sarcomas.

F.6.2 *Foreign-Body Carcinogenesis in Animals*

The development of connective tissue tumors or sarcomas, associated with the presence of persistent foreign bodies in the subcutis, peritoneum or muscle of experimental animal models, has been recognized since the 1940s (*e.g.*, Turner, 1941; Oppenheimer *et al.*, 1948), and reports of tumors in man have occasionally appeared in the medical literature since the 19th century (Brand *et al.*, 1976). Otherwise referred to as surface carcinogenesis, smooth-surface carcinogenesis and solid-state carcinogenesis, foreign-body carcinogenesis (FBC) remains one of the most enigmatic phenomena in the field of experimental cancer research (Moizhess and Vasiliev, 1989), due at least in part to the impression that the carcinogenic action of foreign bodies is due to its physical presence in tissue, and not to chemical or biochemical interactions.

Most of the current knowledge on the phenomenology of FBC, as well as mechanistic understanding, has come from a substantial body of studies, done mostly in rodent animal models that have defined the parameters of foreign-body size, number, shape and composition, and the pathogenesis of lesion development. The earliest studies reported the development of sarcomas in rats implanted with plastic disks (Turner, 1941), or with 2 to 3 cm square cellulose films (Oppenheimer et al., 1948). The latter study was stimulated by the observation of Oppenheimer et al. (1948) of sarcomas arising at the site of the cellulose films that were wrapped around the kidneys of rats to produce experimental hypertension. These results were later confirmed by Zollinger (1952), who enclosed rat kidneys in acrylic resin plastic capsules to produce hypertension, and observed sarcomas at the capsule site in eight of 21 animals. He also was the first to recognize that the tumors were elicited by the foreign bodies themselves, without the involvement of a chemical carcinogen. At about the same time, Druckrey et al. (1952; 1956) called attention to the importance of the form of the implant in the etiology of FBC.

In 1955, Nothdurft concluded that the chemical nature of the implant was irrelevant to the production of the tumor, but that the cancerous process was involved in the formation of the enveloping capsule (summarized in Bischoff and Bryson, 1964). His studies showed that plastic disks were significantly more effective in producing sarcomas in rats than were equivalent masses of powder. This was true for both s.c. and intraperitoneal implantation sites. Additionally, Nothdurft (1955) showed that plastic disks with contiguous smooth surfaces were more carcinogenic than dishes of equivalent size but having perforated holes throughout.

Bischoff and Bryson (1964) have summarized the early work on FBC. Researchers implanted materials including, but not limited to polystyrene, cellulose hydrate, polyvinyl chloride, polyethylene, polymethylmethacrylate, silk, polyvinyl pyrrolidone, carbon polymers, gold, silver, tantalum, platinum, tin, asbestos, glass, quartz, silicone rubber, and dextrans of various molecular weights. These materials were implanted in various combinations of different physical forms such as sticks, balls, powders, bristles, foils (rigid and flexible), disks (with and without perforations), colloids, and fibers.

The results of the studies done through the early 1960s were unclear because of the bewildering array of variables, factors and cofactors that might or might not have played a role in the observed incidences of tumors. Not only were physical variables such as implant surface characteristics, size of implant, number of implants per animal and implant shape, implicated in the efficiency of producing foreign-body tumors, but other factors such as the presence of contaminants on the surface of the implant, the biological solubility or insolubility of the material, chemical reactivity at the surface, including free radical induction, all needed to be considered in the genesis of FBC. To deal with the issue of FBC, Bischoff and Bryson (1964) found it necessary to eliminate much of the testing data because of the presence of impurities or unknown constitution of the test materials, as well as decomposition of the implants, lack of reproducibility in results and inadequate control populations. Based on the response to highly unreactive substances such as gold, platinum, polyethylene, and a few other stable materials, they concluded that:

"There is a type of nonspecific carcinogenesis in rodents which is dependent upon a minimum surface requirement. This type of carcinogenesis is also dependent upon the development of a comparatively nonreactive fibrous capsule around the implant. As far as the subcutaneous site is concerned, the evidence completely justifies this assertion. The degree of smoothness of a surface and the exact meaning of smoothness are matters of comparative value among researchers. The threshold size applies not only to minimum overall dimensions, but also to minimal size irregularities (ridges, pores, etc.). Surface area is of greater significance that is surface texture."

Thus, it was clearly demonstrated that the physical presence of the implant was sufficient to result in tumorigenesis. As new plastic and metal materials were being increasingly introduced in human surgery for anatomical, functional or cosmetic reasons, implant-related basic research became focused on issues of biocompatibility and toxicity. However, FBC was not completely ignored, despite the evidence in people that the risk of developing implant-related tumors was low. In particular, Brand *et al.* (1975; 1976) investigated some of the mechanistic aspects of FBC.

F.7 Radiation Effects

The deterministic effects of radiation exposure of skin and s.c. tissue are well known for large fields, progressing through epilation, erythema, dry desquamation, moist desquamation, and ulceration at threshold doses of 3, 6, 10, 15 and 25 Gy, respectively (Mettler, 1990). However, there is considerable uncertainty about the effects of radiation on small volumes of tissue, as would be the case from a contaminated wound. NCRP (1999) suggested in Report No. 130 that for external exposure of skin to "hot particles," doses be limited so as to preclude the development of ulcers that would compromise the integrity of the skin as a barrier to infection. Presumably the same goal should apply to contaminated wounds, so that deterministic radiation effects do not hinder the healing process, and so that the stochastic risk of tumor formation is minimized. In this Section, the response of skin and s.c. tissue to external irradiation and to embedded radioactive materials is reviewed.

F.7.1 *Soft-Tissue Responses in Humans*

F.7.1.1 *Acute Local Injury.* There is an extensive literature on the response of the skin to acute external irradiation (*e.g.*, Barabanova, 2001; ICRP, 1991b; Mettler, 1990). For completeness, a brief review is in order in this Report. In many respects, the response of the skin to high radiation doses is similar to its response to thermal injury (Section F.5); the depth of tissue injury is the key parameter, which in turn depends on the penetrating ability of the incident radiation. Although the cellular damage occurs promptly, the expression of the injury occurs over a prolonged time, and is usually not immediately apparent, because the outer horny layer of the epidermis is not affected. The time course of injury expression is a function of absorbed dose, absorbed dose rate, radiation energy and quality (*i.e.*, its penetrating ability or linear energy transfer), dose distribution within the irradiated tissue, and the size and location of the irradiated tissue (Barabanova, 2001).

After initial, and usually transient, erythema, there is a latent period with no clinical manifestations of injury, much as occurs in the acute radiation syndrome, and for the same reason; stem cells have been destroyed, but severe injury does not appear until the mature cells they normally replace have died off. Again as in the acute radiation syndrome, the length of the latent period is a function of dose and dose rate. Secondary erythema typically appears at two to three weeks post-exposure, but may appear sooner with higher doses, or later with lower doses. The erythema results from increased vascular permeability much as occurs in the zone of hyperemia in thermal burns. About a week after the appearance of secondary erythema, dry desquamation appears at absorbed doses of 10 Gy or more, as dead epithelium separates from its supporting structures. At doses of 15 to 20 Gy, edema, bullae formation, and moist desquamation occur at three to four weeks or more post-exposure. Reepithelialization and wound healing can still occur at this stage, but at absorbed doses of 25 Gy or more, there is frequently a cycle of reepithelialization followed by breakdown, due to injury to the supporting vasculature. Small ulcers may develop at absorbed doses >25 Gy, and may heal by scar formation, as described in Section F.4 above. At absorbed doses well in excess of 30 Gy, tissue necrosis appears, and the probability of healing depends to a large extent on the area and depth of tissue irradiated (Barabanova, 2001). Various methods of skin grafting have been used in the treatment of radiation injury, but their success has been highly variable, again depending on the absorbed dose and area involved (Peter *et al.*, 2001; Zaharia *et al.*, 2001).

F.7.1.2 *Stochastic Effects.* Although the skin is relatively resistant to cancer induction by ionizing radiation, skin cancers have been observed as a complication of deterministic effects (Barabanova, 2001). However, the more common skin cancers, squamous- and basal-cell carcinomas, are rarely fatal. There is little evidence that malignant melanoma, which if not promptly treated has a high mortality rate, is associated with ionizing radiation exposure, whereas the dominant factor for non-melanoma skin cancer is exposure to ultraviolet radiation (ICRP, 1991b). The risk factor for ionizing radiation-induced skin cancer, based on an additive risk model and averaged over the whole body is taken to be 8.7×10^{-4} Sv^{-1} person-y^{-1} (ICRP, 1991b).

F.7.1.3 *Wound Cases.* Many wounds contaminated with radioactive materials have occurred over the years in nuclear weapons production workers, and the vast majority of these involved plutonium. However, there are few descriptions of the pathological changes that occur in plutonium-containing wounds. Lushbaugh *et al.* (1967) reported on eight accidental cases of intradermal contamination with metallic plutonium, with wound content of from 0.09 to 6.8 MBq ^{239}Pu (0.04 to 3.1 g plutonium). In some cases, the wounds were immediately debrided, but subsequent measurement showed remnants of plutonium metal. In others, millimeter-sized intradermal nodules appeared at the previously debrided wound sites. The nodules sometimes were painful and became progressively more superficial and prominent. The size of the lesions depended on the dispersion of the plutonium particles. The largest nodule was 2 mm in its greatest dimension. At six months, the typical histologic reaction was a fibrous granuloma located in the dermis. Described as a foreign-body reaction to the plutonium particles, it was an inflammatory reaction dominated by macrophages, lymphoid infiltrates, and fibrosis with extensive collagen (Section F.6). After a year or two, no cellular reactions were found, but dense collagenous fibromas formed that became increasingly sparse of nuclei. With time, the fibrous encapsulation continued to change from collagenous fibrils, which were arranged in concentric swirls around the metal deposits, to become more fibrillar and particulate after ~5 y. The final stage was complete liquefaction of the collagen surrounding the plutonium particles. These findings imply that encapsulation of the plutonium in the wound isolates it. However, an apparent breakdown of these capsules with a subsequent reforming of nodules at the wound site has been reported in some cases (Hammond and Putzier, 1964). Such a breakdown could result in plutonium being released into the bloodstream. This observation indicates the desirability of complete removal of plutonium whenever possible.

Preneoplastic lesions associated with embedded radioactive materials have been reported. Lushbaugh and Langham (1962) described a preneoplastic lesion in the skin overlying a plutonium metal fragment embedded in the palm of a machinist. At the time of wounding, a radioactive foreign body was removed from the hand. About 4 y later, a nodule developed at the site and was excised. Autoradiographs of the excised tissue showed dense alpha tracks (evidence of plutonium decays) in the area of maximum damage in the dermis and penetration into the basal layer of the epidermis. Histologically, the reaction at the site was characterized as a chronic radiodermatitis consisting of collagenous degeneration of the corium and epidermal cytological changes, raising the question of the fate of the lesion if the nodule had not been removed.

Despite these reports of preneoplastic lesions, no neoplasms in man have been described associated with embedded radioactive fragments, perhaps due to the usual surgical excision of such wounds.

F.7.1.4 *Thorotrast® Cases.* Intravenous injections of Thorotrast® for radiographic visualization of local circulation were not always completely successful, and small amounts of Thorotrast® were occasionally deposited extravascularly (Section 3.3; Appendix B.6.6). In some cases, a progressively enlarging and calcifying tissue reaction, known as a Thorotrast® granuloma or thorotrastoma, developed 8 to 20 y after deposition in the s.c. tissues. Thorotrast® injections into the carotid artery were apparently most difficult, and Blomberg *et al.* (1963) estimated that in a few percent of the carotid artery injections for cerebral angiography, significant amounts of Thorotrast® were deposited extravascularly. Of 91 cases of thorotrastoma identified in an epidemiological survey in Portugal in 1966, 67 were located in the cervical region (da Horta, 1967b). The development and subsequent behavior of these granulomas depended on the amount of Thorotrast® extravasated, the post-injection interval, and the functional importance of the affected structures; da Horta (1967b) described these lesions as very dense connective tissue in which Thorotrast® was found both free and in phagocytes. With time, the collagenous component underwent hyalinization, fibrinoid transformation softening, and calcification. The central zones, where collagen disintegration was greater, had few cells and contained little Thorotrast®. The periphery, "the invasive zone of the granuloma," was cellular, with many large macrophages containing engulfed Thorotrast®.

Dahlgren (1967a) and da Horta (1967b) reported five cases of malignant connective tissue neoplasms arising at the edges of thorotrastomas ~10 y after the first appearance of the thorotrastoma itself; three spindle-cell sarcomas and two neurofibrosarcomas in the cervical region. Another report (Leiberman *et al.*, 1995) noted a metastasizing soft-tissue sarcoma in a patient 30 y after injection. Thus, in three case series of thorotrastomas in the cervical region, six cases of malignant soft-tissue tumors were seen in 222 patients after a latent period of ~20 y.

F.7.1.5 *Site-Specific Effects: Eyes.* NCRP Report No. 130 (NCRP, 1999) provided a review of the anatomy and physiology of the eye in view of possible exposures to "hot particles" that could become lodged in one of the structures of the eye. That report made the important point that radiation exposure (including contaminated wounds) to the eye may present a more serious situation medically than a corresponding mechanical injury with no contamination, since radiation damage to the progenitor cells of the various structures of the eye may preclude healing of the injury. For example, the corneal endothelium consists of a layer of non-mitotic cells that repair injury by the spreading of surviving adjacent cells. If cell survival is compromised by radiation injury, the repair of mechanical injury could also be inhibited.

In addition, if the lens is involved, or lies within the range of radiations emitted from the wound site, some degree of local opacification may ensue. It is well known that radiation exposure to the eye can result in cataract formation, but such effects have been thought to be solely deterministic, with a threshold of several gray. Evidence described in NCRP Report No. 130 (NCRP, 1999) indicates that the basic cellular damage resulting in opacification is a stochastic process, rather than a deterministic one, since epithelial cells in the germinative zone of the lens have been shown to be the progenitors of the abnormal fiber cells that constitute the cataract (Merriam and Worgul, 1983; Worgul and Rothstein, 1977) These cells differentiate abnormally due to radiation damage to their deoxyribonucleic acid (Worgul *et al.*, 1989). Irradiation of fewer than 1 % of the epithelial cells can be cataractogenic (Worgul *et al.*, 1993) but the expression of opacity may require a substantial portion of the lifespan. Furthermore, partial exposure of the lens to a given dose results in less opacity than if the entire lens had been irradiated (Leinfelder and Riley, 1956). Consequently, localized irradiation from a contaminated wound may cause little or no degradation of vision.

As an example, consider the accident that occurred at the Hanford, Washington site in 1976 (Breitenstein and Palmer, 2001; Thompson, 1983). An ion-exchange column in a glove box exploded, showering a worker with nitric acid and glass shards containing or contaminated with an estimated 40 to 180 GBq of ^{241}Am. Initial medical appraisal revealed nitric-acid burns to the face, including the eyes, and multiple small lacerations and embedded fragments, although not within the eyeballs. The patient complained of stickiness and discomfort in his eyes, with photophobia. Ophthalmologic examination on day 22 after the accident resulted in removal of a small superficial foreign body in the right cornea; removal of two other small fragments noted in the left cornea was delayed as healing of the acid burns was progressing. A small erosion of the left cornea developed over the next 40 d and was treated conservatively. On day 322 iritis was noticed, and another ophthalmologic exam on day 350 noted a 90 % mature cataract of the left lens with corneal scarring over the central area of each cornea; the left cataract was removed on day 547, and it was shown to contain ~18 mBq of ^{241}Am. On day 1,030 post-accident, the patient underwent a right cataract extraction with removal of five foreign bodies from the conjunctiva and cornea (Breitenstein, 1983). External radiation measurements over the left eyeball were able to detect ^{241}Am *in vivo* (Palmer *et al.*, 1983). However, the attending ophthalmologist was of the opinion that the cataracts were induced by trauma rather than by radiation (Breitenstein and Palmer, 1989).

Dose calculation for the eyes proceeds as in any other case, with some determination (or assumption) as to the geometrical relation between the source and the target structures, and the use of point kernels, or Monte-Carlo methods, to estimate the dose. In the Hanford case, the dose was calculated by assuming a constant, uniform distribution of ^{241}Am throughout the lens, determining the alpha radiation dose rate, and integrating the dose rate from the time of exposure to the time of cataract removal; the calculated dose to the lens of the left eye was 0.4 Gy, while that to the lens of the right eye was 0.8 Gy (Filipy *et al.*, 1995).

F.7.1.6 *Site-Specific Effects: Testes.* Even though genetic effects of radiation have never been observed in humans, irradiation of the testes is a continuing concern, with the risk for severe genetic effects taken to be 6×10^{-3} Sv^{-1} (ICRP, 1991a). A reduction in the number of spermatogonia occurs at doses as low as 80 mGy, producing a reduction in sperm count in 30 to 60 d. Temporary sterility may result from doses as low as 150 mGy, and a single dose of 5 to 6 Gy may cause permanent sterility (Mettler and Upton, 1995). However, it is difficult to envision a contaminated wound situation that would produce radiation doses to the testes sufficient to cause sterility, primarily because the entire organs would not be irradiated at high enough levels, although a small portion may be locally irradiated.

F.7.2 *Soft-Tissue Responses in Animals*

The biologic effects of wounding with radioactive materials have been extensively studied in animals. Lisco and Kisieleski (1953) described the tissue reactions in rabbits and rats s.c. implanted with plutonium metal fragments (0.6 to 0.8 mg; 1.3 to 4 MBq ^{239}Pu). Local skin reactions such as erythema or edema were not noted during the course of the study, nor was hair affected. The initial local reactions were described as granulomatous, with increased cellularity at the wound site and the formation of a fibrous capsule. This encapsulation continued with time, gradually replacing the granulomatous features, leading ultimately to calcification of the fibrous capsule surrounding the fragment. The process took 2 to 3 y. Of note was the complete absence at early times of a discernable inflammatory reaction with exudate or edema. The authors noted that the plutonium metal tended to fragment into smaller particles, a phenomenon that occurred as early as 1 d after implantation. No tumors were noted.

In the 1960s, Brues *et al.* (1963; 1964; 1965) conducted a series of studies in which ^{239}Pu(VI) nitrate or polymeric ^{239}Pu was s.c. implanted into rats, with or without accompanying inert foreign bodies. Plutonium-239 nitrate injected into rats caused some tumors at the injection site, but more frequently in the skeleton. This result reflected the relative solubility of the ^{239}Pu in the injection solution and its translocation to the skeleton. In contrast, no local tumors occurred in mice that received similar injections, suggesting a species-specific response.

In rats i.m. injected with polymeric ^{239}Pu, 80 % retention was noted at the injection site after six months. Local sarcomas began appearing at this time. At the end of the 2 y study, 20 to 25 % of the injected dose remained at the wound site, and 2 to 9 % of the rats developed wound-site sarcomas. Mice, in contrast, developed no tumors at the wound sites, nor did dogs or swine that were followed up for at least 8 y after similar s.c. injections. This result also suggests the confounding factor of species-specificity in the interpretation of wound-site carcinogenesis.

Buldakov *et al.* (1971) noted the occurrence of benign and malignant neoplasms as well as focal fibrosis at sites where rats were injected with ^{239}Pu citrate or ammonium ^{239}Pu pentacarbonate, both soluble compounds of ^{239}Pu. The incidence of scar formation ranged from 8 to 30 % depending on the amount of injected ^{239}Pu (2 to 37 kBq). The highest incidence of malignant tumors was ~2.5 %. Bazhin *et al.* (1983) applied ^{239}Pu onto the abraded skin of rats and studied the retention of ^{239}Pu at the wound site, its translocation to systemic deposition sites, and the influence of chelation therapy on the biological effects of the plutonium. Although chelation therapy was shown effective in reducing the incidence of osteosarcoma by a factor of six, it did not affect the incidence of pathological changes in the wound sites. At lower dosages (40 to 180 kBq cm^{-2}) only nonmalignant changes occurred in skin; at higher dosages (722 kBq cm^{-2}) both tumors and fibrosarcomas were seen, but at low incidence (1 to 2 %). These data contrasted with the high tumor incidences observed by Siniakov *et al.* (1988) in rats i.m. injected with ^{239}Pu nitrate. In that study, fibrosarcomas, angiosarcomas, mesenchymomas, fibromas, rhabdomyosarcomas, squamous-cell carcinomas and basilomas were all observed, indicating that many different cell populations (epithelial and mesenchymal) were at risk to the carcinogenic action of ^{239}Pu alpha-particle radiation.

One study has demonstrated the carcinogenicity of DU metal fragments in the soft tissues of rats (Hahn *et al.*, 2002). A lifespan carcinogenesis and bioassay study with i.m.-implanted DU metal (alloyed with 0.75 % titanium) was designed to determine the carcinogenic potential of DU. The sizes and shapes of DU used were similar to the range of sizes and shapes of DU fragments embedded in soldiers wounded in the Gulf War. The mass of DU used varied by a factor of 20 and the surface area varied by a factor of 10. Four implants were made per rat. Fragments of tantalum were used as a negative control. Thorotrast® was used as a positive carcinogenic control. Six groups of 50 male, Wistar rats were treated with one of the following: DU (2 × 1 mm diameter), DU (2.5 × 2.5 × 1.5 mm), DU (5 × 5 × 1.5 mm), Thorotrast® injection (0.050 mL), tantalum (5 × 5 × 1.1 mm), or sham surgery. The fragments were implanted into the biceps femoris muscle of each hind leg. Thorotrast® was injected into the same muscle. The radiographic appearance of the

328 / APPENDIX F

implanted DU fragments changed markedly during the first year. At the time of implantation, the fragments were smooth with sharp edges. At 21 d after implantation, small, radiographically dense blebs extended from the edges of the fragments. At 1 y after implantation, the radiographic profiles of the fragments were rounded. At the time of death, many were enlarged up to 1.5 times. These radiographic changes were indicative of surface corrosion of the DU and capsule formation. The profiles of the tantalum fragments were smooth at all times.

The implants of DU or tantalum were encapsulated with connective tissue at the time of death. Some of the fragments were located in the muscles where they were originally implanted, but some had migrated to the loose connective tissues between the muscles of the leg. The injected Thorotrast® did not induce capsule formation, but localized in and around the muscles. The tantalum fragments were smooth and slipped easily from the capsules. The DU fragments, however, were difficult to remove from the capsules because of corrosion on the surfaces. The capsules around the DU implants were characterized histologically by fibrosis, inflammation, degeneration, and mineralization. Soft-tissue tumors of various types were present in association with many of the implants. The most commonly found were malignant fibrous histiocytoma and fibrosarcoma. The incidence of the tumors was significantly increased in the rats with the largest DU implants when compared with the sham or negative (tantalum) controls of the same size. In addition, there was a dose-related response in the DU treated rats. The response could not be explained by surface area alone. There was a correlation with the initial surface alpha activity. These findings clearly indicate that DU fragments of sufficient size are carcinogenic in rats.

Beta-emitting particles implanted under the skin have been shown to induce skin tumors in mice (Lang *et al.*, 1993). The particles were uranium irradiated with slow neutrons. They measured 300 to 700 m and contained 60 to 300 kBq of beta-emitting radionuclides per particle. Of 13 hairless mice followed for nine months, two developed squamous-cell carcinomas. Epithelial hyperplasia was strong in about half of the mice. These findings illustrate that the penetration of the beta emissions results in skin tumors; neither beta nor alpha-emitting radionuclides produce soft-tissue tumors in mice.

F.8 Summary

The presence of radioactive material in a wound further complicates a very involved process of tissue response and repair. Clearly, very high local radiation doses can impair wound healing by destroying the stem cells necessary to produce new tissue, but in a typical wound, such dose levels are not reached, or are only limited to a very small region, and so do not materially affect the healing process. There is clear evidence for carcinogenic responses to embedded radioactive materials, including plutonium and DU in rats, beta-emitting particles in mice, and Thorotrast® in humans. Embedded plutonium fragments have produced preneoplastic lesions in humans, but the lesions have been excised before any progression to a neoplasm. In addition, there is a low incidence of cancer induction arising from metallic implants in humans, but in most cases, foreign-body reactions in humans are limited to granuloma or fibroma production. In animal models, foreign-body carcinogenesis depends on the type of material embedded, as well as its size and shape, and is species-specific. The preponderance of the evidence seems to indicate that the most likely biological effect of a contaminated wound involving embedded radioactive material in a human will be a foreign-body reaction, with the activity having primarily the effect of driving the breakdown of fibrous capsules and subsequent reencapsulation (Section 3.2).

Glossary[12]

absorbed dose (*D*): Quotient of $d\bar{\epsilon}$ by d*m*, where $d\bar{\epsilon}$ is the mean energy imparted by ionizing radiation to matter in a volume element and d*m* is the mass of matter in that volume element: $D = d\bar{\epsilon}/dm$. For purposes of radiation protection and assessing dose or risk to humans in general terms, the quantity normally calculated is the mean absorbed dose in an organ or tissue (T): $D_T = \bar{\epsilon}_T/m_T$, where $\bar{\epsilon}$ is the total energy imparted in an organ or tissue of mass m_T. The SI unit of absorbed dose is the joule per kilogram (J kg^{-1}), and its special name is the gray (Gy). In conventional units often used by federal and state agencies, absorbed dose is given in rad; 1 rad = 0.01 Gy.

accident: An unintentional or unexpected happening that is undesirable or unfortunate, especially one resulting in injury, damage, harm or loss.

actinide: Element with atomic number from 90 through 103; a member of the actinide series of rare earths.

activity: Rate of transformation (or "disintegration" or "decay") of radioactive material. The SI unit of activity is the reciprocal second (s^{-1}), and its special name is the becquerel (Bq). In conventional units often used by federal and state agencies, activity is given in curies (Ci); 1 Ci = 3.7×10^{10} Bq.

adenocarcinoma: A malignant neoplasm of epithelial cells in a glandular or gland-like pattern.

adenoma: A benign epithelial tumor in which the cells form recognizable glandular structures or in which the cells are derived from glandular epithelium.

adenomatous: Pertaining to adenoma or to nodular hyperplasia of a gland.

adiabatic shear: An instability in metal deformation where the rate of thermal softening exceeds the rate of work hardening associated with the deformation.

adipose: Fatty.

administration (of radioactive material): Introduction of radioactive material directly into the body by injection, oral administration, or by some other route.

adnexal: Pertaining to accessory organs, as of the eye.

alpha radiation: Energetic nuclei of helium atoms, consisting of two protons and two neutrons, emitted spontaneously from nuclei in the decay

[12]Definitions of medical terms are taken from Miller and Keane (1987).

of some radionuclides. Alpha radiation is weakly penetrating, and can be stopped by a sheet of paper or the outer dead layer of skin. Also called alpha particle and sometimes shortened to alpha (*e.g.*, alpha-emitting radionuclide).

angiogenesis: Development of blood vessels in the embryo or into a solid tumor from surrounding tissue.

angiography: X-ray imaging of the blood or lymph vessels.

angiosarcoma: Malignant tumor of vascular tissue; also known as hemangiosarcoma.

anion: Negatively charged ion.

apoptosis: Genetically-programmed or externally-induced self-destruction of a cell.

apotransferrin: Transferrin not bound to iron (see **transferrin**).

aqueous: Watery; prepared with water.

arachidonic acid: A polyunsaturated omega-6 fatty acid that is present in the phospholipids of membranes of the body's cells.

atomic number (Z) (low-Z, high-Z): The atomic number of a nucleus is the number of protons contained in the nucleus. Low-Z describes nuclei with $Z \leq 26$. High-Z describes nuclei with $Z > 26$.

autoradiograph: Image of the distribution of activity in a tissue created by the emitted radiations.

axilla: The underarm area containing lymph nodes and channels, blood vessels, nerves, muscle, and fat; its anterior border is the *pectoralis major* muscle and its posterior border is the *latissimus dorsi* muscle.

basal cell: Cells that form a single row along basement membrane and are responsible for the pseudostratified appearance of the epithelium.

basement membrane: Very thin membrane beneath the epithelium.

becquerel (Bq): The SI special name for the unit of activity. 1 Bq equals one disintegration per second. 37 MBq (megabecquerel) = 1 mCi (millicurie) (see **curie**).

benign: A noncancerous condition that does not spread to other parts of the body.

beta radiation: Energetic electrons or positrons (positively charged electrons) emitted spontaneously from nuclei in decay of some radionuclides. Also called beta particle and sometimes shortened to beta (*e.g.*, beta-emitting radionuclide).

bioassay: A technique used to identify, quantify and/or specify the location of radionuclides in the body by direct (*in vivo*) measurements or indirect (*in vitro*) analysis of tissues or excretions from the body.

biokinetic model: Model describing the time course of absorption, distribution, metabolism and excretion of a substance introduced into the body of an organism.

bioligand: A biologic material that acts as a ligand (see **ligand**).

biopsy: Removal of an entire abnormality (excisional biopsy) or a sampling or portion of an abnormality (core biopsy and incisional biopsy) for microscopic examination in order to diagnose a problem.

bulla: A blister, usually >5 mm in diameter.

calibration: For an instrument intended to measure dose or dose rate related quantities calibration is the determination of the instrument response in a specified radiation field delivering a known dose (rate) at the instrument location; calibration normally involves the adjustment of instrument controls to read the desired dose (rate) and typically requires response determination on all instrument ranges. For instruments designed to measure radioactive surface contamination, calibration may be the determination of the detector reading per unit surface activity or the reading per unit radiation emission rate per unit surface area, or the reading per unit activity.

carcinogenesis: Induction of cancer by radiation or any other agent (a somatic effect).

carcinoma: Malignant tumor made up of epithelial cells, tending to infiltrate surrounding tissues and give rise to metastases.

cation: Positively charged ion.

chelate: Chemical compound in which the central atom (usually a metal ion) is attached to neighboring atoms by at least two bonds in such a way as to form a ring structure.

chelation: Formation of a chelate; therapeutic administration of a chelating agent.

chemotactic: Pertaining to movement of a motile organism in response to chemical stimulation.

cholangiocarcinoma: Adenocarcinoma of the bile ducts.

cholangiography: Radiographic examination of the bile ducts employing a contrast medium.

chondroitin: A mucopolysaccharide widespread in connective tissue, particularly cartilage, and in the cornea.

chromatid: Either of two parallel filaments joined at the centromere that comprise a chromosome.

collagen: A fibrous structural protein that constitutes the protein of the white fibers (collangenous fibers) of skin, tendon, bone cartilage, and all other connective tissues.

collagenase: An enzyme that catalyzes the degradation of collagen.

colloid: Small, insoluble and nondiffusible particle (as a single large molecule or mass of smaller molecules) in solid, liquid or gaseous form that remains in suspension in a surrounding solid, liquid or gaseous medium of different matter.

committed (dose): Integral of an internal dose rate parameter over a specified period of time following an acute intake of a radionuclide by ingestion, inhalation or dermal absorption. Time period over which committed doses are calculated normally is 50 y for intakes by adults or from age at intake to age 70 for intakes by other age groups.

contamination (radioactive): A radioactive substance dispersed in materials or places where it is undesirable.

cornea: Transparent epithelial structure forming the anterior part of the external covering of the eye.

creatinine: Nitrogenous compound formed as the end product of creatine metabolism.

curie (Ci): The conventional special name for the unit of activity equal to 3.70×10^{10} becquerel (or disintegrations per second) (see **becquerel**).

cyst: A fluid-filled sac that may be felt on physical examination or depicted by ultrasonography.

cytokines: Hormone-like low molecular weight proteins that regulate the intensity and duration of immune responses, and play a role in cell-to-cell communication.

cytotoxicity: Ability of a substance to induce degenerative changes in cells that may lead to cell death.

debride: Remove foreign objects and contaminated and devitalized tissue from or adjacent to a wound or lesion until surrounding healthy tissue is exposed.

decontamination: Treatment process that reduces or eliminates the presence of a harmful substance, such as a radioactive material, toxic chemical, or infectious agent.

depleted uranium (DU): Uranium with an isotopic content of <0.7 % ^{235}U; typically DU contains ~0.2 % ^{235}U.

dermis: Layer of the skin between the epidermis and the subcutis, composed of the papillary and reticular layers.

desquamation: Loss of the epithelial elements of the skin.

deterministic effects: Effects in organisms for which the severity varies with the dose of radiation (or other toxic substance), and for which a threshold usually exists.

diethylene triamine pentaacetic acid (DTPA): Chelating substance that binds metal ions. DTPA is rapidly excreted from the body by the kidneys.

diffusion: Spreading out of a material in a medium, due to thermal or mechanical agitation, in response to a concentration gradient.

divalent: Having a valence of two.

dose: General term used to denote mean absorbed dose, equivalent dose, effective dose, or effective equivalent dose, and to denote dose received or committed dose. Particular meaning of the term should be clear from context in which it is used.

dose coefficient: (1) For ingestion or inhalation of radionuclides, committed dose per unit activity intake; or (2) for external exposure to radionuclides in the environment, dose rate per unit concentration in an environmental medium.

dose equivalent (H): Absorbed dose (D) at a point in tissue weighted by quality factor (Q) for type and energy of the radiation causing the dose: $H = D \times Q$. For purposes of radiation protection and assessing health risks in general terms, and especially prior to introduction of the equivalent dose and as used by federal and state agencies, dose equivalent often refers to mean **absorbed dose** in an organ or tissue (T) weighted by average quality factor ($\bar{Q}$) for the particular type of radiation: $H_T = D_T \times \bar{Q}$. The SI unit of dose equivalent is the joule per kilogram (J kg^{-1}), and its special name is the sievert (Sv). In conventional units often used by federal and state agencies, dose equivalent is given in rem; 1 rem = 0.01 Sv.

dosimetric model: (1) For intakes of radionuclides into the body, model that estimates the dose in various organs and tissues per disintegration of a radionuclide in a specified source organ (site of deposition or transit in the body). (2) For external exposure, model that estimates the dose rate in organs and tissues per unit activity concentration of a radionuclide in an environmental medium.

dosimetry: The science or technique of determining radiation dose.

edema: Abnormal accumulation of fluid in the intercellular spaces of the body.

effective dose (E): Sum over specified organs and tissues (T) of **equivalent dose** in each tissue weighted by **tissue weighting factor** (w_T): $E = \Sigma w_T \times H_T$, where $\Sigma w_T \equiv 1$ (ICRP, 1991a) (supersedes **effective dose equivalent**).

effective dose equivalent (H_E): Sum over specified organs and tissues (T) of mean dose equivalent in each tissue weighted by tissue weighting factor (w_T): $H_E = \Sigma w_T \times H_T$, $\Sigma w_T \equiv 1$ (now superseded by **effective dose**, but often used by federal and state agencies).

elastin: A yellow protein that is the essential constituent of elastic connective tissue.

electron: Subatomic charged particle. Negatively charged particles are parts of stable atoms. Both negatively and positively charged electrons may be expelled from the radioactive atom when it disintegrates (see **beta particle**).

electron volt (eV): A unit of energy equal to the kinetic energy gained in a vacuum by a particle having one electronic charge when it passes through a potential difference of 1 volt; 1 eV = 1.6×10^{-19} joule or 1.6×10^{-12} erg.

element: Any substance that cannot be separated into different substances by ordinary chemical methods. Elements are distinguished by the number of protons in the nucleus of atoms.

emergency: A sudden, urgent, usually unforeseen occurrence or occasion requiring immediate action.

encapsulation: Incorporation of a foreign body in a fibrous cyst, resulting in isolation from the rest of the body.

endothelial: Pertaining to the endothelium, the layer of epithelial cells that lines the cavities of the heart, of the blood and lymph vessels, and the serous cavities of the body.

enterocolitis: Inflammation of the small intestine and colon.

eosinophil: A granular leukocyte with a nucleus that usually has two lobes connected by a thread of chromatin, and cytoplasm containing coarse, round granules of uniform size.

epidermis: Outer layer of the skin, consisting of the stratum corneum, stratum lucidum, stratum granulosum, stratum spinosum, and stratum basale.

epilation: Loss of body hair.

epithelial: Pertaining to or composed of epithelium, the cellular covering of internal and external surfaces of the body.

equivalent dose (H_T): Quantity developed for purposes of radiation protection and assessing health risks in general terms, defined as mean **absorbed dose** in an organ or tissue (T) weighted by radiation weighting factor (w_R) for type and energy of the radiation causing the dose: $H_T = D_T \times w_R$ (ICRP, 1991a). The SI unit of equivalent dose is the joule per kilogram (J kg^{-1}), and its special name is the sievert (Sv). In conventional units often used by federal and state agencies, equivalent dose is given in rem; 1 rem = 0.01 Sv (see **dose equivalent**).

erythema: A redness of the skin.

eschar: A slough produced by a thermal burn, a radiation burn, a corrosive application, or by gangrene.

excreta: Waste material (perspiration, urine, stools) eliminated by the body.

extravasation: Discharge or escape, as of blood, from a vessel into the tissues.

fascia: A sheet or band of fibrous tissue that lies deep to the skin or invests muscles and various body organs.

fibrin: An insoluble protein essential to the clotting of blood, formed from fibrinogen by action of thrombin.

fibroblast: An immature fiber-producing cell of connective tissue capable of differentiating into a cell specialized for producing various connective tissues such as cartilage or bone.

fibroma: Tumor composed mainly of fibrous or fully developed connective tissue.

fibronectin: An adhesive glycoprotein; one form circulates in plasma, another is a cell-surface protein that mediates cellular adhesive interactions.

fibroplasia: The formation of fibrous tissue, as in wound healing.

fibrosarcoma: A malignant neoplasm derived from deep fibrous tissue characterized by bundles of immature proliferating fibroblasts that invade locally and metastasize *via* the blood stream.

fission product (FP): Atom, either stable or radioactive, produced by splitting apart of an atomic nucleus, either spontaneously or when induced by absorption of a neutron.

free radicals: Highly reactive molecules containing an odd number of electrons.

gamma radiation: Electromagnetic radiation emitted in de-excitation of atomic nuclei, and frequently occurring in decay of radionuclides. Also called gamma ray and sometimes shortened to gamma (*e.g.*, gamma-emitting radionuclide) (see **photon** and **x ray**).

Geiger-Mueller counter: A gas-filled radiation detector most often used to detect the presence of low dose rate beta particles, x rays, or gamma rays. The detector is not appropriate for use with pulsed radiation sources or when the type or energy of the radiation is to be determined.

geometric mean: The geometric mean of a set of n values is the nth root of the product of the n values. To take a simple case, the geometric mean of (a,b) is the square root (second root) of a times b, which is written $(ab)^{1/2}$.

geometric mean diameter (GMD): Median diameter of a lognormal distribution of particle diameters.

glomerular: Pertaining to a small tuft or cluster, or to a small convoluted mass of capillaries, especially in the kidney.

glycoprotein: Any of a class of conjugated proteins consisting of a compound of protein with a carbohydrate group.

granulation: Process of forming granulation tissue or cytoplasmic granules.

granulomatous: Composed of granulomas (*i.e.*, small nodular delimited aggregation of mononuclear inflammatory cells).

gray (Gy): The SI special name for the unit of the quantities absorbed dose and air kerma. 1 Gy = 1 J kg^{-1}.

half-life ($T_{1/2}$): Time over which half the atoms of a particular radionuclide decay to another nuclear form.

health physicist: A person qualified by training and experience to be professionally engaged in the practice of health physics.

health physics: The profession devoted to the protection of humans and their environment from potential radiation hazards, identifying potential beneficial effects of radiation and assisting in the development of beneficial effects of ionizing and nonionizing radiation.

hemangiosarcoma: Malignant neoplasm originating from blood vessels and involving endothelial and fibroblastic tissue.

hematoma: Localized collection of extravasated blood, usually clotted, in an organ, space or tissue.

hemosiderin: Insoluble form of storage iron, visible microscopically both with and without the use of special stains.

hemostasis: Arrest of the escape of blood by either natural (clot formation or vessel spasm) or artificial (compression or ligation) means.

hepatobiliary: Pertaining to the liver-bile-gall bladder system.

hepatoma: Any tumor of the liver.

hexavalent: Having a valence of six.

high-fired oxide: A highly insoluble metal oxide, usually of uranium or plutonium, commonly produced by combustion in air.

histiocytoma: Tumor containing histiocytes (*i.e.*, macrophages).

histopathology: Pathologic histology (*i.e.*, that dealing with the minute structure, composition and function of diseased tissues).

homeostasis: The tendency of biological systems to maintain relatively constant conditions in the internal environment while continuously interacting with and responding to changes originating within or outside the system.

hyaluronic acid: A mucopolysaccharide found in lubricating proteoglycans of synovial fluid, vitreous humor, cartilage, blood vessels, and skin.

hydrolysis: Cleavage of a compound by the addition of water, the hydroxyl group being incorporated into one fragment and the hydrogen atom in the other.

hydrophilic: Having a strong affinity for water; absorbing water.

hyperemia: An excess of blood in a part of the body.

hyperkeratosis: Hypertrophy of the horny layer of the skin, or any disease characterized by it.

hyperplasia: Abnormal increase in volume of a tissue or organ caused by the formation and growth of new normal cells.

hypocellular: Having an abnormal decrease in the number of cells present.

hypodermis: (see **subcutis**).

indirect bioassay: The assessment of radioactive material deposited in the body by detection of activity in material excreted or removed from the body (*in vitro* measurement).

***in situ*:** Confined to site of origin, not having invaded adjoining tissues or metastasized to other parts of the body (*e.g.*, intraductal).

intake: The amount of radioactive material taken into the body by inhalation, absorption through the skin, ingestion or through wounds.

intake retention fraction: Ratio of the activity measured in the body, or in excreta, to the intake.

integrin: Any one of many membrane proteins in the plasma membrane of cells.

internal dose: Dose to organs or tissues of an organism due to intakes of radionuclides (*e.g.*, by ingestion, inhalation or dermal absorption).

intradermal: Within the dermis.

intramuscular (i.m.): Within muscle tissue.

intraperitoneal: Within the peritoneal cavity.

intravenous (i.v.): Within a vein.

***in vitro*:** From Latin "in glass"; refers to a procedure done outside the body (*e.g.*, in a test tube), as opposed to *in vivo*.

***in vivo*:** From Latin "in life"; refers to a procedure carried out in the living body, as opposed to *in vitro*.

isomer: Compound capable of existing in two or more geometrical configurations.

isotope: Form of a particular chemical element determined by the number of neutrons in the atomic nucleus. An element may have many stable or unstable (radioactive) isotopes.

keratin: Scleroprotein that is the primary component of epidermis, hair, nails, horny tissues, and the organic matrix of tooth enamel.

lanthanide: Element with atomic number from 58 through 71; a member of the lanthanide series of rare earths.

leukocyte: A colorless blood corpuscle (white blood cell) capable of ameboid movement. Granular leukocytes include neutrophils, eosinophils and basophils; nongranular leukocytes include lymphocytes and monocytes.

ligand: Atom, group of atoms with similar chemical properties, ion, radical or molecule that forms a coordination complex with a central atom or ion.

lipophilic: Having an affinity for fat.

lymph: A transparent, usually slightly yellow, often opalescent liquid found within the lymphatic vessels, and collected from tissues in all parts of the body and returned to the blood *via* the lymphatic system. It is ~95 % water, with the remainder consisting of plasma proteins. Its cellular component consists chiefly of lymphocytes.

lymphatic system: Complex network of capillaries, vessels, valves, ducts and organs involved in producing, filtering and conveying lymph and producing various blood cells.

lymph nodes: Kidney bean-shaped structures scattered along vessels of the lymphatic system seen in the axilla or sometimes in the breast itself; act as filters, collecting bacteria or cancer cells that may travel through the lymph system (also called lymph glands).

lymphocyte: Any of the mononuclear, nonphagocytic leukocytes found blood, lymph, and lymphoid tissues which comprise the body's immunocompetent cells and their precursors.

lysis: Destruction or decomposition, especially by enzymatic digestion.

lysosome: One of the minute bodies occurring in many types of cells, containing various types of hydrolytic enzymes and normally involved in the process of localized intracellular digestion.

macrophage: Any of the large, mononuclear, highly phagocytic cells derived from monocytes that occur in the walls of blood vessels and in loose connective tissue.

malignant: Cancerous; a growth of cancer cells.

mast cell: A connective tissue cell that elaborates granules containing histamine or heparin.

mean: Sum of the measured values divided by the number of measurements. The mean value is also often called the (arithmetic) average value. The mean of a distribution is the weighted average of the possible values of the random variable.

mean diameter: Average diameter of the particles (sum of all diameters divided by the number of particles).

medulla: The central or inner portion of an organ.

mesenchymal: Pertaining to the meshwork of embryonic connective tissue in the mesoderm from which are formed the connective tissues of the body and also the blood vessels and lymph vessels.

mesenchymoma: A mixed mesenchymal tumor composed of two or more cellular elements that are not commonly associated, exclusive of fibrous tissue.

metacarpal: Any of the bones extended from the carpals in the wrist to the phalanges of the fingers in humans, or corresponding structures in animals.

mixed oxide (MOX): Combined uranium and plutonium oxides used as nuclear fuels.

model: Mathematical or physical representation of an environmental or biological system, sometimes including specific numerical values for parameters of the system.

monocyte: A mononuclear, phagocytotic leukocyte, 13 to 25 μm in diameter.

monodisperse: Pertaining to particles with a very narrow range of sizes, so that all have the same deposition characteristics when inhaled.

monomer: A simple molecule of low molecular weight, capable of combining *via* covalent bonds to form a polymer.

monovalent: Having a valence of one.

mucoepidermoid: Composed of mucus-producing epithelial cells.

mucopolysaccharide: A group of polysaccharides containing hexosamine that form many of the mucins when dispersed in water.

nanoparticles: Particles having mean diameters in the nanometer range.

necrosis: The morphological changes indicative of cell death caused by enzymatic degradation.

neovascularization: New blood vessel formation.

neurofibrosarcoma: A malignant peripheral nerve sheath tumor.

neutrophil: A granular leukocyte having a nucleus with 3 to 5 lobes.

nuclide: A species of atom having specied numbers of neutrons and protons in its nucleus.

organ dose equivalent ($\bar{H}_T$)**:** The mean dose equivalent for an organ or tissue, obtained by integrating or averaging dose equivalents at points in the organ or tissue. It is the practice in the space radiation protection community to obtain point values of **absorbed dose** (D) and **dose equivalent** (H) using the accepted quality factor-LET (linear energy transfer) relationship [$Q(L)$], and then to average the point quantities over the organ or tissue of interest by means of computational models to obtain the organ dose equivalent ($\bar{H}_T$). For space radiations, NCRP adopted the organ dose equivalent as an acceptable approximation for equivalent dose (H_T) for **stochastic effects**.

osteosarcoma: Malignant tumor of the connective tissue of the bone.

oxidation: Any reaction in which one or more electrons are removed from a chemical species.

oxidation state: Net positive charge on an atom due to loss of electrons to other atoms in a compound.

parenchyma: The essential or functional elements of an organ, as distinguished from its stroma or framework.

parenteral: Not through the alimentary canal (*e.g.*, by subcutaneous, intramuscular, intrasternal or intravenous injection).

partition coefficient: The fraction of a substance retained with a particular rate constant in a multi-component retention equation (*i.e.*, if

$$R(t) = \sum_i A_i e^{-\lambda_i t} \text{ the } A_i \text{ are the partition coefficients}).$$

pathobiology: The structural and functional manifestations of a disease or injury.

pentavalent: Having a valence of five.

percutaneous: Performed through the skin.

pH: Symbol for degree of acidity or alkalinity of a solution.

phagocytic cells: Cells with the ability to engulf solid material.

phagocytosis: The engulfing of microorganisms or other cells and foreign particles by phagocytes.

phalanx: Any bone of a finger or toe (plural: phalanges).

photon: Quantum of electromagnetic radiation, having no charge or mass, that exhibits both particle and wave behavior, especially a gamma or x ray.

plasminogen activator: An enzyme such as urokinase that catalyzes the activation of plasminogen to plasmin.

platelet: The smallest formed element of blood; disk-shaped, non-nucleated cells that adhere to uneven or damaged surfaces and participate in clot formation; also called thrombocytes.

polydisperse: Mixture composed of particles with a range of sizes.

polymer: Compound, usually of high molecular weight, formed by the combination of simpler molecules (monomers).

polymorphonuclear: Having a nucleus so deeply lobed or so divided as to appear to be multiple.

popliteal: Pertaining to the area behind the knee.

preneoplastic: Preceding the formation of a malignancy.

prolactin: Hormone secreted by the anterior pituitary that promotes the growth of breast tissue and stimulates and sustains milk production in postpartum mammals.

prostacyclin: An intermediate in the metabolic pathway of arachidonic acid; it is a potent vasodilator and inhibitor of platelet aggregation.

protease: Any proteolytic enzyme.

rad: The special name for the conventional unit of absorbed dose. 1 rad = 0.01 J kg^{-1}. In the SI system of units, it is replaced by the special name gray (Gy). 1 Gy = 100 rad.

radioactive decay: The spontaneous transformation of one nuclide into a different nuclide or into a different energy state of the same nuclide. The process results in a decrease, with time, of the number of the radioactive atoms in a sample. Decay generally involves the emission from the nucleus of alpha particles, beta particles or gamma rays.

radioanalysis: Measurement of activity content.

radionuclide: Naturally occurring or artificially produced radioactive element or isotope.

rare earth: A member of the lanthanide series (atomic number 58 through 71) or, more rarely of the actinide series (atomic number 90 through 103).

rate constant: A constant (units of inverse time) that relates the number of entities (*e.g.*, atoms), that decay or leave a compartment per unit time to the number present in the compartment.

rem: The special name for the conventional unit numerically equal to the absorbed dose (D) in rad, modified by a quality factor (Q). 1 rem = 0.01 J kg^{-1}. In the SI system of units, it is replaced by the special name sievert (Sv), which is numerically equal to the absorbed dose (D) in gray modified by a radiation weighting factor (w_R). 1 Sv = 100 rem.

reticuloendothelial: Pertaining to the reticuloendothelium, a network of cells and tissues with both endothelial and reticular attributes, found throughout the body, but especially in the blood, connective tissue, spleen, liver, lungs, bone marrow, and lymph nodes.

rhabdomyosarcoma: A highly malignant tumor arising in striated muscle or in embryonal mesenchymal cells.

Ringer's Lactate: Intravenous solution containing sodium chloride, potassium chloride, calcium chloride, and sodium lactate.

sabot: A collar surrounding a munition to fit it to the bore diameter of the weapon.

saline, isotonic: A solution of sodium chloride in purified water of the same osmotic pressure as blood serum.

saline, physiological: A 0.9 % solution of sodium chloride in water that is isotonic.

sarcoma: A tumor, often highly malignant, composed of cells derived from connective tissue such as bone, cartilage, muscle, blood vessel, or lymphoid tissue.

scintillator: A material that emits visible light upon absorption of radiation.

sebaceous: Oily or oil-containing.

shallow dose: The absorbed dose calculated at a depth of 0.07 mm in a sphere of soft tissue of density 1.0 and diameter of 300 mm. Presumed to be the dose received by the basal layer of the epidermis.

sievert (Sv): Special name for the SI unit of **dose equivalent, equivalent dose**, and **effective dose**. 1 Sv = 100 rem.

spall: Small particles of armor plate dispersed by an armor-piercing munition.

spallation: A nuclear reaction in which an incoming particle causes a target to fragment into many pieces.

spallation products: Fragments resulting from a spallation reaction.

specific activity: Activity of a radionuclide per unit mass of the radionuclide; also may refer to activity of a radionuclide per unit mass of material in which the radionuclide is dispersed.

squamous: Scaly or plate-like; flattened.

standard deviation (SD): Square root of the variance.

standard deviation of the mean: The square root of the variance divided by the number of observations: $(s^2 / n)^{1/2}$. An equivalent definition is that the standard deviation of the mean is the standard deviation divided by the square root of the number of observations: $s / n^{1/2}$.

standard error: The standard deviation of an estimate considered as a random variable. The standard deviation of the mean is often known as the standard error.

stasis: Stoppage or diminution of flow, as of blood or other body fluids.

stochastic effects: Adverse effects in biological organisms for which the probability, but not the severity, is assumed to be a function of dose of ionizing radiation (or other contaminant) without threshold.

stratum corneum: The outermost layer of the epidermis.

stroma: The tissue forming the ground substance, framework, or matrix of an organ.

subcutis: Loose connective tissue between the skin and muscle.

survey meter: An instrument or device, usually portable, for monitoring the level of radiation or of radioactive contamination in an area or location.

suspension: A chemical mixture in which particles are dispersed in a medium.

Systeme Internationale (SI): A system of scientific units designed to foster uniformity in measurements. In nuclear medicine the SI units of becquerel, gray and sievert have replaced the conventional units of curie, rad and rem.

systemic: Pertaining to or affecting the body as a whole.

tetravalent: Having a valence of four.

thorium: A naturally radioactive element. Thorium-232 is the parent of one radioactive series, and specific thorium nuclides are members of the three naturally-occurring radionuclide series.

Thorotrast®: A proprietary contrast medium for roentgenography that contained a colloidal suspension of thorium dioxide (VanHeyden Company, Dresden-Radebeul, Germany).

thorotrastoma: A granuloma at the site of Thorotrast® injection; frequently associated with a malignancy such as sarcoma.

thrombin: An enzyme resulting from activation of prothrombin, which catalyzes the conversion of fibrinogen to fibrin.

thromboxane: An intermediate in the metabolic pathway of arachidonic acid, released from stimulated platelets; one form, thromboxane A_2 is a potent inducer of platelet aggregation and constrictor of arterial smooth muscle.

tissue weighting factor (w_T): A factor that indicates the ratio of the risk of stochastic effects attributable to irradiation of a given organ or tissue (T) to the total risk when the whole body is uniformly irradiated.

transferrin: A serum globulin that binds and transports iron.

transition: A nuclear change from one energy state to another, generally accompanied by the emission of particles or photons. Often called a decay, or disintegration.

transition group metal: Any of the 38 elements in groups 3 through 12 of the periodic table (*i.e.*, atomic numbers 21 through 30, 39 through 48, 72 through 80, and 104 through 112).

transuranic: Having an atomic number greater than that of uranium (92); same as transuranium.

trivalent: Having a valence of three.

ultrafilterable: Small enough to pass though a micropore filter.

uptake: Quantity of a radionuclide taken up by the systemic circulation (*e.g.*, by absorption from compartments in the respiratory or gastrointestinal tracts).

uranium: A naturally radioactive element. In natural ores, it consists of 0.7 % ^{235}U, 99.3 % ^{238}U, and a small amount of ^{234}U.

variance: The variance of a set of measurements is the average value of the squares of the deviations of individual values from the mean value. The individual deviations from the mean: $(x_1 - m)$, $(x_2 - m)$,

$(x_3 - m)$, $(x_n - m)$. When all the deviations are squared, added together, and divided by $(n - 1)$, the result is the variance, usually denoted s^2.

vasoactive: Exerting an effect on the caliber of blood vessels.

vitronectin: A glycoprotein found in blood plasma, associated with hemostasis.

x ray: (1) Electromagnetic radiation emitted in de-excitation of bound atomic electrons, and frequently occurring in decay of radionuclides, referred to as characteristic x rays, (2) electromagnetic radiation produced in deceleration of energetic charged particles (*e.g.*, beta radiation) in passing through matter, referred to as continuous x rays or bremsstrahlung (gamma ray and photon), or (3) a medical radiograph.

Z; low-Z, high-Z: The symbol for the atomic number of a nucleus (*i.e.*, the number of protons contained in the nucleus). Low-Z describes nuclei with $Z < 26$. High-Z describes nuclei with $Z > 26$. Very high-Z describes nuclei with $Z > 73$.

Acronyms and Symbols

% ID	percent of the injected dosage
A	activity (becquerel)
A_i	partition coefficient for retention component i
A_r	isotopic weight (g mol^{-1})
$B(t)$	activity in blood volume at time t
CIS	colloid and intermediate state
cps	counts per second
CsI(Tl)	thallium-activated cesium iodide
dpm	disintegrations per minute
DTPA	diethylene triamine pentaacetic acid
DU	depleted uranium
$\bar{\varepsilon}$	mean energy of radiation emitted per transformation
e	electron charge (1.609×10^{-19} Coulomb)
e	committed dose coefficient
E	committed effective dose
ECW	extracellular water
e/r	charge/radius ratios
FBC	foreign-body carcinogenesis
FP	fission products
FU^{-1}	fecal to urinary excretion ratio
GI	gastrointestinal
GMD	geometric mean diameter
h_T	committed equivalent dose coefficient for tissue T
H_T	committed equivalent dose to tissue T
i.m.	intramuscular, intramuscularly
i.v.	intravenous, intravenously
K_{sp}	solubility product constant
λ_i	rate constant for retention component i
LAXLN	left axillary lymph node
log	logarithm (base 10)
LSCLN	left superficial cervical lymph node
m	injected mass (micrograms)

$m(t)$	intake retention fraction at time t
mol	mole (gram molecular weight)
MOX	mixed oxide
M^{n+}	concentration of cation (mol L^{-1})
N	number of atoms
NaI(Tl)	thallium-activated sodium iodide
N_A	Avogadro constant (6.022×10^{23} mol^{-1})
PABS	particles, aggregates and bound state
PDGF	platelet-derived growth factor
$R(t)$	retention at time t (percent of injected amount)
REAC/TS	Radiation Emergency Assistance Center/ Training Site
s.c.	subcutaneous, subcutaneously
SD	standard deviation
Si(Li)	lithium-drifted silicon
t	time (days)
TGF-β	transforming growth factor beta
TNF-α	tumor necrosis factor alpha
TPA	trapped particles and aggregates
$T_{1/2}$	radiological half-life (seconds)
$U(t)$	daily urinary excretion at time t
UCRL	University of California Radiation Laboratory
V	injected volume (liters)
VAMC	Veterans' Affairs Medical Center

References

ABBATT, J.D. (1967). "Leukemia and other fatal blood dyscrasias in thorium dioxide patients," Ann. NY Acad. Sci. **145**(3), 767–775.

AEPI (1995). U.S. Army Environmental Policy Institute. *Health and
Environmental Consequences of Depleted Uranium Use in the
U.S. Army: Technical Report*, http://www.fas.org/man/dod-101/sys/land/
docs/techreport.html (accessed July 24, 2007) (U.S. Department of
Defense, Washington).

AFRRI (2007). *Armed Forces Radiobiology Research Institute*. http://
www.afrri.usuhs.mil (accessed July 24, 2007) (Armed Forces Radiobiology Research Institute, Bethesda, Maryland).

AHRLAND, S. (1986). "Solution chemistry and kinetics of ionic reactions,"
pages 1480 to 1546 in *The Chemistry of the Actinide Elements*, 2nd ed.,
Katz, J.J., Seaborg, G.T. and Morss, L.R., Eds. (Chapman and Hall
Ltd., New York).

ALLEN, R.C. (1949). *The Effects of Uranium Dioxide Powder Applied Subcutaneously Through an Incision in the Skin of Rabbits*, U.S. Atomic
Energy Commission Report AECD-2709 (National Technical Information Service, Springfield, Virginia).

ALTMAN, P.L. and KATZ, D.D. (1961). *Blood and Other Body Fluids* (Fed-
eration of American Societies for Experimental Biology, Bethesda,
Maryland).

ANDERSSON, M., VYBERG, M., VISFELDT, J., CARSTENSEN, B. and
STORM, H.H. (1994). "Primary liver tumors among Danish patients
exposed to Thorotrast," Radiat. Res. **137**(2), 262–273.

ANSEL, J.C., TIESMAN, J.P., OLERUD, J.E., KRUEGER, J.G., KRANE,
J.F., TARA, D.C., SHIPLEY, G.D., GILBERTSON, D., USUI, M.L. and
HART, C.E. (1993). "Human keratinocytes are a major source of cuta-
neous platelet-derived growth factor," J. Clin. Invest. **92**(2), 671–678.

ARTURSON, G. (1983). "Arachidonic acid metabolism and prostaglandin
activity following burn injury," page 57 in *Traumatic Injury: Infection
and Other Immunologic Sequelae*, Ninnemann, J.L., Ed. (University
Park Press, Baltimore, Maryland).

ATHERTON, D.R., MAYS, C.W. and STOVER, B.J. (1958). "Radionuclide
distribution in adult beagle bones," pages 118 to 125 in *Radiobiology
Laboratory, College of Medicine, Semi-Annual Progress Report*, Report
COO-217 (University of Utah, Salt Lake City, Utah).

BAES, C.F., JR. and MESMER, R.E. (1976). *The Hydrolysis of Cations*
(John Wiley and Sons, New York).

BAGGIOLINI, M., DEWALD, B. and MOSER, B. (1994). "Interleukin-8
and related chemotactic cytokines—CXC and CC chemokines," Adv.
Immunol. **55**, 97–179.

346

BAILEY, A.J., BAZIN, S., SIMS, T.J., LE LOUS, M., NICHOLETIS, C. and DELAUNAY, A. (1975). "Characterization of the collagen of human hypertrophic and normal scars," Biochem. Biophys. Acta. **405**(2), 412–421.

BAILEY, B.R., ECKERMAN, K.F. and TOWNSEND, L.W. (2003). "An analysis of a puncture wound case with medical intervention," Radiat. Prot. Dosim. **105**(1–4), 509–512.

BAIR, W.J., BALLOU, J.E., PARK, J.F. and SANDERS, C.L. (1973). "Plutonium in soft tissues with emphasis on the respiratory tract," pages 501 to 568 in *Uranium, Plutonium, Transplutonic Elements*, Hodge, H.C., Stannard, J.N. and Hursh, J.B., Eds. (Springer-Verlag, New York).

BARABANOVA, A.V. (2001). "Local radiation injury," pages 223 to 240 in *Medical Management of Radiation Accidents*, 2nd ed., Gusev, I.A., Guskova, A.K. and Mettler, F.A., Jr., Eds. (CRC Press, Boca Raton, Florida).

BARRATT, T.M. and WALSER, M. (1969). "Extracellular fluid in individual tissues and in whole animals: The distribution of radiosulfate and radiobromide," J. Clin. Invest. **48**(1), 56–66.

BARRETT, P.H.R., BELL, B.M., COBELLI, C., GOLDE, H., SCHUMITZKY, A., VICINI, P. and FOSTER, D.M. (1998). "SAAM II: Simulation, analysis, and modeling software for tracer and pharmacokinetic studies," Metabolism **47**(4), 484–492.

BARRY, W.J. and ROMINGER, C.J. (1964). "Thorotrast granulomas," Am. J. Roentgenol. Ther. Nucl. Med. **92**, 584–590.

BATTEGAY, E.J., RUPP, J., IRUELA-ARISPE, L., SAGE, E.H. and PECH, M. (1994). "PDGF-BB modulates endothelial proliferation and angiogenesis *in vitro via* PDGF β-receptors," J. Cell. Biol. **125**(4), 917–928.

BAZHIN, A.G., LIUBCHANSKII, E.R., NIFATOV, A.N. and SINIAKOV, E.G. (1983). "Behavior and biological effect of ^{239}Pu on entry into a skin abrasion," Med. Radiol. (Mosk.) **28**(2), 46–51 [in Russian].

BAZHIN, A.G., LIUBCHANSKII, E.R., NIFATOV, A.P. and SINIAKOV, E.G. (1984). "Behavior and biological action of ^{239}Pu administered intramuscularly during complexon therapy," Radiobiologiia **24**(1), 129–132 [in Russian].

BAZHIN, A.G., KHOKHRIAKOV, V.F. and SHEVKUNOV, V.A. (1994). "Wounds and burns of the skin polluted by alpha irradiation in personnel of radiochemistry enterprises," Gig. Sanit. (9), 27–29 [in Russian].

BEAMISH, M.R. and BROWN, E.B. (1974). "The metabolism of transferrin-bound ^{111}In and ^{59}Fe in the rat," Blood **43**(5), 693–701.

BEITER, H., GIBB, F.R. and MORROW, P.E. (1975). "Intramuscular retention of UO_3 and UO_2," Health Phys. **29**(2), 273–277.

BERGER, M.J. (1971). "Distribution of absorbed dose around point sources of electrons and beta particles in water and other media," MIRD Pamphlet No. 7, J. Nucl. Med. (Suppl.) **5**, 5–23.

BERGER, C.D. and LANE, B.H. (1984). *Calibration of a Large Hyperpure Germanium Detector Array for Actinide Lung Counting with a Tissue-Equivalent Torso Phantom*, Report ORNL/TM-8723 (Oak Ridge National Laboratory, Oak Ridge, Tennessee).

BERGER, M.E. and SADOFF, R.L. (2002). "Psychological support of radiation-accident patients, families, and staff," pages 191 to 200 in *The Medical Basis for Radiation-Accident Preparedness: The Clinical Care of Victims. Proceedings of the Fourth International REAC/TS Conference*, Ricks, R.C., Berger, M.E. and O'Hara, F.M., Eds. (Parthenon Publishing Group, New York).

BERLINER, R.W. (1973). "The excretion of urine," pages 5-1 to 5-57 in *Best and Taylor's Physiological Basis of Medical Practice*, 9th ed., Brobeck, J.R., Ed. (Williams and Wilkins, Baltimore, Maryland).

BISCHOFF, F. and BRYSON G. (1964). "Carcinogenesis through solid state surfaces," Prog. Exp. Tumor Res. **14**, 85–133.

BISTLINE, R.W. (1973). *Translocation Dynamics of 239-Plutonium*, U.S. Energy Research and Development Administration Report No. COO-1781-20 (National Technical Information Service, Springfield, Virginia).

BISTLINE, R.W., WATTERS, R.L. and LEBEL, J.L. (1972). "A study of translocation dynamics of plutonium and americium from simulated puncture wounds in beagle dogs," Health Phys. **22**(6), 829–831.

BISTLINE, R.W., LEBEL, J.L. and DAGLE, G.E. (1976). "Translocation dynamics of $Pu(NO_3)_4$ and PuO_2 from puncture wounds to lymph nodes and major organs of beagles," pages 10 to 18 in *Radiation and the Lymphatic System, Proceedings of the Fourteenth Annual Hanford Biology Symposium*, Ballou, J.E., Ed., U.S. Atomic Energy Commission Report CONF-740930 (National Technical Information Service, Springfield, Virginia).

BLEISE, A., DANESI, P.R. and BURKART, W. (2003). "Properties, use and health effects of depleted uranium (DU): A general overview," J. Environ. Radioact. **64**(2–3), 93–112.

BLOMBERG, R., LARSSON L.E., LINDELL, B. and LINDGREN, E. (1963). "Late effects of Thorotrast in cerebral angiography," Acta Radiol. Diagn. **11**, 995–1006.

BOYKIN, J.V., ERIKSSON, E. and PITTMAN, R.N. (1980). "*In vivo* microcirculation of a scald burn and the progression of postburn dermal ischemia," Plast. Reconstr. Surg. **66**(2), 191–198.

BRADBERRY, S.M., FELDMAN, M.A., BRAITHWAITE, R.A., SHORTLAND-WEBB, W. and VALE, J.A. (1996). "Elemental mercury-induced skin granuloma: A case report and review of the literature," J. Toxicol. Clin. Toxicol. **34**(2), 209–216.

BRAND, K.G. (1994). "Do implanted medical devices cause cancer?" J. Biomater. Appl. **8**(4), 325–343.

BRAND, K.G., BUOEN, L.C., JOHNSON, K.H. and BRAND, I. (1975). "Etiological factors, stages, and the role of the foreign body in foreign body tumorigenesis: A review," Cancer Res. **35**(2), 279–286.

BRAND, K.G., JOHNSON, K.H. and BUOEN, L.C. (1976). "Foreign body tumorigenesis," CRC Crit. Rev. Toxicol. **4**(4), 353–394.

BREITENSTEIN, B.D., JR. (1983). "1976 Hanford americium exposure incident: Medical management and chelation therapy," Health Phys. **45**(4), 855–866.

BREITENSTEIN, B.D., JR. and PALMER, H.E. (1989). "Lifetime follow-up of the 1976 americium accident victim," Rad. Prot. Dosim. **26**(1), 317–322.

BREITENSTEIN, B.D., JR. and PALMER, H.E. (2001). "Lifetime follow-up of the 1976 americium accident victim," pages 337 to 343 in *Medical Management of Radiation Accidents*, 2nd ed., Gusev, I.A., Guskova, A.K. and Mettler, F.A. Jr., Eds. (CRC Press, Boca Raton, Florida).

BROWN, G.L., NANNEY, L.B., GRIFFEN, J., CRAMER, A.B., YANCEY, J.M., CURTSINGER. L.J., HOLTZIN, L., SCHULTZ, G.S., JURK-IEWICZ, M.J. and LYNCH, J.B. (1989). "Enhancement of wound healing by topical treatment with epidermal growth factor," N. Eng. J. Med. **321**(2), 76–79.

BRUENGER, F.W., ATHERTON, D.R., STEVENS, W. and STOVER, B.J. (1971). "Interaction between blood constituents and some actinides," pages 212 to 227 in *Research in Radiobiology, Annual Report of Work in Progress in the Internal Irradiation Program*, Dougherty, T.F., Ed., University of Utah College of Medicine Report No. COO-219-244 (National Technical Information Service, Springfield, Virginia).

BRUES, A.M., AUERBACH, H. and DEROCHE, G. (1963). "Effects of plutonium injected subcutaneously in the rat and mouse," pages 81 to 85 in *Biological and Medical Research Division Semiannual Report, January Through June 1963*, ANL-6823 (Argonne National Laboratory, Argonne, Illinois).

BRUES, A.M., AUERBACH, H., DEROCHE, G. and PILARSKI, L.M. (1964). "Mechanisms of carcinogenesis," pages 47 to 48 in *Biological and Medical Research Division Annual Report, 1964*, ANL-6971 (Argonne National Laboratory, Argonne, Illinois).

BRUES, A.M., AUERBACH, H., DEROCHE, G. and GRUBE, D.D. (1965). "Mechanisms of carcinogenesis," pages 164 to 166 in *Biological and Medical Research Division Annual Report, 1965*, ANL-7136 (Argonne National Laboratory, Argonne, Illinois).

BRUES, A.M., AUERBACH, H., DEROCHE, G. and GRUBE, D.D. (1966). "Mechanisms of carcinogenesis," pages 132 to 134 in *Biological and Medical Research Division Annual Report, 1966*, ANL-7278 (Argonne National Laboratory, Argonne, Illinois).

BRUES, A.M., AUERBACH, H., DEROUCHE, G.M. and GRUBE, D.D. (1968). "Mechanisms of carcinogenesis," pages 115 to 119 in *Biological and Medical Research Division, 1968*, ANL-7535 (Argonne National Laboratory, Argonne, Illinois).

BUDKO, L.N. (1961). "Strontium-90 absorption through the intact skin of rats," pages 105 to 107 in *Distribution, Biological Effects, and Migration of Radioactive Isotopes*, Ledbedinskii, A.V. and Moskalev, Y.I., Eds. U.S. Atomic Energy Commission Report No. AEC-TR-7512 (National Technical Information Service, Springfield, Virginia).

BUGGE, T.H., KOMBRINCK, K.W., FLICK, M.J., DAUGHERTY, C.C., DANTON, M.J.S. and DEGEN, J.L. (1996). "Loss of fibrinogen rescues mice from the pleiotropic effects of plasminogen deficiency," Cell **87**(4), 709–719.

BULDAKOV, L.A., NIFATOV, A.P., EROKHIN, R.A. and FILLIPOVA, L.G. (1971). "Plutonium-239 biological impact at hypodermic and intradermic injection," pages 350 to 355 in *Long-Term Sequelae of Radiation Lesions* (Atomizdat, Moscow).

BUSHBERG, J.T. and MILLER, K.L. (2004). "Hospital responses to radiation casualties," pages 445 to 462 in *Public Protection from Nuclear, Chemical, and Biological Terrorism*, Brodsky, A., Johnson, R.H. Jr. and Goans, R.E., Eds. (Medical Physics Publishing, Madison, Wisconsin).

CABLE, J.W., HORSTMAN, V.G., CLARKE, W.J. and BUSTAD, L.K. (1962). "Effects of intradermal injections of plutonium in swine," Health Phys. **8**, 629–634.

CARBAUGH, E.H., DECKER, W.A. and SWINT, M.J. (1989). "Medical and health physics management of a plutonium wound," Radiat. Prot. Dosim. **26**(1), 345–349.

CARRIGAN, R.H. (1967). "Manufacture of thorium dioxide suspension (Thorotrast)," Ann. NY Acad. Sci. **145**(3), 530–532.

CARRITT, J., FRYXELL, R., KLEINSCHMIDT, J., KLEINSCHMIDT, R., LANGHAM, W., SAN PIETRO, A., SCHAFFER, R. and SCHNAP, B. (1947). "The distribution and excretion of plutonium administered intravenously to the rat," J. Biol.Chem. **171**, 273–283.

CASPER, J. (1967). "The introduction in 1928–29 of thorium dioxide in diagnostic radiology," Ann. NY Acad. Sci. **145**(3), 527–529.

CDC (1982). Centers for Disease Control and Prevention. *Reports of the Epidemiology and Surveillance of Injuries* (Centers for Disease Control and Prevention, Atlanta).

CDC (2007). *Centers for Disease Control and Prevention. Your Online Source for Credible Health Information.* http://www.cdc.gov (accessed July 24, 2007) (Centers for Disease Control and Prevention, Atlanta, Georgia).

CHAPTINEL, Y., DURAND, F., PIECHOWSKI, J. and MENOUX, B. (1988). *Dosimetrie et Therapeutique des Contaminations Cutanees*, Report CEA-R-5441 (Commissariat a l'Energie Atomique, Gif-sur-Yvette, France).

CLARK, R.A.F. (1996). *The Molecular and Cellular Biology of Wound Repair* (Plenum Press, New York).

CLARK, R.A.F. and SINGER, A.J. (2000). "Wound repair: Basic biology to tissue engineering," pages 857 to 878 in *Principles of Tissue Engineering*, 2nd ed., Lanza, R.P., Langer, R. and Vacati, J.P., Eds. (Academic Press, San Diego, California).

CLARK, R.A.F., LANIGAN, J.M., DELLAPELLE, P., MANSEAU, E., DVORAK, H.F. and COLVIN, R.B. (1982). "Fibronectin and fibrin provide a provisional matrix for epidermal cell migration during wound reepithelialization," J. Invest. Dermatol. **79**(5), 264–269.

CLARK, R.A.F., FOLKVORD, J.M., HART, C.E., MURRAY, M.J. and MCPHERSON, J.M. (1989). "Platelet isoforms of platelet-derived growth factor stimulate fibroblasts to contract collagen matrices," J. Clin. Invest. **84**(3), 1036–1040.

CLARK, R.A.F., NIELSEN, L.D., WELCH, M.P. and MCPHERSON, J.M. (1995). "Collagen matrices attenuate the collagen-synthetic response of cultured fibroblasts to TGF-β," J. Cell Sci. **108**(Part 3), 1251–1261.

CLEVELAND J.M. (1970). *The Chemistry of Plutonium* (Gordon and Beach, New York).

COLE, L., WRIGHT, T.W. and PREWETT, S.V. (1988). "A case study of the discovery of an imbedded uranium fragment in the chest of a worker at a depleted uranium manufacturing facility," (abstract), Health Phys. **52** (Suppl. 1), S60.

COLLART, F.R., HORIO, M., SCHLENKER, R.A., KATHREN, R.L. and HUBERMAN, E. (1992). "Alteration of the c-*fms* gene in a blood sample from a Thorotrast individual," Health Phys. **63**(1), 27–32.

CONKLIN, J.J., WALKER, R.I. and HIRSCH, E.F. (1983) "Current concepts in the management of radiation injuries and associated trauma," Surg. Gynecol. Obstet. **156**(6), 809–829.

COTTON, F.A. and WILKINSON, G. (1980). *Advanced Inorganic Chemistry: A Comprehensive Text*, 4th ed. (John Wiley and Sons, New York).

CRCPD (2007). *Conference of Radiation Control Program Directors, Inc.* http://www.crcpd.org (accessed July 24, 2007) (Conference of Radiation Control Program Directors, Inc., Frankfort, Kentucky).

CRONKITE, E.P. (1973). "Blood and lymph," pages 4-1 to 4-129 in *Best and Taylor's Physiological Basis of Medical Practice*, Brobeck, J.R., Ed. (Williams and Wilkins, Baltimore, Maryland).

CROWLEY, J.F., HAMILTON, J.G. and SCOTT, K.G. (1949). "The metabolism of carrier-free radioberyllium in the rat," J. Biol. Chem. **177**, 975–984.

CUNNINGHAM, B.B. (1954). "Preparation and properties of the compounds of plutonium," pages 371 to 434 in *The Chemistry of the Actinide Elements*, Seaborg, G.T. and Katz, J.J., Eds. (McGraw-Hill, New York).

DAGLE, G.E., PHEMISTER, R.D., LEBEL, J.L., JAENKE, R. and WATTERS, R.L. (1975). "Plutonium-induced popliteal lymphadenitis in beagles," Radiat. Res. **61**(2), 239–250.

DAGLE, G.E., BISTLINE, R.W., LEBEL, J.L. and WATTERS, R.L. (1984). "Plutonium-induced wounds in beagles," Health Phys. **47**(1), 73–84.

DAHLGREN, S. (1967a). "Late effects of thorium dioxide on the liver of patients in Sweden," Ann. NY Acad. Sci. **145**, 718–723.

DAHLGREN, S. (1967b). "Effects of locally deposited colloidal thorium dioxide," Ann. NY Acad. Sci. **145**(3), 786–790.

DA HORTA, J.S. (1967a). "Late effects of Thorotrast on the liver and spleen, and their efferent lymph nodes," Ann. NY Acad. Sci. **145**(3), 676–699.

DA HORTA, J.S. (1967b). "Effects of colloidal thorium dioxide extravasates in the subcutaneous tissues of the cervical regions in man," Ann. NY Acad. Sci. **145**(3), 776–785.

DAVIS, S. and YANCOPOULOS, G.D. (1999). "The angiopoietins: Yin and yang in angiogenesis," Curr. Top. Microbiol. Immunol. **237**, 173–185.

DAXON, E. (1994). "Desert Storm casualties: Impact of depleted uranium," pages 139 to 148 in: *Proceedings of the Depleted Uranium Health and Safety Information Exchange Meeting*, U.S. Department of Energy Report No.Y/AMT-71 (National Technical Information Service, Springfield, Virginia).

DE REY, B.M., LANFRANCHI, H.E. and CABRINI, R.L. (1984). "Deposition pattern and toxicity of subcutaneously implanted uranium dioxide in rats," Health Phys. **46**(3), 688–692.

DOBSON, E.L., GOFMAN, J.W., JONES, H.B., KELLY, L.S. and WALKER, L.A. (1949). "Studies with colloids containing radioisotopes of yttrium, zirconium, columbium, and lanthanum II: The controlled selective localization of radioisotopes of yttrium, zirconium, and columbium in the bone marrow, liver, and spleen," J. Lab. Clin. Med. **34**, 305–312.

DOUNCE, A.L. (1949). "The mechanism of action of uranium compounds in the animal body," pages 951 to 992 in *Pharmacology and Toxicology of Uranium Compounds*, Voegtlin, C. and Hodge, H.C., Eds. (McGraw-Hill, New York).

DOUNCE, A.L. and LAN, T.H. (1949). "The action of uranium on enzymes and proteins," pages 759 to 888 in *Pharmacology and Toxicology of Uranium Compounds*, Voegtlin, C. and Hodge, H.C., Eds. (McGraw-Hill, New York).

DRUCKREY, H. and SCHMAHL, D. (1952). "Carcerogene wirkung von kunststoff-folien," Z. Naturforsch. 7b, 353–361.

DRUCKREY, H., SCHMAHL, D. and MECKE, R. JR. (1956). "Carcerogene wirkung von gummi nach implantation in ratten," Z. Krebsforsch. **61**(1), 55–64.

DUCOUSSO, R., CAUSSE, A. and PASQUIER, C. (1974). "A study of the translocation of radiostrontium from wounds and therapy by local insolubilization," pages 1418 to 1421 in *Proceedings of 3rd International Congress of the International Radiation Protection Association*, Snyder, W.S. Ed., U.S. Atomic Energy Commission Report No. CONF-730907-P2 (National Technical Information Service, Springfield, Virginia).

DUDLEY, R.A. (1967). "A survey of radiation dosimetry in thorium dioxide cases," Ann. NY Acad. Sci. **145**(3), 595–607.

DUFFIELD, J.R. and TAYLOR, D.M. (1986). "The biochemistry of the actinides," pages 129 to 157 in *Handbook on the Physics and Chemistry of the Actinides* (Elsevier Science, New York).

DURBIN, P.W. (1960). "Metabolic characteristics within a chemical family," Health Phys. **2**, 225–238.

DURBIN, P.W. (1962). "Distribution of the transuranic elements in mammals," Health Phys. **8**(6), 665–671.

DURBIN, P.W. (1973). "Metabolism and biological effects of the transplutonium elements," pages 739 to 908 in *Uranium, Plutonium, Transplutonic Elements, Volume 36*, Hodge, H.C., Stannard, J.N. and Hursh, J.B., Eds. (Springer-Verlag, New York).

DURBIN, P.W. (2006). "Bioinorganic chemistry of the actinides: Metabolism in mammals, chemical and radiation toxicity, and therapeutic decorporation," pages 3339 to 3440 in *The Chemistry of the Actinide and Transactinide Elements*, 3rd ed., Vol. 5, Morss, L.R., Edelstein, N.M., Fuger, J. and Katz, J.J., Eds. (Springer, New York).

DURBIN, P.W. and WRENN, M.E. (1975). "Metabolism and effects of uranium in animals," pages 67 to 129 in *Conference on Occupational Health Experience with Uranium*, Wrenn, M.E., Ed., U.S. Energy Research and Development Administration Report CONF-750445 (National Technical Information Service, Springfield, Virginia).

DURBIN, P.W., WILLIAMS, M.H., GEE, M., NEWMAN, R.H. and HAMILTON, J.G. (1956). "Metabolism of the lanthanons in the rat," Proc. Soc. Exp. Biol. Med. **91**(1), 78–85.

DURBIN, P.W., SCOTT, K.G. and HAMILTON, J.G. (1957). "The distribution of radioisotopes of some heavy metals in the rat," Univ. of Calif. Publ. Pharmacol. **3**(1), 1–34.

DURBIN, P.W., ASLING, C.W., JEUNG, N., WILLIAMS, M.H., POST, J.F., JOHNSTON, M.E. and HAMILTON, J.G. (1958). *The Metabolism and Toxicity of Radium-223 in Rats*, University of California Radiation Laboratory, UCRL-8189 (National Technical Information Service, Springfield, Virginia).

DURBIN, P.W., JEUNG, N., KULLGREN, B. and CLEMONS, G.K. (1992). "Gross composition and plasma and extracellular water volumes of tissues of a reference mouse," Health Phys. **63**(4), 427–442.

DURHAM, J.S. (1991). "Hot particle dose calculations using the computer code VARSKIN MOD 2," Radiat. Prot. Dosim. **39**, 75–78.

DURHAM, J.S. (1992). *VARSKIN MOD 2 and SADDE MOD2: Computer Codes for Assessing Skin Dose from Skin Contamination*, NUREG/CR-5873 (National Technical Information Service, Springfield, Virginia).

DURHAM, J.S. (2006). *VARSKIN3: A Computer Code for Assessing Skin Dose from Skin Contamination*, NUREG/CR-6918 (National Technical Information Service, Springfield, Virginia).

DURHAM, J.S., REECE, W.D. and MERWIN, S.E. (1991). "Modelling three dimensional beta sources for skin dose calculations using VARSKIN MOD 2," Radiat. Prot. Dosim. **37**(2), 89–94.

ECKERMAN, K.F., WOLBARST, A.B. and RICHARDSON, C.B. (1988). *Limiting Values of Radionuclide Intake and Air Concentration and Dose Conversion Factors for Inhalation, Submersion, and Ingestion.* Federal Guidance Report No. 11, EPA-520/1-88-020 (U.S. Environmental Protection Agency, Washington).

EIDSON, A.F. (1980a). "*In vitro* solubility of aerosols of industrial uranium and plutonium mixed-oxide nuclear fuel materials," pages 19 to 33 in *Radiation Dose Estimates and Hazard Evaluations for Inhaled Airborne Radionuclides*, Annual Progress Report Lovelace Biomedical and Environmental Research Institute, NUREG/CR-1458 (National Technical Information Service, Springfield, Virginia).

EIDSON, A.F. (1980b). "Infrared spectra of industrial uranium and plutonium mixed-oxide nuclear fuel materials," pages 1 to 17 in *Radiation
Dose Estimates and Hazard Evaluations for Inhaled Airborne Radionuclides*, Annual Progress Report Lovelace Biomedical and Environmental Research Institute, NUREG/CR-1458 (National Technical
Information Service, Springfield, Virginia).

ENTINE, G. (1976). "Nuclear applications of CdTe detectors," pages 68 to
70 in *Proceedings of ERDA Symposium on X- and Gamma-Ray Sources
and Applications*, U.S. Energy Research and Development Administration, CONF-760539 (National Technical Information Service, Springfield, Virginia).

EVERETT, N.B., SIMMONS, B. and LASHER, E.P. (1956). "Distribution
of blood (^{59}Fe) and plasma (^{131}I) volumes of rats determined by liquid
nitrogen freezing," Circ. Res. **4**(4), 419–424.

FABER, M. (1962). "Thorotrast in man—the carrier state and the
sequelae," pages 473 to 498 in *Some Aspects of Internal Irradiation,
Proceedings of a Symposium*, Dougherty, T.F., Jee, W.S.S., Mays, C.W.
and Stover, B.J., Eds. (Pergamon Press, New York).

FABER, M. (1985). "Observations on the Danish Thorotrast patients,"
Strahlentherapie **80**, 140–142.

FABER, M. and JOHANSEN, C. (1967). "Leukemia and other hematologi-
cal diseases after Thorotrast," Ann. NY Acad. Sci. **145**(3), 755–758.

FALK, R.B., DAUGHERTY, N.M., ALDRICH, J.M., FURMAN, F.J. and
HILMAS, D.E. (2006). "Application of multi-compartment wound mod-
els to plutonium-contaminated wounds incurred by former workers at
Rocky Flats," Health Phys. **91**(2), 128–143.

FDA (2007). *U.S. Food and Drug Administration*. http://www.fda.gov
(accessed July 24, 2007) (U.S. Food and Drug Administration, Rockville, Maryland).

FIGGINS, P.E. (1961). *The Radiochemistry of Polonium*, National Academy of Sciences/National Research Council, Subcommittee on Radiochemistry, NAS-NS 3037 (National Technical Information Service,
Springfield, Virginia).

FILIPY, R.E., TOOHEY, R.E., KATHREN, R.L. and DIETERT, S.E.
(1995). "Deterministic effects of ^{241}Am exposure in the Hanford americium accident case," Health Phys. **69**(3), 338–345.

FINKEL, M.P. and BISKIS, B.O. (1962). "Toxicity of plutonium in mice,"
Health Phys. **8**(6), 565–579.

FINKLE, R.D., JACOBSON, L.O., KISIELESKI, W., LAWRENCE, B.,
SIMMONS, E.L. and SNYDER, R.H. (1946). *The Toxicity and Metabo-
lism of Plutonium in Laboratory Animals*, U.S. Atomic Energy
Commission, CH-3783 (National Technical Information Service,
Springfield, Virginia).

FLEISCHER, R.L. and RAABE, O.G. (1977). "Fragmentation of respirable
PuO_2 particles in water by alpha decay — a mode of 'dissolution',"
Health Phys. **32**(4), 253–257.

FOLKMAN, J. and KLAGSBRUN, M. (1987). "Angiogenic factors," Science
235(4787), 442–447.

FREILING, E.C. (1961). "Fractionation in surface bursts," pages 25 to 46 in *Proceedings of the Conference on Radioactive Fallout from Nuclear Weapons Tests*, Klement, A.W., Jr., Ed., U.S. Atomic Energy Commission Report TID-7632 (National Technical Information Service, Springfield, Virginia).

GAMBLE, J.L. (1954). *Chemical Anatomy, Physiology and Pathology of Extracellular Fluid; A Lecture Syllabus* (Harvard University Press, Cambridge, Massachusetts).

GANZ, T. and LEHRER, R.L. (1995). "Biochemistry and function of monocytes and macrophages," pages 869 to 884 in *Williams Hematology*, 5th. ed., Beutler, E., Lichtman, M.A., Coller, B.S. and Kipps, T.J., Eds. (McGraw-Hill, New York).

GARRISON, W.M. and HAMILTON, J.G. (1951). "Production and isolation of carrier-free radioisotopes," Chem. Rev. **49**(2), 237–272.

GERBER, G.B. and THOMAS, R.G., Eds. (1992). *Guidebook for the Treatment of Accidental Internal Radionuclide Contamination of Workers*, Rad. Prot. Dosim. **41**(1), 1–49.

GINDLER, J.E. (1973). "Physical and chemical properties of uranium," pages 69 to 164 in *Uranium, Plutonium, Transplutonic Elements, Volume 36*, Hodge, H.C., Stannard, J.N. and Hursh, J.B., Eds. (Springer-Verlag, New York).

GLASSTONE, S., Ed. (1962). *The Effects of Nuclear Weapons* (rev.), U.S. Atomic Energy Commission (U.S. Government Printing Office, Washington).

GRAHAM, S.G. and KIRKHAM, S.J. (1983). "Identification of ^{241}Am in the auxiliary lymph nodes with an intrinsic germanium detector," Health Phys. **44** (Suppl. 1), 343–352.

GRAHAM, S.J., HEATON, R.B., GARVIN, D.F. and COTELINGAM, J.D. (1992). "Whole-body pathologic analysis of a patient with Thorotrast-induced myelodysplasia," Health Phys. **63**(1), 20–26.

GRAMPA, G. (1967). "Liver distribution of colloidal thorium dioxide and development of liver epithelial tumors in rats," Ann. NY Acad. Sci. **145**(3), 738–747.

GRAY, A.J., BISHOP, J.E., REEVES, J.T. and LAURENT, G.J. (1993). "Aα and Bβ chains of fibrinogen stimulate proliferation of human fibroblasts," J. Cell Sci. **104**(Part 2), 409–413.

GRAY, S.A., STRADLING, G.N., PEARCE, M.J., WILSON, I., MOODY, J.C., BURGADA, R., DURBIN, P.W. and RAYMOND, K.N. (1994). "Removal of plutonium and americium from the rat using 3,4,3-LIHOPO and DTPA after simulated wound contamination: Effect of delayed administration and mass of plutonium," Radiat. Prot. Dosim. **53**(1), 319–322.

GREILING, D. and CLARK, R.A.F. (1997). "Fibronectin provides a conduit for fibroblast transmigration from a collagenous stroma into fibrin clot provisional matrix," J. Cell Sci. **110**(Part 7), 861–870.

GRIGORYAN, K.V. (1966). "Buildup dynamics of chronically administered ^{144}Ce in the organism of animals," pages 61 to 66 in *Distribution and Biological Effects of Radioactive Isotopes*, Moskalev, Y.I., Ed., U.S. Atomic Energy Commission Report No. AEC-tr-6944 (rev.) (National Technical Information Service, Springfield, Virginia).

GRONDAHL-HANSEN, J., LUND, L.R., RALFKIAER, E., OTTE-VANGER, V. and DANO, K. (1988). "Urokinase- and tissue-type plasminogen activators in keratinocytes during wound reepithelialization *in vivo*," J. Invest. Dermatol. **90**(6), 790–795.

GUILMETTE, R.A. and MAYS, D., Eds. (1992). "Total-body evaluation of a Thorotrast patient," Health Phys. **63**(1), 1–123.

GUILMETTE. R.A., GILLETT, N.A., EIDSON, A.F., GRIFFITH, W.C. and BROOKS, A.L. (1989). "The influence of nonuniform alpha irradiation of Chinese hamster liver on chromosome damage and the induction of cancer," pages 142 to 148 in *Proceedings of a Workshop on Risks from Radium and Thorotrast*, Taylor, D.M., Mays, C.W., Gerber, G.B. and Thomas, R.G., Eds. (British Institute of Radiology, London).

GUILMETTE, R.A., HAHN, F.F. and DURBIN, P.W. (2005). "Biokinetics and dosimetry of depleted uranium (DU) in rats implanted with DU metal fragments," pages 174 to 178 in *Proceedings of the 9th International Conference on Health Effects of Incorporated Radionuclides: Emphasis on Radium, Thorium, Uranium and Their Daughter Products*, Oeh, U., Roth, R. and Paretzke, H.G., Eds., http://www.gsf.de/heir/ProceedingsHEIR2004_ebook.pdf (accessed July 24, 2007) (Institut fur Strahlenschutz, GSF, Neuherberg).

GURD, F.R.N. and WILCOX, P.E. (1956). "Complex formation between metallic cations and proteins, peptides and amino acids," Adv. Protein Chem. **48**(11), 311–427.

GUSEV, I.A., GUSKOVA, A.K. and METTLER, F.A., JR., Eds. (2001). *Medical Management of Radiation Accidents*, 2nd ed. (CRC Press, Boca Raton, Florida).

HAHN, F.F. (2000). *Carcinogenesis of Depleted Uranium Fragments*, Final Report to the U.S. Army Medical Research and Materiel Command (National Technical Information Service, Springfield, Virginia).

HAHN, F.F., GUILMETTE, R.A. and HOOVER, M.D. (2002). "Implanted depleted uranium fragments cause soft tissue sarcomas in the muscles of rats," Environ. Health Perspect. **110**(1), 51–59.

HAM, A.W. (1974). *Histology*, 7th ed. (J.B. Lippincott, Philadelphia).

HAMILTON, J.G. (1943). *Metabolism of Fission Products, Progress Report for Month Ending March 15, 1943*, U.S. Atomic Energy Commission Report No.CH-554 [declassified report issued as Report No. MDDC-1142 (1947)] (National Technical Information Service, Springfield, Virginia).

HAMILTON, J.G. (1947a). "Metabolic properties of plutonium and allied materials," pages 2 to 6 in *Technical Progress Report on the Metabolic Properties of Plutonium and Allied Materials for July 1947*, University of California Radiation Laboratory Report No. BP-115 (University of California, Berkeley, California).

HAMILTON, J.G. (1947b). "The metabolism of the fission products and the heaviest elements," Radiology **49**, 325–343.

HAMILTON, J.G. (1948a). "The metabolic properties of the fission products and actinide elements," Rev. Mod. Phys. **20**(4), 718–728.

HAMILTON, J.G. (1948b). "The metabolic properties of plutonium and allied materials," pages 4 to 28 in *Medical and Health Divisions Quarterly Report, October 1947 to January 1948*, University of California Radiation Laboratory, UCRL-41 (University of California, Berkeley, California).

HAMILTON, J.G. (1948c). "Metabolic properties of plutonium and allied materials," pages 4 to 20 in *Medical and Health Division Quarterly Report March 1948*, University of California Radiation Laboratory, UCRL-98 (University of California, Berkeley, California).

HAMILTON, J.G. (1948d). "Metabolic properties of plutonium and allied materials," pages 4 to 24 in *Medical and Health Division Quarterly Report June 1948*, University of California Radiation Laboratory, UCRL-150 (University of California, Berkeley, California).

HAMILTON, J.G. (1948e). "Metabolic properties of plutonium and allied materials," pages 4 to 19 in *Medical and Health Division Quarterly Report September 1948*, University of California Radiation Laboratory, UCRL-193 (University of California, Berkeley, California).

HAMILTON, J.G. (1948f). "Metabolic properties of plutonium and allied materials," pages 4 to 16 in *Medical and Health Division Quarterly Report December 1948*, University of California Radiation Laboratory, UCRL-270 (University of California, Berkeley, California).

HAMILTON, J.G. (1949a). "The metabolism of the radioactive elements created by nuclear fission," New England J. Med. **240**, 863–870.

HAMILTON, J.G. (1949b). "Metabolic properties of plutonium and allied materials," pages 4 to 24 in *Medical and Health Division Quarterly Report March 1949*, University of California Radiation Laboratory, UCRL-332 (University of California, Berkeley, California).

HAMILTON, J.G. (1949c). "Metabolic properties of plutonium and allied materials," pages 4 to 24 in *Medical and Health Division Quarterly Report June 1949*, University of California Radiation Laboratory, UCRL-414 (University of California, Berkeley, California).

HAMILTON, J.G. (1949d). "Metabolic properties of plutonium and allied materials," pages 4 to 36 in *Medical and Health Division Quarterly Report September 1949*, University of California Radiation Laboratory, UCRL-480 (University of California, Berkeley, California).

HAMILTON, J.G. (1949e). "Metabolic properties of plutonium and allied materials," pages 4 to 22 in *Medical and Health Division Quarterly Report December 1949*, University of California Radiation Laboratory, UCRL-587 (University of California, Berkeley, California).

HAMILTON, J.G. (1950a). "Metabolic properties of plutonium and allied materials," pages 4 to 21 in *Medical and Health Division Quarterly Report June 1950*, University of California Radiation Laboratory, UCRL-806 (University of California, Berkeley, California).

HAMILTON, J.G. (1950b). "Metabolic properties of plutonium and allied materials," pages 4 to 40 in *Medical and Health Division Quarterly Report September 1950*, University of California Radiation Laboratory, UCRL-960 (University of California, Berkeley, California).

HAMILTON, J.G. (1950c). "The metabolic properties of various elements," pages 4 to 41 in *Medical and Health Division Quarterly Report December 1950*, University of California Radiation Laboratory, UCRL-1143 (University of California, Berkeley, California).

HAMILTON, J.G. (1951a). "The metabolic properties of various materials," pages 4 to 32 in *Medical and Health Division Quarterly Report March 1951*, University of California Radiation Laboratory, UCRL-1282 (University of California, Berkeley, California).

HAMILTON, J.G. (1951b). "The metabolic properties of various materials," pages 4 to 22 in *Medical and Health Division Quarterly Report June 1951*, University of California Radiation Laboratory, UCRL-1437 (University of California, Berkeley, California).

HAMILTON, J.G. (1951c). "The metabolic properties of various materials," pages 4 to 21 in *Medical and Health Division Quarterly Report September 1951*, University of California Radiation Laboratory, UCRL-1561 (University of California, Berkeley, California).

HAMILTON, J.G. (1952). "The metabolic properties of various materials," pages 6 to 16 in *Medical and Health Division Quarterly Report AUGUST 1952*, University of California Radiation Laboratory, UCRL-1922 (University of California, Berkeley, California).

HAMILTON, J.G. (1954a). "The metabolic properties of various materials," pages 24 to 30 in *Medical and Health Physics Quarterly Report April 1954*, University of California Radiation Laboratory, UCRL-2553 (University of California, Berkeley, California).

HAMILTON, J.G. (1954b). "The metabolic properties of various materials," pages 3 to 8 in *Medical and Health Physics Quarterly Report May 1954*, University of California Radiation Laboratory, UCRL-2605 (University of California, Berkeley, California).

HAMMOND, S.E. and PUTZIER, E.A. (1964). "Observed effects of plutonium in wounds over a long period of time," Health Phys. **10**(6), 399–406.

HAMPTON, J.C. and ROSARIO, B. (1967). "The distribution of colloidal thorium dioxide in mouse liver after intravenous injection," Ann. NY Acad. Sci. **145**(3), 533–544.

HARRIS, W.R., CARRANO, C.J., PECORARO, V.L. and RAYMOND, K.N. (1981). "Siderophilin metal coordination. 1. Complexation of thorium by transferrin: Structure-function implications," J. Am. Chem. Soc. **103**, 2231–2237.

HARRISON, J.D. and DAVID, A.J. (1977). "A comparison of the translocation of different chemical forms of plutonium from simulated wound sites in rats and hamsters and the effect of diethylenetriaminepentaacetate (DTPA) on clearance," pages 68 to 70 in *Annual Research and Development Report 1976* (Health Protection Agency, London).

HARRISON, J.D. and DAVID, A.J. (1978). "The use of DTPA to limit the systemic burden of plutonium after wound contamination," pages 91 to 93 in *Annual Research and Development Report 1977* (Health Protection Agency, London).

HARRISON, J.D., DAVID, A.J. and STATHER, J.W. (1977a). "The translocation of plutonium-239 from simulated wound sites in the rat after deposition as the nitrate," pages 63 to 65 in *Annual Research and Development Report 1976* (Health Protection Agency, London).

HARRISON, J.D., DAVID, A.J. and STATHER, J.W. (1977b). "The translocation of plutonium-238 and plutonium-239 deposited as the nitrates in a simulated wound site in the rat," pages 66 to 67 in *Annual Research and Development Report 1976* (Health Protection Agency, London).

HARRISON, J.D., DAVID, A.J. and STATHER, J.W. (1978a). "The wound clearance and comparative metabolism of plutonium, americum, and curium in rodents," pages 88 to 90 in *Annual Research and Development Report 1977* (Health Protection Agency, London).

HARRISON, J.D., DAVID, A.J. and STATHER, J.W. (1978b). "Experimental studies of the translocation of plutonium from simulated wound sites in the rat," Int. J. Radiat. Biol. Relat. Stud. Phys. Chem. Med. **33**(5), 457–472.

HARRISON, J.D., HODGSON, A., HAINES, J.W. and STATHER, J.W. (1990). *Biokinetics of Plutonium-239 and Americium-241 in the Rat after Subcutaneous Deposition of Contaminated Particles from the Former Nuclear Weapons Test Site at Maralinga: Implications for Human Exposure*, NRPB-M198 (Health Protection Agency, London).

HARRISON, J.D., HODGSON, A., HAINES, J.W. and STATHER, J.W. (1993). "The biokinetics of plutonium-239 and americium-241 in the rat after subcutaneous deposition of contaminated particles from the former nuclear weapons site at Maralinga: Implications for human exposures," Hum. Exp. Toxicol. **12**(4), 303–321.

HASTY, K.A., HIBBS, M.S., KANG, A.H. and MAINARDI, C.L. (1986). "Secreted forms of human neutrophil collagenase," J. Biol. Chem. **261**(12), 5645–5650.

HATCH, G.E., GARDNER, D.E. and MENZEL, D.B. (1980). "Simulation of oxidant production in alveolar macrophages by pollutant and latex particles," Environ. Res. **23**(1), 121–136.

HAVEN, F.L. and HODGE, H.C. (1949). "Toxicity following the parenteral administration of certain soluble uranium compounds," pages 281 to 308 in *Pharmacology and Toxicology of Uranium Compounds*, Voegtlin, C. and Hodge, H.C., Eds. (McGraw-Hill, New York).

HEBDA, P.A., KLINGBEIL, C.K., ABRAHAM, J.A. and FIDDES, J.C. (1990). "Basic fibroblast growth factor stimulation of epidermal wound healing in pigs," J. Invest. Dermatol. **95**(6), 626–631.

HEGGERS, J.P., LOY, G.L., ROBSON, M.C. and DEL BECCARO, E.J. (1980). "Histological demonstration of prostaglandins and thromboxanes in burned tissue," J. Surg. Res. **28**(2), 110–117.

HEID, K.R. and JECH, J.J. (1969). "Assessing the probable severity of plutonium inhalation cases," Health Phys. **17**(3), 433–447.

HELDIN, C.H. and WESTERMARK, B. (1996). "Role of platelet-derived growth factor *in vivo*," pages 249 to 274 in *The Molecular and Cellular Biology of Wound Repair*, Clark, R.A.F., Ed. (Plenum Press, New York).

HELFINSTINE, S.Y., GUILMETTE, R.A. and SCHLAPPER, G.A. (1992). "*In vitro* dissolution of curium oxide using a phagolysosomal simulant solvent system," Environ. Health Perspect. **97**, 131–137.

HENGE-NAPOLI, M.H., ANSOBORLO, E., DONNADIEU-CLARAZ, M., BERRY, J.P., GILBERT, R., MONDAN, A. and PRADAL, B. (1994). "Solubility and transferability of several industrial forms of uranium oxides," Radiat. Prot. Dosim. **53**(1), 157–161.

HENGE-NAPOLI, M.H., STRADLING, G.N. and TAYLOR, D.M., Eds. (2000). "Preface: Decorporation of radionuclides from the human body," Radiat. Prot. Dosim. **87**(1), 9–10.

HINDMAN, J.C. (1954). "Ionic and molecular species of plutonium in solution," pages 301 to 370 in *The Chemistry of the Actinide Elements*, Seaborg, G.T. and Katz, J.J., Eds. (McGraw-Hill, New York).

HOLBROOK, K.A. and WOLFF, K. (1993). "The structure and development of skin," pages 97 to 145 in *Dermatology in General Medicine*, Fitzpatrick, T.B., Eisen, A.Z., Wolff, K., Freedberg, I.M. and Austen, K.F., Eds. (McGraw Hill, New York).

HONMA, T. and HAMASAKI, T. (1996). "Ultrastructure of multinucleated giant cell apoptosis in foreign-body granuloma," Virchows. Arch. **428**(3), 165–176.

HOOPER, F.J., SQUIBB, K.S., SIEGEL, E.L., MCPHAUL, K. and KEOGH, J.P. (1999). "Elevated urine uranium excretion by soldiers with retained uranium shrapnel," Health Phys. **77**(5), 512–519.

HUNT, T.K., Ed. (1980). *Wound Healing and Wound Infection: Theory and Surgical Practice* (Appleton-Century-Crofts, New York).

HURSH, J.B. (1967). "Loss of thorium daughters by thorium dioxide patients," Ann. NY Acad. Sci. **145**(3), 634–641.

HYMAN, C. and PALDINO, R.L. (1967). "Influence of sex hormones and tissues on colloidal thorium dioxide distribution and effects in rabbits," Ann. NY Acad. Sci. **145**(3), 576–584.

IAEA (1964). International Atomic Energy Agency. *Thorotrast. A Bibliography of Its Diagnostic Use and Biological Effects*, Report WP/42 (International Atomic Energy Agency, Vienna).

IAEA (1978). International Atomic Energy Agency. *Treatment of Incorporated Transuranium Elements*, Technical Report Series No. 184 (International Atomic Energy Agency, Vienna).

IAEA (1996a). International Atomic Energy Agency. *International Basic Safety Standards for Protection Against Ionizing Radiation and for the Safety of Radiation Sources*. Safety Series No. 115 (International Atomic Energy Agency, Vienna).

IAEA (1996b). International Atomic Energy Agency. *Assessment and Treatment of External and Internal Radionuclide Contamination*, TECDOC-869 (International Atomic Energy Agency, Vienna).

IAEA (2004). International Atomic Energy Agency. *Methods for Assessing Occupational Radiation Doses Due to Intakes of Radionuclides*, Safety Series Report No. 37 (International Atomic Energy Agency, Vienna).

ICRP (1959). International Commission on Radiological Protection. *Report of Committee II on Permissible Dose for Internal Radiation*, ICRP Publication 2 (Elsevier Science, New York).

ICRP (1972). International Commission on Radiological Protection. *The Metabolism of Compounds of Plutonium and Other Actinides*, ICRP Publication 19 (Elsevier Science, New York).

ICRP (1975). International Commission on Radiological Protection. *Reference Man: Anatomical, Physiological and Metabolic Characteristics*, ICRP Publication 23 (Elsevier Science, New York).

ICRP (1979). International Commission on Radiological Protection. *Limits for Intakes of Radionuclides by Workers Part 3*, ICRP Publication 30, Ann. ICRP **6**(2–3) (Elsevier Science, New York).

ICRP (1986). International Commission on Radiological Protection. *The Metabolism of Plutonium and Related Elements*, ICRP Publication 48, Ann. ICRP **16**(2–3) (Elsevier Science, New York).

ICRP (1989). International Commission on Radiological Protection. *Age-Dependent Doses to Members of the Public from Intake of Radionuclides: Part 1*, ICRP Publication 56, Ann. ICRP **20**(2) (Elsevier Science, New York).

ICRP (1991a). International Commission on Radiological Protection. *1990 Recommendations of the International Commission on Radiological Protection*, ICRP Publication 60, Ann. ICRP **21**(1–3) (Elsevier Science, New York).

ICRP (1991b). International Commission on Radiological Protection. *The Biological Basis for Dose Limitation in the Skin*, ICRP Publication 59, Ann. ICRP **22**(2) (Elsevier Science, New York).

ICRP (1993). International Commission on Radiological Protection. *Age-Dependent Doses to Members of the Public from Intake of Radionuclides: Part 2. Ingestion Dose Coefficients*, ICRP Publication 67, Ann. ICRP **23**(3–4) (Elsevier Science, New York).

ICRP (1994a). International Commission on Radiological Protection. *Human Respiratory Tract Model for Radiological Protection*, ICRP Publication 66, Ann. ICRP **24**(1–3) (Elsevier Science, New York).

ICRP (1994b). International Commission on Radiological Protection. *Dose Coefficients for Intakes of Radionuclides by Workers*, ICRP Publication 68, Ann. ICRP **24**(2) (Elsevier Science, New York).

ICRP (1995a). International Commission on Radiological Protection. *Age-Dependent Doses to Members of the Public from Intake of Radionuclides: Part 3. Ingestion Dose Coefficients*, ICRP Publication 69, Ann. ICRP **25**(1) (Elsevier Science, New York).

ICRP (1995b). International Commission on Radiological Protection. *Age-Dependent Doses to Members of the Public from Intake of Radionuclides: Part 4. Inhalation Dose Coefficients*, ICRP Publication 71, Ann. ICRP **25**(3) (Elsevier Science, New York).

ICRP (1997). International Commission on Radiological Protection. *Individual Monitoring for Internal Exposure of Workers*, ICRP Publication 78, Ann. ICRP **27**(3–4) (Elsevier Science, New York).

ICRP (2002a). International Commission on Radiological Protection. *Supporting Guidance 3. Guide for the Practical Application of the ICRP Human Respiratory Tract Model*, Ann. ICRP **32**(1–2). (Elsevier Science, New York).

ICRP (2002b). International Commission on Radiological Protection. *Basic Anatomical and Physiological Data for Use in Radiological Protection: Reference Values*, ICRP Publication 89, Ann. ICRP **32**(3–4). (Elsevier Science, New York).

ICRU (1993). International Commission on Radiation Units and Measurements. *Quantities and Units in Radiation Protection Dosimetry*, ICRU Report 51 (Oxford University Press, Oxford, United Kingdom).

ICRU (1996). International Commission on Radiation Units and Measurements. *Dosimetry of External Beta Rays for Radiation Protection*, ICRU Report 56 (Oxford University Press, Oxford, United Kingdom).

ILYIN, L.A. (2001). "Skin wounds and burns contaminated by radioactive substances (metabolism, decontamination, tactics, and techniques of medical care)," pages 363 to 419 in *Medical Management of Radiation Accidents*, 2nd ed., Gusev, I.A., Guskova, A.K. and Mettler, F.A., Jr., Eds. (CRC Press, Boca Raton, Florida).

ILYIN, L.A. and IVANNIKOV, A.T. (1979). *Radioactive Substances and Wounds* (Atomizdat, Moscow) [in Russian].

ILYIN, L.A., IVANNIKOV, A.T., PARFENOV, Y.D. and STOLYAROV, V.P. (1975). "Strontium absorption through damaged and undamaged human skin," Health Phys. **29**(1), 75–80.

ILYIN, L.A., IVANNIKOV, A.T., BAZHIN, A.G., KONSTANTINOVA, T.P. and ALTUKHOVA, G.A. (1977). "Intake of Po-210 into the body through the damaged skin and efficiency of some methods in preventing its absorption," Health Phys. **32**(2), 107–111.

ILYIN, L.A., IVANNIKOV, A.T., BELIAEV, I.K., BAZHIN, A.G. and ALTUKHOVA, G.A. (1982). "Percutaneous [239]Pu uptake in rats with skin burns from nitric acid," Gig. Sanit. (1), 26–29.

JECH, J.J., HEID, K.R. and LARSON, H.V. (1969). "Prompt assessments and mitigatory action after accidental intake of plutonium," pages 77 to 93 in *Handling of Radiation Accidents*, Proceedings Series STI/PUB/229 (International Atomic Energy Agency, Vienna).

JENNINGS, T.A., PETERSON, L., AXIOTIS, C.A., FRIEDLAENDER, G.E., COOKE, R.A. and ROSAI, J. (1988). "Angiosarcoma associated with foreign body material. A report of three cases," Cancer **62**(11), 2436–2444.

JOHANSEN, C. (1967). "Tumors in rabbits after injection of various amounts of thorium dioxide," Ann. NY Acad. Sci. **145**(3), 724–727.

JOHNSON, L.J. (1969). *Relative Translocation and Distribution of Pu and Am from Experimental PuO$_2$ Subcutaneous Implants in Beagles*, U.S. Atomic Energy Commission Report No. COO-1787-6 (National Technical Information Service, Springfield, Virginia).

JOHNSON, L.J. and LAWRENCE, J.N.P. (1974). "Plutonium contaminated wound experience and assay techniques at the Los Alamos Scientific Laboratory," Health Phys. **27**(1), 55–59.

JOHNSON, L.J., BULL, E.H., LEBEL, J.L. and WATTERS, R.L. (1970a). "Kinetics of lymph node activity accumulation from subcutaneous PuO_2 implants," Health Phys. **18**(4), 416–418.

JOHNSON, L.J., WATTERS, R.L., LAGERQUIST, C.R. and HAMMOND, S.E. (1970b). "Relative distribution of plutonium and americium following experimental PuO_2 implants," Health Phys. **19**(4), 743–749.

JOHNSON, L.J., WATTERS, R.L., LEBEL, J.L., LAGERQUIST, C.R. and HAMMOND, S.E. (1972). "The distribution of Pu and Am: Subcutaneous administration of PuO_2 and the effect of chelation therapy," pages 213 to 220 in *Radiobiology of Plutonium*, Stover, B.J. and Jee, W.S.S., Eds. (J.W. Press, Salt Lake City, Utah).

JULIANO, R.L. and HASKILL, S. (1993). "Signal transduction from the extracellular matrix," J. Cell Biol. **120**(3), 577–585.

KALISTRATOVA, V.S., KOGAN, A.G. and KOZLOVA, M.D. (1968). "Effect of certain factors on the behavior of ^{111}Ag in the organism of animals," pages 188 to 193 in *Distribution and Biological Effects of Radioactive Isotopes*, Moskalev, Y.I., Ed., AEC-tr-6944 (rev.) (National Technical Information Center, Springfield, Virginia).

KATHREN, R.L. (1995). "The United States transuranium and uranium registries: 1968–1993," Radiat. Prot. Dosim. **60**(4), 349–354.

KATHREN, R.L. and HILL, R.L. (1992). "Distribution and dosimetry of Thorotrast in USUR case 1001," Health Phys. **63**(1), 72–88.

KATZ, J.H. (1970). "Transferrin and its functions in the regulation of iron metabolism," pages 539 to 577 in *Regulation of Hematopoiesis*, Vol. I, Gordon, A.S., Ed. (Appleton-Century-Crofts, New York).

KATZIN, L.L. (1957). The chemistry of thorium," pages 66 to 102 in *The Chemistry of the Actinide Elements*, Seaborg, G.T. and Katz, J.J., Eds. (McGraw-Hill, New York).

KAWIN, B., COPP, D.H. and HAMILTON, J.G. (1950). *Studies of the Metabolism of Certain Fission Products and Plutonium*, University of California Radiation Laboratory, UCRL-812 (University of California, Berkeley, California).

KECK, P.J., HAUSER, S.D., KRIVI, G., SANZO, K., WARREN, T., FEDER, J. and CONNOLLY, D.T. (1989). "Vascular permeability factor, an endothelial cell mitogen related to PDGF," Science **246**(4935), 1309–1312.

KELSEY, C.A., METTLER, F.A. JR., BREWER, M., STEPHANSON, L., GRAHAM, J.J., TELAPK, R.J., DOEZEMA, D. and HARTSHORNE, M.F. (1998). "$^{192}IrCl$ acid skin burn: Case report and review of the literature," Health Phys. **74**(5), 610–612.

KEOUGH, R.F. and POWERS, G.J. (1970). "Determination of plutonium in biological materials by extraction and liquid scintillation counting," Anal. Chem. **42**(3), 419–421.

KISIELESKI, W. and WOODRUFF, L. (1947). "Studies on the distribution of plutonium in the rat," pages 86 to 103 in *Argonne National Laboratory Biology Division Quarterly Report*, Report No. ANL-4108, Brues, A.M., Ed (Argonne National Laboratory, Argonne, Illinois).

KOBZIK, L., GODLESKI, J.J. and BRAIN, J.D. (1990). "Oxidative metabolism in the alveolar macrophage: Analysis by flow cytometry," J. Leukoc. Biol. **47**(4), 295–303.

KOCHER, D.C. (1981). *Radioactive Decay Data Tables. A Handbook of Decay Data for Application to Radiation Dosimetry and Radiological Assessments*, DOE/TIC-11026 (National Technical Information Service, Springfield, Virginia).

KOCHER, D.C. and ECKERMAN, K.F. (1987). "Electron dose-rate conversion factors for external exposure of the skin from uniformly deposited activity on the body surface," Health Phys. **53**(2), 135–141.

KRAWCZYK, W.S. (1971). "A pattern of epidermal cell migration during wound healing," J. Cell Biol. **49**, 247–263.

KREUGER, M.R., TAMES, D.R. and MARIANO, M. (1998). "Expression of NO-synthase in cells of foreign-body and BCG-induced granulomata in mice: Influence of L-NAME on the evolution of the lesion," Immunology **95**(2), 278–282.

KREYLING, W.G. and SCHEUCH, G. (2000). "Clearance of particles deposited in the lungs," pages 323 to 376 in *Particle-Lung Interactions*, Gehr, P. and Heyder, J., Eds. (Marcel Dekker, New York).

KUSAMA, T., ITOH, S. and YOSHIZAWA, Y. (1986). "Absorption of radionuclides through wounded skin," Health Phys. **51**(1), 138–141.

LAFUMA, J., NENOT, J.C. and MORIN, M. (1971). "Experimental research into the treatment of contamination by transplutonium elements," pages 249 to 257 in *Radiation Protection Problems Relating to Transuranium Elements* (Commission of the European Communities, Luxembourg).

LAGERQUIST, C.R., HAMMOND, S.E. and HYLTON, D.B. (1972). "Distribution of plutonium and americium in the body 5 years after an exposure *via* contaminated puncture wound," Health Phys. **22**(6), 921–924.

LANG, S., KOSMA, V.M., SERVOMAA, K., RUUSKANEN, J. and RYTOMAA, T. (1993). "Tumour induction in mouse epidermal cells irradiated by hot particles," Int. J. Radiat. Biol. **63**(3), 375–381.

LANGHAM, W.H., LAWRENCE, J.N.P., MCCLELLAND, J. and HEMPELMANN, L.H. (1962). "The Los Alamos Scientific Laboratory's experience with plutonium in man," Health Phys. **8**(6), 753–760.

LANZ, H., SCOTT, K.G., CROWLEY, J. and HAMILTON, J.G. (1946). *Metabolism of Thorium, Protactinium, and Neptunium in the Rat*, Metallurgical Laboratory Report No. CH-3606 (reprinted as Manhattan District Declassified Document No. MDDC-648) (National Technical Information Service, Springfield, Virginia).

LANZ, H., JR., WALLACE, P.C. and HAMILTON, J.G. (1950). "The metabolism of arsenic in laboratory animals using ^{74}As as a tracer," pages 263 to 282 in *University of California Publications in Pharmacology*, Anderson, H.H., Alles, G.A. and Daniels, T.C., Eds., Vol. 2, No. 20 (University of California Press, Berkeley, California).

LATIMER, W. (1952). *The Oxidation States of the Elements and Their Potentials in Aqueous Solutions*, 2nd ed. (Prentice Hall, New York).

LAURER, G.R. and EISENBUD, M. (1968). "*In vivo* measurements of nuclides emitting soft penetrating radiations," pages 189 to 207 in *Proceedings of the Symposium on Diagnosis and Treatment of Deposited Radionuclides*, Kornberg, H.A. and Norwood, W.D., Eds. (Exerpta Medical Foundation, New York).

LEACH, L.J., MAYNARD, E.A., HODGE, H.C., SCOTT, J.K., YUILE, C.L., SYLVESTER, G.E. and WILSON, H.B. (1970). "A five-year inhalation study with natural uranium dioxide (UO_2) dust—I. Retention and biologic effect in the monkey, dog and rat," Health Phys. **18**(6), 599–612.

LEBEL, J.L., BISTLINE, R.W., SCHALLBERGER, J.A., DAGLE, G.E. and GOMEZ, L.S. (1976). "Studies of plutonium and the lymphatic system: Six years of progress at Colorado State University," pages 2 to 9 in *Hanford Biology Symposium on Radiation and the Lymphatic System*, Ballou, J.E., Ed., CONF-740930 (National Technical Information Service, Springfield, Virginia).

LEHNERT, B.E. and MORROW, P.E. (1985). "The initial lag in phagocytic rate by macrophages in monolayer is related to particle encounters and binding," Immunol. Invest. **14**(6), 515–521.

LEINFELDER, P.J. and RILEY, E.F. (1956). "Further studies of effects of x-radiation on partially shielded lens of rabbit," AMA Arch. Ophthalmol. **55**(1), 84–86.

LESSARD, E.T., YIHUA, X., SKRABLE, K.W., CHABOT, G.E., FRENCH, C.S., LABONE, T.R., JOHNSON, J.R., FISHER, D.R., BELANGER, R. and LIPSZTEIN, J.L. (1987). *Interpretation of Bioassay Measurements*, NUREG/CR-4884 (U.S. Nuclear Regulatory Commission, Washington).

LEVENSON, S.M., GEEVER, E.F., CROWLEY, L.V., OATES, J.F., III, BERARD, C.W. and ROSEN, H. (1965). "The healing of rat skin wounds," Ann. Surg. **161**, 293–308.

LEWIS, G.P. (1969). "Changes in the composition of rabbit hind limb lymph after thermal injury," J. Physiol. **205**(3), 619–634.

LEWIS, G.P. and YATES, C. (1972). "Flow and composition of lymph collected from the skeletal muscle of the rabbit hind limb," J. Physiol. **226**(2), 57P–58P.

LIEBERMANN, D., LUEHRS, H. and VAN KAICK, G. (1995) "Late effects of paravascular Thorotrast deposits," pages 271 to 274 in *Health Effects of Internally Deposited Radionuclides: Emphasis on Radium and Thorium*, van Kaick, G., Karaoglou, A. and Kellerer, A.M., Eds. (World Scientific, Hackensack, New Jersey).

LINDEMAN, G., MCKAY, M.J., TAUBMAN, K.L. and BILOUS, A.M. (1990) "Malignant fibrous histiocytoma developing in bone 44 years after shrapnel trauma," Cancer **66**(10), 2229–2232.

LINDEN, M.A., MANTON, W.I., STEWART, R.M., THAL, E.R. and FEIT, H. (1982). "Lead poisoning from retained bullets: Pathogenesis, diagnosis, and management," Ann. Surg. **195**(3), 305–313.

LINDENBAUM, A. and WESTFALL, W. (1965). "Colloidal properties of plutonium in dilute aqueous solution," Int. J. Radiat. Appl. Isotopes **16**, 545–553.

LIPSZTEIN, J.L., MELO, D.R., OLIVEIRA, C.A.N., BERTELLI, L. and RAMALHO, A.T. (1998). "The Goiania ^{137}Cs accident—a review of the internal and cytogenic dosimetry," Radiat. Prot. Dosim. **79**(1), 149–154.

LISCO, H. and KISIELESKI, W.E. (1953). "The fate and pathologic effects of plutonium metal implanted into rabbits and rats," Am. J. Pathol. **29**(2), 305–321.

LLOYD, R.D., TAYLOR, G.N., MAYS, C.W., MCFARLAND, S.S. and ATHERTON, D.R. (1975). "DTPA therapy of [241]Am from a simulated wound site," Health Phys. **29**(5), 808–811.

LOEVINGER, R., BUDINGER, T.F. and WATSON, E.E. (1991). *MIRD Primer for Absorbed Dose Calculations* (rev.) (Society of Nuclear Medicine, New York).

LUCKEY, T.D. and VENUGOPAL, B. (1977). *Metal Toxicity in Mammals* (Plenum Press, New York).

LUK, C.K. (1971). "Study of the nature of the metal-binding sites and estimate of the distance between the metal-binding sites in transferrin using trivalent lanthanide ions as fluorescent probes," Biochemistry **10**(15), 2838–2843.

LUKACS, N.W., CHENSUE, S.W., STRIETER, R.M., WARMINGTON, K. and KUNKEL, S.L. (1994). "Inflammatory granuloma formation is mediated by TNF-alpha-inducible intercellular adhesion molecule-1," J. Immunol. **152**(12), 5883–5889.

LUSHBAUGH, C.C. and LANGHAM, J. (1962). "A dermal lesion from implanted plutonium," Arch. Dermatol. **86**, 461–464.

LUSHBAUGH, C.C., CLOUTIER, R.J., HUMASON, G., LANGHAM, J. and GUZAK, S. (1967). "Histopathological study of intradermal plutonium metal deposits: Their conjectured fate," Ann. NY Acad. Sci. **145**(3), 791–797.

LYNCH, S.E., COLVIN, R.B. and ANTONIADES, H.N. (1989). "Growth factors in wound healing. Single and synergistic effects on partial thickness porcine skin wounds," J. Clin. Invest. **84**(2), 640–646.

MACK, C. (1967). *Essentials of Statistics for Scientists and Technologists* (Plenum Press, New York).

MADRI, J.A., SANKAR, S. and ROMANIC, A.M. (1996). "Angiogenesis," pages 355 to 372 in *The Molecular and Cellular Biology of Wound Repair*. Clark, R.A.F., Ed. (Plenum Press, New York).

MANTON, W.I. and THAL, E.R (1986). "Lead poisoning from retained missiles. An experimental study," Ann. Surg. **204**(5), 594–599.

MARIEB, E.N. (1992). *Human Anatomy and Physiology*, 2nd ed. (Benjamin Cummings Publishing, Redwood City, California).

MARTELL, A.E. and SMITH, R.M. (1976). *Critical Stability Constants, Volume 4. Inorganic Complexes* (Plenum Press, New York).

MARTELL, A.E. and SMITH, R.M. (1982). *Critical Stability Constants, Volume 5, First Supplement* (Plenum Press, New York).

MATSUOKA, O., KASHIMA, M., JOSHIMA, H. and NODA, Y. (1972). "Whole-body autoradiographic studies on plutonium metabolism as affected by its physio-chemical state and route of administration," Health Phys. **22**(6), 713–722.

MCCLAIN, D.E., BENSON, K.A., DALTON, T.K., EJNIK, J., EMOND, C.A., HODGE, S.J., KALINICH, J.F., LANDAUER, M.A., MILLER, A.C., PELLMAR, T.C., STEWART, M.D., VILLA, V. and XU, J. (2001). "Biological effects of embedded depleted uranium (DU): Summary of Armed Forces Radiobiology Research Institute research," Sci. Total Environ. **274**(1–3), 115–118.

MCCLANAHAN, B.J. and KORNBERG, H.A. (1967). "Treatment of plutonium contaminated wounds with diethylenetriaminepentaacetic acid in rats," pages 395 to 402 in *Proceedings of the Symposium on Diagnosis and Treatment of Deposited Radionuclides*, Kornberg, H.A. and Norwood, W.D., Eds. (Excerpta Medica Foundation, Amsterdam).

MCCLANAHAN, B.J. and RAGAN, H.A. (1967). "Plutonium-contaminated wound studies in swine," pages 101 to 103 in *Battelle Pacific Northwest Laboratory Annual Report*, BNWL-480 (Vol. 1) (Pacific Northwest Laboratory, Richland, Washington).

MCCLANAHAN, B.J., WOOD, D.H., HORSTMAN, V.G., RAGAN, H.A. and BUSTAD, L.K. (1964). "Effects of plutonium in swine skin and its removal," pages 120 to 122 in *Hanford Biology Research Annual Report*, Kornberg, H.A. and Sweza, E.G., Eds., HW-80500 (Pacific Northwest Laboratory, Richland, Washington).

MCDIARMID, M.A., HOOPER, F.J., SQUIBB, K. and MCPHAUL, K. (1999). "The utility of spot collection for urinary uranium determinations in depleted uranium exposed Gulf War veterans," Health Phys. **77**(3), 261–264.

MCDIARMID, M.A., KEOGH, J.P., HOOPER, F.J., MCPHAUL, K., SQUIBB, K., KANE, R., DIPINO, R., KABAT, M., KAUP, B., ANDERSON, L., HOOVER, D., BROWN, L., HAMILTON, M., JACOBSON-KRAM, D., BURROWS, B. and WALSH, M. (2000). "Health effects of depleted uranium on exposed Gulf War veterans," Environ. Res. **82**(2), 168–180.

MCDIARMID, M.A., ENGELHARDT, S.M. and OLIVER, M. (2001). "Urinary uranium concentrations in an enlarged Gulf War veteran cohort," Health Phys. **80**(3), 270–273.

MCDIARMID, M.A., SQUIBB, K. and ENGELHARDT, S.M. (2004). "Biologic monitoring for urinary uranium in Gulf War I veterans," Health Phys. **87**(1), 51–56.

MCINROY, J.L., GONZALES, E.R. and MIGLIO, J.J. (1992). "Measurement of thorium isotopes and ^{228}Ra in soft tissues and bones of a deceased Thorotrast patient," Health Phys. **63**(1), 54–71.

MENETRIER, F., GRAPPIN, L., RAYNAUD, P., COURTAY, C., WOOD, R. JOUSSINEAU, S., LIST, V., STRADLING, G.N., TAYLOR, D.M., BERARD, P., MORCILLO, M.A. and RENCOVA, J. (2005). "Treatment of accidental intakes of plutonium and americium: Guidance notes" Appl. Radiat. Isot. **62**(6), 829–846.

MERRIAM, G.R., JR. and WORGUL, B.V. (1983). "Experimental radiation cataract—its clinical relevance," Bull. NY Acad. Med. **59**(4), 372–392.

METTLER, F.A. (1990). "Assessment and management of local radiation injuries," pages 127 to 150 in *Medical Management of Radiation Accidents*, Mettler, F.A. Jr., Kelsey, C.A. and Ricks, R.C., Eds. (CRC Press, Boca Raton, Florida).

METTLER, F.A. and UPTON, A.C. (1995). "Direct effects of radiation," pages 256 to 260 in *Medical Effects of Ionizing Radiation,* 2nd ed. (W.B. Saunders, Philadelphia).

MILLER, B.F. and KEANE, C.B., Eds. (1987). *Encyclopedia and Dictionary of Medicine, Nursing, and Allied Health*, 4th ed. (W.B. Saunders, Philadelphia).

MOIZHESS, T.G. and VASILEV, J.M. (1989). "Early and late stages of foreign-body carcinogenesis can be induced by implants of different shapes," Int. J. Cancer **44**(3), 449–453.

MORGAN, R.W. and ELCOCK, M. (1995). "Artificial implants and soft tissue sarcomas," J. Clin. Epidemiol. **48**(4), 545–549.

MORI, T., MACHINAMI, R., HATAKEYAMA, S., FUKUTOMI, K., KATO, Y., AKASHI, M., FUKUMOTO, M. and AOKI, I. (2005). "The 2002 results of the first series of follow-up studies on Japanese Thorotrast patients and their relationships to autopsy series," pages 31 to 46 in *Proceedings of the 9th International Conference on Health Effects of Incorporated Radionuclides: Emphasis on Radium, Thorium, Uranium and Their Daughter Products*, Oeh, U., Roth, P. and Paretzke, H.G., Eds., http://www.gsf.de/heir/ProceedingsHEIR2004_ebook.pdf (accessed July 24, 2007) (Institut fur Strahlenschutz, GSF, Neuherberg).

MORIN, M., NENOT, J.C. and LAFUMA, J. (1972). "Metabolic and therapeutic study following administration to rats of ^{238}Pu nitrate—a comparison with ^{239}Pu," Health Phys. **23**(4), 475–480.

MORIN, M., NENOT, J.C. and LAFUMA, J. (1973a). "The behavior of ^{237}Np in the rat," Health Phys. **24**(3), 311–315.

MORIN, M., SKUPINSKI, W., NENOT, J.C. and LAFUMA, J. (1973b). "Experimental research on the treatment of contaminations by actinide solutions," pages 317 to 320 in *Health Physics Problems of Internal Contamination, Proceedings of the IRPA Second European Congress on Radiation Protection*, Bujdoso, E. Ed. (Akademiai Kiado, Budapest, Hungary).

MORROW, P.E. (1988). "Possible mechanisms to explain dust overloading of the lungs," Fundam. Appl. Toxicol. **10**(3), 369–384.

MORROW, P.E., GIBB, F.R and JOHNSON, L. (1964). "Clearance of insoluble dust from the lower respiratory tract," Health Phys. **10**, 543–555.

MORROW, P.E., GIBB, F.R., DAVIES, H. and FISHER, M. (1968). "Dust removal from the lung parenchyma: An investigation of clearance stimulants," Toxicol. Appl. Pharmacol. **12**(3), 372–396.

MOSKALEV, Y.I. (1961a). "Distribution of lanthanum-140 in the animal organism," pages 45 to 59 in *Distribution, Biological Effects and Migration of Radioactive Isotopes*, Ledbedinskii, A.V. and Moskalev, Y.I., Eds. (Medgiz, Moscow).

MOSKALEV, Y.I. (1961b). "Distribution of cesium-137 in the animal organism," pages 4 to 19 in *Distribution, Biological Effects and Migration of Radioactive Isotopes*, Ledbedinskii, A.V. and Moskalev, Y.I., Eds. (Medgiz, Moscow).

MOSKALEV, Y.I. (1961c). "Distribution of barium-140 in the animal organism," pages 29 to 83 in *Distribution, Biological Effects and Migration of Radioactive Isotopes*, Ledbedinskii, A.V. and Moskalev, Y.I. Eds. (Medgiz, Moscow).

MOSKALEV, Y.I. (1961d). "Influence of an isotope carrier on distribution of cerium-144," pages 185 to 191 in *Distribution, Biological Effects and Migration of Radioactive Isotopes*, Ledbedinskii, A.V. and Moskalev, Yu.I , Eds. (Medgiz, Moscow).

MUELLER, H.L., ROBINSON, B., MUGGENBURG, B.A., GILLETT, N.A. and GUILMETTE, R.A. (1990). "Particle distribution in lung and lymph node tissues of rats and dogs and the migration of particle-containing alveolar cells *in vitro*," J. Toxicol. Environ. Health **30**(3), 141–165.

MUSIKAS, C. (1976). "Contribution to the study of U(V) ions and pentavalent transuranics in aqueous solution," J. Inorg. Nucl. Chem. (Suppl. 1976) 171–177.

NBS (1953). National Bureau of Standards. *Maximum Permissible Amounts of Radioisotopes in the Human Body and Maximum Permissible Concentrations in Air and Water*, NBS Handbook 52 (U.S. Department of Commerce, Washington).

NCRP (1980). National Council on Radiation Protection and Measurements. *Management of Persons Accidentally Contaminated with Radionuclides*, NCRP Report No. 65 (National Council on Radiation Protection and Measurements, Bethesda, Maryland).

NCRP (1985). National Council on Radiation Protection and Measurements. *A Handbook of Radioactivity Measurements Procedures*, 2nd ed., NCRP Report No. 58 (National Council on Radiation Protection and Measurements, Bethesda, Maryland).

NCRP (1989). National Council on Radiation Protection and Measurements. *Limit for Exposure to "Hot Particles" on the Skin*, NCRP Report No.106 (National Council on Radiation Protection and Measurements, Bethesda, Maryland).

NCRP (1991). National Council on Radiation Protection and Measurements. *Developing Radiation Emergency Plans for Academic, Medical or Industrial Facilities*, NCRP Report No. 111 (National Council on Radiation Protection and Measurements, Bethesda, Maryland).

NCRP (1993). National Council on Radiation Protection and Measurements. *Limitation of Exposure to Ionizing Radiation*, NCRP Report No. 116 (National Council on Radiation Protection and Measurements, Bethesda, Maryland).

NCRP (1997). National Council on Radiation Protection and Measurements. *Deposition, Retention and Dosimetry of Inhaled Radioactive Substances*, NCRP Report No. 125 (National Council on Radiation Protection and Measurements, Bethesda, Maryland).

NCRP (1999). National Council on Radiation Protection and Measurements. *Biological Effects and Exposure Limits for "Hot Particles,"* NCRP Report No. 130 (National Council on Radiation Protection and Measurements, Bethesda, Maryland).

NCRP (2001a). National Council on Radiation Protection and Measurements. *Scientific Basis for Evaluating the Risks to Populations from Space Applications of Plutonium*, NCRP Report No. 131 (National Council on Radiation Protection and Measurements, Bethesda, Maryland).

NCRP (2001b). National Council on Radiation Protection and Measurements. *Management of Terrorist Events Involving Radioactive Material*, NCRP Report No. 138 (National Council on Radiation Protection and Measurements, Bethesda, Maryland).

NENOT, J.C. and STATHER, J.W. (1979). *The Toxicity of Plutonium, Americium, and Curium* (Pergamon Press, New York).

NENOT, J.C., MASSE, R., MORIN, M. and LAFUMA, J. (1972a). "An experimental comparative study of the behavior of ^{237}Np, ^{238}Pu, ^{239}Pu, ^{241}Am and ^{242}Cm in bone," Health Phys. **22**(6), 657–665.

NENOT, J.C., MORIN, M., SKUPINSKI, W. and LAFUMA, J. (1972b). "Experimental removal of ^{144}Ce, ^{241}Am, ^{242}Cm and ^{238}Pu from the rat skeleton," Health Phys. **23**(5), 635–640.

NEUMAN, W.F. and NEUMAN, M.W. (1958). *The Chemical Dynamics of Bone Mineral* (University of Chicago Press, Chicago).

NEWMAN, S.L., HENSON, J.E. and HENSON, P.M. (1982). "Phagocytosis of senescent neutrophils by human monocyte-derived macrophages and rabbit inflammatory macrophages," J. Exp. Med. **156**, 430–442.

NORWOOD, W.D. and FUQUA, P.A. (1969). "Medical care for accidental deposition of plutonium (^{239}Pu) within the body," pages 147 to 161 in *Handling of Radiation Accidents*, STI/PUB/229 (International Atomic Energy Agency, Vienna).

NOTHDURFT, H. (1955) "Uber die sarcomaulosung durch fremdkorper-implantationen bei ratten in abhangigkreit von der form der implantate," Naturwissenschaften, **42**, 106.

OAKLEY, W.D. and THOMPSON, R.C. (1956). "Further studies on percutaneous absorption and decontamination of plutonium in rats," pages 106 to 111 in *Hanford Biology Research Annual Report 1955*, HW-41500 (National Technical Information Services, Springfield, Virginia).

OBERDORSTER, G. (1993). "Lung dosimetry: Pulmonary clearance of inhaled particles," Aerosol Sci. Technol. **18**(3), 279–289.

OHLENSCHLAGER, L. (1970). "Chirurgische versogung der mit alpha-aktivitot kontaminierten verletzung," pages 563 to 583 in *Radiation Problems Relating to Transuranium Elements* (Gesellschaft fur Kernforschung, Karlsruhe, Germany).

OLMAN, M.A., MACKMAN, N., GLADSON, C.L., MOSER, K.M. and LOSKUTOFF, D.J. (1995). "Changes in procoagulant and fibrinolytic gene expression during bleomycin-induced lung injury in the mouse," J. Clin. Invest. **96**(3), 1621–1630.

OPPENHEIMER, B.S., OPPENHEIMER, E.T. and STOUT, A.P. (1948). "Sarcomas induced in rats by implanting cellophane," Proc. Soc. Exp. Biol. Med. **67**, 33–34.

ORCUTT, J.A. (1949). "The toxicology of compounds of uranium following applications to the skin," pages 377 to 414 in *Pharmacology and Toxicology of Uranium Compounds, with a Section on the Pharmacology and Toxicology of Fluorine and Hydrogen Fluoride*, Voegtlin, C. and Hodge, H.C., Eds. (McGraw-Hill, New York).

ORISE (2007). Oak Ridge Institute for Science and Education. *Radiation Emergency Assistance Center/Training Site (REAC/TS)*, http://orise.orau.gov/reacts (accessed July 24, 2007) (Oak Ridge Associated Universities, Oak Ridge, Tennessee).

OSAGWI (2000). Office of the Special Assistant for Gulf War Illness, *Environmental Exposure Report: Depleted Uranium in the Gulf (II)*, http://www.gulflink.osd.mil/du_ii (accessed July 24, 2007) (U.S. Department of Defense, Washington).

PAINTER, E., RUSSELL, E., PROSSER, C.L., SWIFT, M.N., KISIELESKI, W. and SACHER, G. (1946). *Clinical Physiology of Dogs Injected with Plutonium*, AECD-2042 (National Technical Information Services, Springfield, Virginia).

PALMER, H.E., RIEKSTS, G. and ICAYAN, E.E. (1983). "1976 Hanford americium exposure incident: *In vivo* measurements," Health Phys. **45**(4), 893–910.

PAQUET, F., CHAZEL, V., HOUPERT, P., GUILMETTE, R. and MUGGENBURG, B. (2003). "Efficacy of 3,4,3-Li (1,2-HOPO) for decorporation of Pu, Am and U from rats injected intramuscularly with high-fired particles of MOX," Radiat. Prot. Dosim. **105**(1–4), 521–525.

PASSOW, H., ROTHSTEIN, A. and CLARKSON, T.W. (1961). "The general pharmacology of the heavy metals," Pharmacol. Rev. **13**, 185–224.

PECORARO, V.L., HARRIS, W.R., CARRANO, C.J. and RAYMOND, K.N. (1981). "Siderophilin metal coordination. difference ultraviolet spectroscopy of di-, tri-, and tetravalent metal ions with ethylenebis [(o-hydroxyphenyl)glycine]," Biochemistry **20**(24), 7033–7039.

PELLMAR, T.C., FUCIARELLI, A.F., EJNIK, J.W., HAMILTON, M., HOGAN, J., STROCKO, S., EMOND, C., MOTTAZ, H.M. and LANDAUER, M.R. (1999). "Distribution of uranium in rats implanted with depleted uranium pellets," Toxicol. Sci. **49**(1), 29–39.

PERKINS, R.W. and THOMAS, C.W. (1980). "Worldwide fallout," pages 53 to 82 in *Transuranic Elements in the Environment*, Hanson, W.C., Ed., DOE/TIC-22800 (National Technical Information Service, Springfield, Virginia).

PETER, R.U., CARSIN, H., COSSET, J.M., CLOUGH, K., GOURMELON, P. and NENOT, J.C. (2001). "Accident involving abandoned radioactive sources in Georgia, 1997," pages 259 to 268 in *Medical Management of Radiation Accidents*, 2nd ed., Gusev, I.A., Guskova, A.K. and Mettler, F.A., Jr., Eds. (CRC Press, Boca Raton, Florida).

PETROV. R.V., PRAVETSKII, V.N., STEPANOV, YU. S. and SHAL'NOV, M.I. (1963). *Radioactive Fallout*, AEC-TR-6634 (U.S Government Printing Office, Washington).1966).

PIECHOWSKI, J. (1995). "Evaluation of systemic exposure resulting from wounds contaminated by radioactive products," Indian Bull. Rad. Prot. **18**(1–2), 8–14.

PIECHOWSKI, J. and CHAPTINEL, Y. (2004). "Evaluation de la dose locale pour une blessure contaminee," Radioprotection **39**(3), 355–366.

PIECHOWSKI, J., MENOUX, B. and CHAPTINEL, Y. (1992). *Evaluation de l'Exposition Systemique Resultant d'une Blessure Contaminee par des Produits Radioactifs*, Report CEA-R-5583 (Commissariat a l'Energie Atomique, Gif-sur-Yvette, France).

PIERSON, R.N., JR., PRICE, D.C., WANG, J. and JAIN, R.K. (1978). "Extracellular water measurements: Organ tracer kinetics of bromide and sucrose in rats and man," Am. J. Physiol. Renal Physiol. **235**(3), F254-F264.

PILCHER, B.K., DUMIN, J.A., SUDBECK, B.D., KRANE, S.M., WELGUS, H.G. and PARKS, W.C. (1997). "The activity of collagenase-1 is required for keratinocyte migration on a type I collagen matrix," J. Cell Biol. **137**(6), 1445–1457.

PLENT, S., SHAH, S. and WESTMORE, G.A. (1990). "Thorotrast granuloma—a renascence," J. Laryngol. Otol. **104**(4), 355–357.

POLACARZ, S.V., LAING, R.W. and LOOMES, R. (1992). "Thorotrastgranuloma: An unexpected diagnosis," J. Clin. Path. **45**(3), 259–261.

POPPLEWELL, D.S. and BOOCOCK, G. (1967). "Distribution of some actinides in blood serum proteins," pages 45 to 55 in *Proceedings of the Symposium on Diagnosis and Treatment of Deposited Radionuclides*, Kornberg, H.A. and Norwood, W.D., Eds. (Excerpta Medica Foundation, Amsterdam).

POPPLEWELL, D.S., STRADLING, G.N. and HAM, G.J. (1975). "The chemical form of plutonium in urine," Radiat. Res. **62**(3), 513–519.

POSTLETHWAITE, A.E., KESKI-OJA, J., BALIAN, G. and KANG, A.H. (1981). "Induction of fibroblast chemotaxis by fibronectin. Localization of the chemotactic region to a 140,000-molecular weight non-gelatin-binding fragment," J. Exp. Med. **153**(2), 494–499.

RAI, D., RAO, L., WEGER, H.T., FELMY, A.R. and CHOPPIN, G.R. (1998a). *Thermodynamic Data for Predicting Concentrations of Pu(III), Am(III), and Cm(III) in Geologic Environments*, PNWD-2427 (Pacific Northwest National Laboratory, Richland, Washington).

RAI, D., RAO, L., WEGER, H.T., FELMY, A.R. and CHOPPIN, G.R. (1998b). *Thermodynamic Data for Predicting Concentrations of Th(IV), Np(IV), and Pu(IV) in Geological Environments*, PNWD-2428 (Pacific Northwest National Laboratory, Richland, Washington).

REED, M.J., VERNON, R.B., ABRASS, I.B. and SAGE, E.H. (1994). "TGF-beta 1 induces the expression of type I collagen and SPARC, and enhances contraction of collagen gels by fibroblasts from young and aged donors," J. Cell Physiol. **158**(1), 169–179.

RICE, R.H. and COHEN, D.E. (1996). "Toxic responses of the skin," pages 529 to 546 in *Casarett and Doull's Toxicology: The Basic Science of Poisons*, 5th ed., Klaasen, C.D., Ed. (McGraw-Hill, New York).

RICHES, D.W.H. (1996). "Macrophage involvement in wound repair, remodeling, and fibrosis," pages 95 to142 in *The Molecular and Cellular Biology of Wound Repair*, Clark, R.A.F., Ed. (Plenum Press, New York).

RICKS, R.C., BERGER, M.E., HOLLOWAY, E.C. and GOANS, R.E. (2001). "Radiation accidents in the United States," pages 167 to 172 in *Medical Management of Radiation Accidents*, 2nd ed., Gusev, I.A., Guskova, A.K. and Mettler, F.A., Jr., Eds. (CRC Press, Boca Raton, Florida).

RIEDEL, W., DALHEIMER, A., SAID, M., WALTER, U. and KAUL, A. (1983). "Recent results of the German Thorotrast study—dose-relevant physical and biological properties of Thorotrast-equivalent colloids," Health Phys. **44** (Suppl. 1), 293–298.

ROBERTS, A.B. and SPORN, M.B. (1996). "Transforming growth factor-β," pages 275 to 310 in *The Molecular and Cellular Biology of Wound Repair*, Clark, R.A.F., Ed. (Plenum Press, New York).

ROGACHEVA, S.A. (1961). "Cerium-144 absorption through the rat skin and effect of $CaNa_2$-EDTA on absorption," pages 108 to 112 in *Distribution, Biological Effects and Migration of Radioactive Isotopes*, Lebedinskii, A.V. and Moskalev, Yu.I., Eds. (Medgiz, Moscow).

ROTHSTEIN, A. and CLARKSON, T.W. (1959). *The Cell Membrane as the Site of Action of Heavy Metals. Discussion: The Interaction of Metals with Epithelia*, University of Rochester Atomic Energy Project Report UR-549 (National Technical Information Service, Springfield, Virginia).

RUSSELL, J.J., KATHREN, R.L., SHORT, R.A. and MCINROY, J.F. (1995). "Long-term organ retention and pathology in a Thorotrast patient: A preliminary report," pages 215 to 223 in *Health Effects of Internally Deposited Radionuclides: Emphasis on Radium and Thorium*, van Kaick, G., Karaoglou, A. and Kellerer, A.M., Eds. (World Scientific, Singapore).

SAHNI, A., ODRLJIN, T. and FRANCIS, C.W. (1998). "Binding of basic fibroblast growth factor to fibrinogen and fibrin," J. Biol. Chem. **273**(13), 7554–7559.

SANDERS, C.L. (1967). "Phagocytosis and translocation of ^{239}PuO$_2$ particles by peritoneal phagocytes of the rat," pages 81 to 90 in *Proceedings of the Symposium on Diagnosis and Treatment of Deposited Radionuclides*, Kornberg, H.A. and Norwood, W.D., Eds. (Excerpta Medica Foundation, New York).

SBARRA, A.J., SELVARAJ, R.J., PAUL, B.B., POSKITT, P.K., ZGLICZYN-SKI, J.M., MITCHELL, G.W., JR. and LOUIS, F. (1976). "Biochemical, functional, and structural aspects of phagocytosis," Int. Rev. Exp. Pathol. **16**, 249–271.

SCHALLBERGER, J.A. (1974). *Plutonium—Lymph Relationship*, Colorado State University Report COO-1787-24 (National Technical Information Service, Springfield, Virginia).

SCHALLBERGER, J.A., DEWHIRST, M.W. and LEBEL, J.L. (1976). "Lymph transport of soluble and insoluble plutonium," pages 19 to 27 in *Proceedings of the Hanford Biology Symposium on Radiation and the Lymphatic System*, Ballou, J.E., Ed., Energy Research and Development Administration Report CONF-740930 (Battelle Pacific Northwest Laboratory, Richland, Washington).

SCHIRMER, W. and WAECHTER, N. (1968). "Table of specific activities of the nuclides (Z=88 to Z=104)," Actinides Rev. **1**, 125–134.

SCHOFIELD, G.B. (1964). "Absorption and measurement of radionuclides in wounds and abrasions," Clin. Radiol. **15**, 50–54.

SCHOFIELD, G.B., HOWELLS, H., WARD, F., LYNN, J.C. and DOLPHIN, G.W. (1974). "Assessment and management of a plutonium contaminated wound case," Health Phys. **26**(6), 541–554.

SCHUBERT, J. and CONN, E.E. (1949). "Radiocolloidal behavior of some fission products," Nucleonics **4**, 2–11.

SCHWARTZ, M.A., SCHALLER, M.D. and GINSBERG, M.H. (1995). "Integrins: Emerging paradigms of signal transduction," Ann. Rev. Cell. Dev. Biol. **11**, 549–599.

SCHWIETZER, G.K. (1956). "The radiocolloidal properties of the rare earth elements," pages 31 to 34 in *Rare Earths in Biochemical and Medical Research: A Conference Sponsored by the Medical Division, Oak Ridge Institute of Nuclear Studies*, Kyker, G.C. and Anderson, E.B., Eds., Oak Ridge Institute of Nuclear Studies Report ORINS-12 (National Technical Information Service, Springfield, Virginia).

SCOTT, K.G. and HAMILTON, J.G. (1950). "The metabolism of silver in the rat with radiosilver used as an indicator," Univ. Calif. Pub. Pharmacol. **2**, 241–262.

SCOTT, K.G., OVERSTREET, R., JACOBSON, L., HAMILTON, J.G., FISHER, H., CROWLEY, J., CHAIKOFF, I.L., ENTENMAN, C., FISHLER, M., BARBER, A.J. and LOOMIS, F. (1947). *The Metabolism of Carrier-Free Fission Products in the Rat*, Manhattan District Declassified Document, MDDC-1275 (National Technical Information Service, Springfield, Virginia).

SCOTT, K.G., AXELROD, D.J., FISHER, H., CROWLEY, J.F. and HAMILTON, J.G (1948a). "The metabolism of plutonium in rats following intramuscular injection," J. Biol. Chem. **176**(1), 283–293.

SCOTT, K.G., COPP, D.H., AXELROD, D.J. and HAMILTON, J.G. (1948b). "The metabolism of americium in the rat," J. Biol. Chem. **175**(2), 691–703.

SCOTT, K.G., AXELROD, D.S. and HAMILTON, J.G. (1949). "The metabolism of curium in the rat," J. Biol. Chem. **177**(1), 325–335.

SCOTT, K.G., HAMILTON, J.G. and WALLACE, P.C. (1951). *The Deposition of Carrier-Free Radio-Vanadium in the Rat Following Intravenous Administration*, University of California Radiation Laboratory, UCRL-1318 (University of California, Berkeley, California).

SHANNON, R.D. (1976). "Revised effective ionic radii and systematic studies of interatomic distances in halides and chalcogenides," Acta Cryst. **A32**, 751–767.

SHAW, R.J., DOHERTY, D.E., RITTER, A.G., BENEDICT, S.H. and CLARK, R.A.F. (1990). "Adherence-dependent increase in human monocyte PDGF(B) mRNA is associated with increases in c-*fos*, c-*jun*, and EGF2 mRNA," J. Cell Biol. **111**(5), 2139–2148.

SHERMAN, I.S., STRAUSS, M.G. and PEHL, R.H. (1984). "A Si(Li)-NaI(Tl) detector for direct measurement of plutonium *in vivo*," Health Phys. **47**(5), 711–721.

SHULTIS, J.K. and FAW, R.E. (1996). *Radiation Shielding* (Prentice Hall, Upper Saddle River, New Jersey).

SILLEN, L.G. and MARTELL, A.E. (1964). "Stability constants of metal-ion complexes," pages 50 to 51 in *Chemical Society of London*, Special Publication No. 17 (Burlington House, London).

SILLEN, L.G. and MARTELL, A.E. (1971). "Stability constants of metal-ion complexes," pages 21 to 22 in *Chemical Society of London*, Special Publication No. 25 (Burlington House. London).

SIMPSON, M.E., ASLING, C.W. and EVANS, H.M. (1950). "Some endocrine influences on skeletal growth and differentiation," Yale J. Biol. Med. **23**(1), 1–27.

SINGER, A.J. and CLARK, R.A.F. (1999). "Cutaneous wound healing," N. Engl. J. Med. **341**(10), 738–746.

SINGER, I.I., KAWKA, D.W., KAZAZIS, D.M. and CLARK, R.A.F. (1984). "*In vivo* co-distribution of fibronectin and actin fibers in granulation tissue: Immunofluorescence and electron microscope studies of the fibronexus at the myofibroblast surface," J. Cell Biol. **98**(6), 2091–2106.

SINIAKOV, E.G., NIFATOV, A.P., BAZHIN, A.G. and LIUBCHANSKII, E.R. (1988). "Biological effects of the intramuscular administration of [239]Pu as affected by chelate therapy," Med. Radiol. (Mosk.) **33**(3), 60–63 [in Russian].

SMITH, V.H. (1974). "Distribution and retention of inhaled DTPA," page 108 in *Pacific Northwest Laboratory Annual Report for 1973 to the USAEC Division of Biomedical and Environmental Research*, BNWL-1850, Part 1 (National Technical Information Service, Springfield, Virginia).

SMITH, J.R.H. (2003). "Implications of human nasal clearance studies for the interpretation of nose blow and bioassay sample measurements," Rad. Prot. Dosim. **105**(1–4), 119–122.

SMITH, R.M. and MARTELL, A.E. (1977). *Critical Stability Constants, Volume 3. Other Organic Ligands* (Plenum Press, New York).

SMITH, R.M. and MARTELL, A.E. (1989). *Critical Stability Constants, Volume 6. Second Supplement* (Plenum Press, New York).

SMITH, H., STRADLING, G.N., LOVELESS, B.W. and HAM, G.J. (1977). "The *in vivo* solubility of plutonium-239 dioxide in the rat lung," Health Phys. **33**(6), 539–551.

SNIPES, M.B. (1989). "Long-term retention and clearance of particles inhaled by mammalian species," Crit. Rev. Toxicol. **20**(3), 175–211.

SNIPES, M.B. and CLEM, M.F. (1981). "Retention of microspheres in the rat lung after intratracheal instillation," Environ. Res. **24**(1), 33–41.

SQUIBB, K.S., LEGGETT, R.W. and MCDIARMID, M.A. (2005). "Prediction of renal concentrations of depleted uranium and radiation dose in Gulf War veterans with embedded shrapnel," Health Phys. **89**(3), 267–273.

STABIN, M.G. (1996). "MIRDOSE: Personal computer software for internal dose assessment in nuclear medicine," J. Nucl. Med. **37**(3), 538–546.

STAINO-COICO, L., KRUEGER, J.G., RUBIN, J.S., D'LIMI, S., VALLAT, V.P., VALENTINO, L., FAHEY, T.I. 3rd, HAWES, A., KINGSTON, G., MADDEN, M.R., MATHWICH, M., GOTTLIEB, A.B. and AARONSON, S.A. (1993). "Human keratinocyte growth factor effects in a porcine model of epidermal wound healing," J. Exp. Med. **178**(3), 865–878.

STANLEY, J.A., EIDSON, A.F. and MEWHINNEY, J.A. (1982). "Distribution, retention and dosimetry of plutonium and americium in the rat, dog, and monkey after inhalation of an industrial mixed uranium and plutonium aerosol," Health Phys. **43**(4), 521–530.

STATHER, J.W., SMITH, H., JAMES, A.C. and RODWELL, P. (1976). "The experimental use of aerosol and liposomal forms of CaDTPA as a treatment for plutonium contamination," pages 387 to 400 in *Diagnosis and Treatment of Incorporated Radionuclides*, IAEA Proceedings STI/PUB/411 (International Atomic Energy Agency, Vienna).

STEVENS, W. and BRUENGER, F.W. (1972). "Interaction of ^{249}Cf and ^{252}Cf with constituents of dog and human blood," Health Phys. **22**(6), 679–683.

STEVENS, W., BRUENGER, F.W. and STOVER, B.J. (1968). "*In vivo* studies on the interactions of PuIV with blood constituents," Radiat. Res. **33**(3), 490–500.

STOUGAARD, M., PRAESTHOLM, J. and STOIER, M. (1984). "Late effects of perivascular injection of Thorotrast in the neck," J. Laryngol. Otol. **98**(10), 1003–1007.

STOVER, B.J. (1983). "Effects of Thorotrast in humans," Health Phys. **44** (Suppl. 1), 253–257.

STOVER, B.J., ATHERTON, D.R. and KELLER, N. (1959). "Metabolism of Pu^{239} in adult beagle dogs," Radiat. Res. **10**(2), 130–147.

STOVER, B.J., ATHERTON, D.R., BRUENGER, F.W. and BUSTER, D.S. (1962). "Further studies of the metabolism of ^{239}Pu in adult beagles," Health Phys. **8**(6), 589–597.

STOVER, B.J., BRUENGER, F.W. and STEVENS, W. (1968). "The reaction of PuIV with the iron transport system in human blood serum," Radiat. Res. **33**(2), 381–394.

STRADLING, G.N. and TAYLOR, D.M. (2005) "Decorporation of radionuclides," pages 9.1 to 9.34 in *Radiological Protection (Landhold-Bornstein Numerical Data and Functional Relationships in Science and Technology Group VIII, Vol. 4)*, Kaul, A. and Becker, D., Eds. (Springer, Berlin).

STRADLING, G.N., POPPLEWELL, D.S. and HAM, G.J. (1976). "The chemical form of americium and curium in urine," Health Phys. **31**(6), 517–519.

STRADLING, G.N., HAM, G.J., SMITH, H. and BREADMORE, S.E. (1978). "The mobility of americium dioxide in the rat," Radiat. Res. **76**(3), 549–560.

STRADLING, G.N., GRAY, S.A., MOODY, J.C., PEARCE, M.J., WILSON, I., BURGADA, R., BAILLY, T., LEROUX, Y., RAYMOND, K.N. and DURBIN, P.W. (1993). "Comparative efficacies of 3,4,3,-LIHOPO and DTPA for enhancing the excretion of plutonium and americium from the rat after simulated wound contamination as nitrates," Int. J. Radiat. Biol. **64**(1), 133–140.

STRADLING, G.N., GRAY, S.A., PEARCE, M.J., WILSON, I., MOODY, J.C., BURGADA, R., DURBIN, P.W. and RAYMOND, K.N. (1995a). "Decorporation of ^{228}Th from the rat by 3,4,3-LIHOPO and DTPA after simulated wound contamination," Hum. Exp. Toxicol. **14**(2), 165–169.

STRADLING, G.N., GRAY, S.A., PEARCE, M.J., WILSON, I., MOODY, J.C., HODGSON, A. and RAYMOND, K.N. (1995b). *Efficacy of TREN-(Me-3,2-HOPO), 5-LI(Me-3,2,-HOPO) and DTPA for Removing Plutonium and Americium from the Rat after Inhalation and Wound Contamination as Nitrates*, NRPB-M534 (Health Protection Agency, London).

SUGIYAMA, H., KATO, Y., ISHIHARA, T., HIRASHIMA, K. and KUMATORI, T. (1985). "Late effects of Thorotrast administration: Clinical and pathophysiological studies," Strahlentherapie **80**, 136–139.

SURI, C., JONES, P.F., PATAN, S., BARTUNKOVA, S., MAISONPIERRE, P.C., DAVIS, S., SATO, T.N. and YANCOPOULOS, G.D. (1996). "Requisite role of angiopoietin-1, a ligand for the TIE2 receptor, during embryonic angiogenesis," Cell **87**(7), 1171–1180.

SWARM, R.L. (1967). "Experience with colloidal thorium dioxide," Ann. NY Acad. Sci. **145**(3), 525–526.

TAUBER, W.B. (1992). "Clinical consequences of Thorotrast in a long-term survivor," Health Phys. **63**(1), 13–19.

TAYLOR, D.M. (1967). "The effects of desferrioxamine on the retention of actinide elements in the rat," Health Phys. **13**(2), 135–140.

TAYLOR, D.M. (1969). "The metabolism of plutonium in adult rabbits," Br. J. Radiol. **42**(493), 44–50.

TAYLOR, D.M. (1973a). "Chemical and physical properties of plutonium," pages 323 to 348 in *Uranium, Plutonium, Transplutonic Elements*, Hodge, H.C., Stannard, J.N. and Hursh, J.B., Eds. (Springer-Verlag, New York).

TAYLOR, D.M. (1973b). "Chemical and physical properties of the transplutonium elements," pages 717 to 738 in *Uranium, Plutonium, Transplutonic Elements*, Hodge, H.C., Stannard, J.N. and Hursh, J.B., Eds. (Springer-Verlag, New York).

TAYLOR, D.M. (1998). "The bioinorganic chemistry of actinides in blood," J. Alloys Compounds 271–273, 6–10.

TAYLOR, D.M. and SOWBY, F.D. (1962). "The removal of americium and plutonium from the rat by chelating agents," Phys. Med. Biol. **7**, 83–91.

TAYLOR, D.M., SOWBY, F.D. and KEMBER, N.F. (1961). "The metabolism of americium and plutonium in the rat," Phys Med. Biol. **6**, 73–86.

TESSMER, C.F. and CHANG, J.P. (1967). "Thorotrast localization by light and electron microscopy," Ann. NY Acad. Sci. **145**(3), 545–575.

THOMAS, R.G., MCCLELLAN, R.O., THOMAS, R.L., CHIFFELLE, T.L., HOBBS, C.H., JONES, R.K., MAUDERLY, J.L. and PICKRELL, J.A. (1972). "Metabolism, dosimetry and biological effects of inhaled [241]Am in beagle dogs," Health Phys. **22**(6), 863–871.

THOMPSON, R.C., Ed. (1983). "1976 Hanford americium exposure incident: Overview and perspective," Health Phys. **45**(4), 837–947.

TONRY, L.L. (1993). *Solubility of Depleted Uranium Fragments Within Simulated Lung Fluid*, Master's thesis (University of Massachusetts, Lowell, Massachusetts).

TOOHEY, R.E. (2002). "Role of the health physicist in dose assessment," pages 33 to 43 in *Proceedings of the Fourth International REAC/TS Conference on The Medical Basis for Radiation-Accident Preparedness: The Clinical Care of Victims*, Ricks, R.C., Berger, M.E. and O'Hara, F.M., Jr., Eds. (Parthenon Publishing, New York).

TOOHEY, R.E. (2003a). "Excretion of depleted uranium by Gulf War veterans," Radiat. Prot. Dosim. **105**(1–4), 171–174.

TOOHEY, R.E. (2003b). "Internal dose assessment in radiation accidents," Radiat. Prot. Dosim. **105**(1–4), 329–331.

TOOLE, B.P. (1991). "Proteoglycans and hyaluronan in morphogenesis and differentiation," pages 305 to 341 in *Cell Biology of the Extracellular Matrix*, 2nd ed., Hay, E.D., Ed. (Plenum Press, New York).

TRAUB, R.J., REECE, W.D., SCHERPELZ, R.I. and SIGALLA, L.A. (1987). *Dose Calculations for Contamination of the Skin Using the Computer Code VARSKIN*, NUREG/CR-4418 (National Technical Information Service, Springfield, Virginia).

TURNER, F.C. (1941). "Sarcomas at sites of subcutaneously implanted Bakelite disks in rats," J. Natl. Cancer Inst. **2**, 81–91.

TURNER, G.A. and TAYLOR, D.M. (1968). "The transport of plutonium, americium, and curium in the blood of rats," Phys. Med. Biol. **13**, 535–546.

VAN MIDDLESWORTH, L. (1947). *Study of Plutonium Metabolism in Bone*, Ph.D. Thesis (University of California, Berkeley, California).

VAUGHAN, J. (1973). "Distribution, excretion and effects of plutonium as a bone-seeker," pages 349 to 502 in *Uranium, Plutonium, Transplutonic Elements*, Hodge, H.C., Stannard, J.N. and Hursh, J.B., Eds. (Springer-Verlag, New York).

VEIKKOLA, T. and ALITALO, K. (1999). "VEGFs, receptors and angiogenesis," Semin. Cancer Biol. **9**(3), 211–220.

VIEGAS, S.F. and CALHOUN, J.H. (1986). "Lead poisoning from a gunshot wound to the hand," J. Hand Surg. **11**(5), 729–732.

VOLF, V. (1974a). "Combined effect of DTPA and citrate on an intramuscular ^{239}Pu deposit in rats," Health Phys. **27**(1), 152–153.

VOLF, V. (1974b). "Experimental background for prompt treatment with DTPA of ^{239}Pu-contaminated wounds," Health Phys. **27**(3), 273–277.

VOLF, V. (1975). "The effect of combinations of chelating agents on the translocation of intramusculary deposited ^{239}Pu nitrate in the rat," Health Phys. **29**(1), 61–68.

VOLF, V. (1978). *Treatment of Incorporated Transuranium Elements: A Report Sponsored by WHO and the IAEA*, IAEA Technical Report Series No. 184, STI/DOC/10/184 (International Atomic Energy Agency, Vienna).

VUKICEVIC, S., MARUSIC, A., STAVLJENIC, A., CESNJAJ, M. and IVANKOVIC, D. (1994). "The role of tumor necrosis factor-alpha in the generation of acute phase response and bone loss in rats and talc granulomatosis," Lab. Invest. **70**(3), 386–391.

WEAST, R.C., Ed. (1973). *CRC Handbook of Chemistry and Physics*, 53rd ed. (CRC Press, Boca Raton, Florida).

WEEKS, M.H. and OAKLEY, W.D. (1954). "Absorption of plutonium through the living skin of the rat," pages 102 to 105 in *Hanford Biology Research—Annual Report for 1953*, HW-30437 (National Technical Information Service, Springfield, Virginia).

WEEKS, M.H. and OAKELY, W.D. (1955). "Percutaneous absorption of plutonium solutions in rats," pages 56 to 63 in *Hanford Biology Research—Annual Report for 1954*, HW-35917 (National Technical Information Service, Springfield, Virginia).

WELCH, M.P., ODLAND, G.F. and CLARK, R.A.F. (1990). "Temporal relationships of F-actin bundle formation, collagen and fibronectin matrix assembly, and fibronectin receptor expression to wound contraction," J. Cell Biol. **110**(1), 133–145.

WERNER, S. (1998). "Keratinocyte growth factor: A unique player in epithelial repair processes," Cytokine Growth Factor Rev. **9**(2) 153–165.

WIJEKOON, C.J., WEERASEKERA, K.H. and WEERASINGHE, A.K. (1995). "Sarcoid-like granulomas of the skin seven years after bomb blast injury," Ceylon Med. J. **40**(3) 126–127.

WILLIAMS, T.J. (1988). "Factors that affect vessel reactivity and leukocyte emigration," pages 115 to 183 in *Molecular and Cellular Biology of Wound Repair*, Clark, R.A.F. and Henson, P.M. Eds. (Plenum Press, New York).

WOODLEY, D.T., KALEBEC, T., BANES, A.J., LINK, W., PRUNIERAS, M. and LIOTTA, L. (1986). "Adult human keratinocytes migrating over nonviable dermal collagen produce collagenolytic enzymes that degrade type I and type IV collagen," J. Invest. Dermatol. **86**(4), 418–423.

WORGUL, B.V. and ROTHSTEIN, H. (1977). "On the mechanism of radiation cataractogenesis," Medikon **6**, 5–24.

WORGUL, B.V., MERRIAM, G.R., JR. and MEDVEDOVSKY, C. (1989). "Cortical cataract development—an expression of primary damage to the lens epithelium," Lens Eye Toxic Res. **6**(4), 559–571.

WORGUL, B.V., BRENNER, D.J., MEDVEDOVSKY, C., MERRIAM, G.R., JR. and HUANG, Y. (1993). "Accelerated heavy particles and the lens. VII: The cataractogenic potential of 450 MeV/amu iron ions," Invest. Ophthalmol. Vis. Sci. **34**(1), 184–193.

WRENN, M.E., DURBIN, P. W., HOWARD, B., LIPSZTEIN, J., RUNDO, J., STILL, E.T. and WILLIS, D.L. (1985). "Metabolism of ingested U and Ra," Health Phys. **48**(5), 601–633.

WRENN, M.E., LIPSZTEIN, J. and BERTELLI, L. (1989). "Pharmakinetic models relevant to toxicity and metabolism for uranium in humans and animals," Radiat. Prot. Dosim. **26**(1), 243–248.

XU, J. and CLARK, R.A.F. (1996). "Extracellular matrix alters PDGF regulation of fibroblast integrins," J. Cell Biol. **132**(1–2), 239–249.

ZAHARIA, M., PINILLOS-ASHTON, L., PICON, C. and METTLER, F.A. (2001). "Localized irradiation from an industrial radiography source in San Ramon, Peru," pages 269 to 276 in *Medical Management of Radiation Accidents*, 2nd ed., Gusev, I.A., Guskova, A.K. and Mettler, F.A., Jr., Eds. (CRC Press, Boca Raton, Florida).

ZAWACKI, B.E. (1974). "The natural history of reversible burn injury," Surg. Gynecol. Obstet. **139**(6), 867–872.

ZOLLINGER, H.U. (1952) "Experimentelle Erzeugung maligner Mierenkapseltumoren bei der Ratte durch Druckreiz," Schweiz. Z. Path. Bakt. **15**, 666–671 (in German).

The NCRP

The National Council on Radiation Protection and Measurements is a nonprofit corporation chartered by Congress in 1964 to:

1. Collect, analyze, develop and disseminate in the public interest information and recommendations about (a) protection against radiation and (b) radiation measurements, quantities and units, particularly those concerned with radiation protection.
2. Provide a means by which organizations concerned with the scientific and related aspects of radiation protection and of radiation quantities, units and measurements may cooperate for effective utilization of their combined resources, and to stimulate the work of such organizations.
3. Develop basic concepts about radiation quantities, units and measurements, about the application of these concepts, and about radiation protection.
4. Cooperate with the International Commission on Radiological Protection, the International Commission on Radiation Units and Measurements, and other national and international organizations, governmental and private, concerned with radiation quantities, units and measurements and with radiation protection.

The Council is the successor to the unincorporated association of scientists known as the National Committee on Radiation Protection and Measurements and was formed to carry on the work begun by the Committee in 1929.

The participants in the Council's work are the Council members and members of scientific and administrative committees. Council members are selected solely on the basis of their scientific expertise and serve as individuals, not as representatives of any particular organization. The scientific committees, composed of experts having detailed knowledge and competence in the particular area of the committee's interest, draft proposed recommendations. These are then submitted to the full membership of the Council for careful review and approval before being published.

The following comprise the current officers and membership of the Council:

Officers

President	Thomas S. Tenforde
Senior Vice President	Kenneth R. Kase
Secretary and Treasurer	David A. Schauer

Members

John F. Ahearne
Edward S. Amis, Jr.
Sally A. Amundson
Kimberly E. Applegate
Benjamin R. Archer
Stephen Balter
Steven M. Becker
Joel S. Bedford
Eleanor A. Blakely
William F. Blakely
John D. Boice, Jr.
Wesley E. Bolch
Thomas B. Borak
Andre Bouville
Leslie A. Braby
David J. Brenner
James A. Brink
Antone L. Brooks
Jerrold T. Bushberg
John F. Cardella
Stephanie K. Carlson
Charles E. Chambers
Polly Y. Chang
S.Y. Chen
Kelly L. Classic
Mary E. Clark
Michael L. Corradini
Allen G. Croff
Paul M. DeLuca
David A. Eastmond
Stephen A. Feig
John R. Frazier
Donald P. Frush

Thomas F. Gesell
Ronald E. Goans
Robert L. Goldberg
Raymond A. Guilmette
Roger W. Harms
Kathryn Held
John W. Hirshfeld, Jr.
F. Owen Hoffman
Roger W. Howell
Timothy J. Jorgensen
Kenneth R. Kase
Ann R. Kennedy
William E. Kennedy, Jr.
David C. Kocher
Ritsuko Komaki
Amy Kronenberg
Susan M. Langhorst
Edwin M. Leidholdt
Howard L. Liber
James C. Lin
Jill A. Lipoti
John B. Little
Paul A. Locke
Jay H. Lubin
C. Douglas Maynard
Debra McBaugh
Ruth E. McBurney
Cynthia H. McCollough
Barbara J. McNeil
Fred A. Mettler, Jr.
Charles W. Miller
Donald L. Miller
William H. Miller
William F. Morgan

David S. Myers
Bruce A. Napier
Gregory A. Nelson
Carl J. Paperiello
R. Julian Preston
Jerome C. Puskin
Abram Recht
Allan C.B. Richardson
Henry D. Royal
Michael T. Ryan
Jonathan M. Samet
Thomas M. Seed
Stephen M. Seltzer
Roy E. Shore
Edward A. Sickles
Steven L. Simon
Paul Slovic
Christopher G. Soares
Daniel J. Strom
Thomas S. Tenforde
Julie E.K. Timins
Richard E. Toohey
Lawrence W. Townsend
Fong Y. Tsai
Richard J. Vetter
Chris G. Whipple
Stuart C. White
J. Frank Wilson
Susan D. Wiltshire
Gayle E. Woloschak
Shiao Y. Woo
Andrew J. Wyrobek
Marco A. Zaider

Distinguished Emeritus Members

Warren K. Sinclair, *President Emeritus;* Charles B. Meinhold, *President Emeritus*
S. James Adelstein, *Honorary Vice President*
W. Roger Ney, *Executive Director Emeritus*
William M. Beckner, *Executive Director Emeritus*

Seymour Abrahamson
Lynn R. Anspaugh
John A. Auxier
William J. Bair
Harold L. Beck
Bruce B. Boecker
Robert L. Brent
Reynold F. Brown
Randall S. Caswell
J. Donald Cossairt
James F. Crow
Gerald D. Dodd
Sarah S. Donaldson
William P. Dornsife
Patricia W. Durbin

Keith F. Eckerman
Thomas S. Ely
Richard F. Foster
R.J. Michael Fry
Ethel S. Gilbert
Joel E. Gray
Robert O. Gorson
Arthur W. Guy
Eric J. Hall
Naomi H. Harley
William R. Hendee
Donald G. Jacobs
Bernd Kahn
Charles E. Land
Roger O. McClellan
Kenneth L. Miller

Dade W. Moeller
A. Alan Moghissi
Wesley L. Nyborg
John W. Poston, Sr.
Andrew K. Poznanski
Genevieve S. Roessler
Marvin Rosenstein
Lawrence N. Rothenberg
Eugene L. Saenger
William J. Schull
John E. Till
Robert L. Ullrich
Arthur C. Upton
F. Ward Whicker
Marvin C. Ziskin

Lauriston S. Taylor Lecturers

Patricia W. Durbin (2007) *The Quest for Therapeutic Actinide Chelators*

Robert L. Brent (2006) *Fifty Years of Scientific Research: The Importance of Scholarship and the Influence of Politics and Controversy*

John B. Little (2005) *Nontargeted Effects of Radiation: Implications for Low-Dose Exposures*

Abel J. Gonzalez (2004) *Radiation Protection in the Aftermath of a Terrorist Attack Involving Exposure to Ionizing Radiation*

Charles B. Meinhold (2003) *The Evolution of Radiation Protection: From Erythema to Genetic Risks to Risks of Cancer to ?*

R. Julian Preston (2002) *Developing Mechanistic Data for Incorporation into Cancer Risk Assessment: Old Problems and New Approaches*

Wesley L. Nyborg (2001) *Assuring the Safety of Medical Diagnostic Ultrasound*

S. James Adelstein (2000) *Administered Radioactivity: Unde Venimus Quoque Imus*

Naomi H. Harley (1999) *Back to Background*

Eric J. Hall (1998) *From Chimney Sweeps to Astronauts: Cancer Risks in the Workplace*

William J. Bair (1997) *Radionuclides in the Body: Meeting the Challenge!*

Seymour Abrahamson (1996) *70 Years of Radiation Genetics: Fruit Flies, Mice and Humans*

Albrecht Kellerer (1995) *Certainty and Uncertainty in Radiation Protection*

R.J. Michael Fry (1994) *Mice, Myths and Men*

Warren K. Sinclair (1993) *Science, Radiation Protection and the NCRP*

Edward W. Webster (1992) *Dose and Risk in Diagnostic Radiology: How Big? How Little?*

Victor P. Bond (1991) *When is a Dose Not a Dose?*

J. Newell Stannard (1990) *Radiation Protection and the Internal Emitter Saga*

Arthur C. Upton (1989) *Radiobiology and Radiation Protection: The Past Century and Prospects for the Future*

Bo Lindell (1988) *How Safe is Safe Enough?*

Seymour Jablon (1987) *How to be Quantitative about Radiation Risk Estimates*

Herman P. Schwan (1986) *Biological Effects of Non-ionizing Radiations: Cellular Properties and Interactions*

John H. Harley (1985) *Truth (and Beauty) in Radiation Measurement*

Harald H. Rossi (1984) *Limitation and Assessment in Radiation Protection*

Merril Eisenbud (1983) *The Human Environment—Past, Present and Future*

Eugene L. Saenger (1982) *Ethics, Trade-Offs and Medical Radiation*

James F. Crow (1981) *How Well Can We Assess Genetic Risk? Not Very*

Harold O. Wyckoff (1980) *From "Quantity of Radiation" and "Dose" to "Exposure" and "Absorbed Dose"—An Historical Review*

Hymer L. Friedell (1979) *Radiation Protection—Concepts and Trade Offs*

Sir Edward Pochin (1978) *Why be Quantitative about Radiation Risk Estimates?*

Herbert M. Parker (1977) *The Squares of the Natural Numbers in Radiation Protection*

Currently, the following committees are actively engaged in formulating recommendations:

Program Area Committee 1: Basic Criteria, Epidemiology,
Radiobiology, and Risk
  SC 1-8 Risk to Thyroid from Ionizing Radiation
  SC 1-13 Impact of Individual Susceptibility and Previous Radiation
    Exposure on Radiation Risk for Astronauts
  SC 1-15 Radiation Safety in NASA Lunar Missions'
  SC 1-17 Second Cancers and Cardiopulmonary Effects After Radiotherapy
  SC 85 Risk of Lung Cancer from Radon
Program Area Committee 2: Operational Radiation Safety
  SC 2-3 Radiation Safety Issues for Image-Guided Interventional Medical
    Procedures
  SC 2-4 Self Assessment of Radiation Safety Programs
  SC 46-17 Radiation Protection in Educational Institutions
Program Area Committee 3: Nonionizing Radiation
Program Area Committee 4: Radiation Protection in Medicine
  SC 4-1 Management of Persons Contaminated with Radionuclides
  SC 4-2 Population Monitoring and Decontamination Following a Nuclear/
    Radiological Incident
Program Area Committee 5: Environmental Radiation and
Radioactive Waste Issues
  SC 64-22 Design of Effective Effluent and Environmental Monitoring
    Programs
Program Area Committee 6: Radiation Measurements and
Dosimetry
  SC 6-1 Uncertainties in the Measurement and Dosimetry of External
    Radiation Sources
  SC 6-2 Radiation Exposure of the U.S. Population
  SC 6-3 Uncertainties in Internal Radiation Dosimetry
  SC 6-4 Fundamental Principles of Dose Reconstruction
  SC 6-5 Radiation Protection and Measurement Issues Related to Cargo
    Scanning with High-Energy X Rays Produced by Accelerators
  SC 6-6 Skin Doses from Dermal Contamination
  SC 6-7 Evaluation of Inhalation Doses in Scenarios Involving Resuspension
    by Nuclear Detonations at the Nevada Test Site

In recognition of its responsibility to facilitate and stimulate cooperation
among organizations concerned with the scientific and related aspects of radiation protection and measurement, the Council has created a category of NCRP
Collaborating Organizations. Organizations or groups of organizations that are
national or international in scope and are concerned with scientific problems
involving radiation quantities, units, measurements and effects, or radiation
protection may be admitted to collaborating status by the Council. Collaborating Organizations provide a means by which NCRP can gain input into its
activities from a wider segment of society. At the same time, the relationships
with the Collaborating Organizations facilitate wider dissemination of information about the Council's activities, interests and concerns. Collaborating
Organizations have the opportunity to comment on draft reports (at the time
that these are submitted to the members of the Council). This is intended to
capitalize on the fact that Collaborating Organizations are in an excellent position to both contribute to the identification of what needs to be treated in NCRP

reports and to identify problems that might result from proposed recommendations. The present Collaborating Organizations with which NCRP maintains liaison are as follows:

American Academy of Dermatology
American Academy of Environmental Engineers
American Academy of Health Physics
American Academy of Orthopaedic Surgeons
American Association of Physicists in Medicine
American College of Medical Physics
American College of Nuclear Physicians
American College of Occupational and Environmental Medicine
American College of Radiology
American Conference of Governmental Industrial Hygienists
American Dental Association
American Industrial Hygiene Association
American Institute of Ultrasound in Medicine
American Medical Association
American Nuclear Society
American Pharmaceutical Association
American Podiatric Medical Association
American Public Health Association
American Radium Society
American Roentgen Ray Society
American Society for Therapeutic Radiology and Oncology
American Society of Emergency Radiology
American Society of Health-System Pharmacists
American Society of Radiologic Technologists
Association of Educators in Imaging and Radiological Sciences
Association of University Radiologists
Bioelectromagnetics Society
Campus Radiation Safety Officers
College of American Pathologists
Conference of Radiation Control Program Directors, Inc.
Council on Radionuclides and Radiopharmaceuticals
Defense Threat Reduction Agency
Electric Power Research Institute
Federal Communications Commission
Federal Emergency Management Agency
Genetics Society of America
Health Physics Society
Institute of Electrical and Electronics Engineers, Inc.
Institute of Nuclear Power Operations
International Brotherhood of Electrical Workers
National Aeronautics and Space Administration
National Association of Environmental Professionals
National Center for Environmental Health/Agency for Toxic Substances
National Electrical Manufacturers Association
National Institute for Occupational Safety and Health
National Institute of Standards and Technology

Nuclear Energy Institute
Office of Science and Technology Policy
Paper, Allied-Industrial, Chemical and Energy Workers International
    Union
Product Stewardship Institute
Radiation Research Society
Radiological Society of North America
Society for Cardiovascular Angiography and Interventions
Society for Pediatric Radiology
Society for Risk Analysis
Society of Chairmen of Academic Radiology Departments
Society of Interventional Radiology
Society of Nuclear Medicine
Society of Radiologists in Ultrasound
Society of Skeletal Radiology
U.S. Air Force
U.S. Army
U.S. Coast Guard
U.S. Department of Energy
U.S. Department of Housing and Urban Development
U.S. Department of Labor
U.S. Department of Transportation
U.S. Environmental Protection Agency
U.S. Navy
U.S. Nuclear Regulatory Commission
U.S. Public Health Service
Utility Workers Union of America

NCRP has found its relationships with these organizations to be extremely valuable to continued progress in its program.

Another aspect of the cooperative efforts of NCRP relates to the Special Liaison relationships established with various governmental organizations that have an interest in radiation protection and measurements. This liaison relationship provides: (1) an opportunity for participating organizations to designate an individual to provide liaison between the organization and NCRP; (2) that the individual designated will receive copies of draft NCRP reports (at the time that these are submitted to the members of the Council) with an invitation to comment, but not vote; and (3) that new NCRP efforts might be discussed with liaison individuals as appropriate, so that they might have an opportunity to make suggestions on new studies and related matters. The following organizations participate in the Special Liaison Program:

Australian Radiation Laboratory
Bundesamt fur Strahlenschutz (Germany)
Canadian Nuclear Safety Commission
Central Laboratory for Radiological Protection (Poland)
China Institute for Radiation Protection
Commissariat a l'Energie Atomique (France)
Commonwealth Scientific Instrumentation Research Organization
    (Australia)
European Commission

Health Council of the Netherlands
Health Protection Agency
International Commission on Non-ionizing Radiation Protection
International Commission on Radiation Units and Measurements
Japan Radiation Council
Korea Institute of Nuclear Safety
Russian Scientific Commission on Radiation Protection
South African Forum for Radiation Protection
World Association of Nuclear Operators
World Health Organization, Radiation and Environmental Health

NCRP values highly the participation of these organizations in the Special Liaison Program.

The Council also benefits significantly from the relationships established pursuant to the Corporate Sponsor's Program. The program facilitates the interchange of information and ideas and corporate sponsors provide valuable fiscal support for the Council's program. This developing program currently includes the following Corporate Sponsors:

3M
Duke Energy Corporation
GE Healthcare
Global Dosimetry Solutions, Inc.
Landauer, Inc.
Nuclear Energy Institute

The Council's activities have been made possible by the voluntary contribution of time and effort by its members and participants and the generous support of the following organizations:

3M Health Physics Services
Agfa Corporation
Alfred P. Sloan Foundation
Alliance of American Insurers
American Academy of Dermatology
American Academy of Health Physics
American Academy of Oral and Maxillofacial Radiology
American Association of Physicists in Medicine
American Cancer Society
American College of Medical Physics
American College of Nuclear Physicians
American College of Occupational and Environmental Medicine
American College of Radiology
American College of Radiology Foundation
American Dental Association
American Healthcare Radiology Administrators
American Industrial Hygiene Association
American Insurance Services Group
American Medical Association
American Nuclear Society
American Osteopathic College of Radiology

American Podiatric Medical Association
American Public Health Association
American Radium Society
American Roentgen Ray Society
American Society of Radiologic Technologists
American Society for Therapeutic Radiology and Oncology
American Veterinary Medical Association
American Veterinary Radiology Society
Association of Educators in Radiological Sciences, Inc.
Association of University Radiologists
Battelle Memorial Institute
Canberra Industries, Inc.
Chem Nuclear Systems
Center for Devices and Radiological Health
College of American Pathologists
Committee on Interagency Radiation Research and Policy Coordination
Commonwealth Edison
Commonwealth of Pennsylvania
Consolidated Edison
Consumers Power Company
Council on Radionuclides and Radiopharmaceuticals
Defense Nuclear Agency
Defense Threat Reduction Agency
Eastman Kodak Company
Edison Electric Institute
Edward Mallinckrodt, Jr. Foundation
EG&G Idaho, Inc.
Electric Power Research Institute
Electromagnetic Energy Association
Federal Emergency Management Agency
Florida Institute of Phosphate Research
Florida Power Corporation
Fuji Medical Systems, U.S.A., Inc.
Genetics Society of America
Global Dosimetry Solutions
Health Effects Research Foundation (Japan)
Health Physics Society
ICN Biomedicals, Inc.
Institute of Nuclear Power Operations
James Picker Foundation
Martin Marietta Corporation
Motorola Foundation
National Aeronautics and Space Administration
National Association of Photographic Manufacturers
National Cancer Institute
National Electrical Manufacturers Association
National Institute of Standards and Technology
New York Power Authority
Philips Medical Systems
Picker International

Public Service Electric and Gas Company
Radiation Research Society
Radiological Society of North America
Richard Lounsbery Foundation
Sandia National Laboratory
Siemens Medical Systems, Inc.
Society of Nuclear Medicine
Society of Pediatric Radiology
Southern California Edison Company
U.S. Department of Energy
U.S. Department of Labor
U.S. Environmental Protection Agency
U.S. Navy
U.S. Nuclear Regulatory Commission
Victoreen, Inc.
Westinghouse Electric Corporation

Initial funds for publication of NCRP reports were provided by a grant from the James Picker Foundation.
NCRP seeks to promulgate information and recommendations based on leading scientific judgment on matters of radiation protection and measurement and to foster cooperation among organizations concerned with these matters. These efforts are intended to serve the public interest and the Council welcomes comments and suggestions on its reports or activities.

NCRP Publications

NCRP publications can be obtained online in both hard- and soft-copy (downloadable PDF) formats at http://NCRPpublications.org. Professional societies can arrange for discounts for their members by contacting NCRP. Additional information on NCRP publications may be obtained from the NCRP website (http://NCRPonline.org) or by telephone (800-229-2652, ext. 25) and fax (301-907-8768). The mailing address is:

NCRP Publications
7910 Woodmont Avenue
Suite 400
Bethesda, MD 20814-3095

Abstracts of NCRP reports published since 1980, abstracts of all NCRP commentaries, and the text of all NCRP statements are available at the NCRP website. Currently available publications are listed below.

NCRP Reports

No.   Title

8   *Control and Removal of Radioactive Contamination in Laboratories* (1951)

22 *Maximum Permissible Body Burdens and Maximum Permissible Concentrations of Radionuclides in Air and in Water for Occupational Exposure* (1959) [includes Addendum 1 issued in August 1963]

25 *Measurement of Absorbed Dose of Neutrons, and of Mixtures of Neutrons and Gamma Rays* (1961)

27 *Stopping Powers for Use with Cavity Chambers* (1961)

30 *Safe Handling of Radioactive Materials* (1964)

32 *Radiation Protection in Educational Institutions* (1966)

35 *Dental X-Ray Protection* (1970)

36 *Radiation Protection in Veterinary Medicine* (1970)

37 *Precautions in the Management of Patients Who Have Received Therapeutic Amounts of Radionuclides* (1970)

38 *Protection Against Neutron Radiation* (1971)

40 *Protection Against Radiation from Brachytherapy Sources* (1972)

41 *Specification of Gamma-Ray Brachytherapy Sources* (1974)

42 *Radiological Factors Affecting Decision-Making in a Nuclear Attack* (1974)

44 *Krypton-85 in the Atmosphere—Accumulation, Biological Significance, and Control Technology* (1975)

46 *Alpha-Emitting Particles in Lungs* (1975)

117 *Research Needs for Radiation Protection* (1993)
118 *Radiation Protection in the Mineral Extraction Industry* (1993)
119 *A Practical Guide to the Determination of Human Exposure to Radiofrequency Fields* (1993)
120 *Dose Control at Nuclear Power Plants* (1994)
121 *Principles and Application of Collective Dose in Radiation Protection* (1995)
122 *Use of Personal Monitors to Estimate Effective Dose Equivalent and Effective Dose to Workers for External Exposure to Low-LET Radiation* (1995)
123 *Screening Models for Releases of Radionuclides to Atmosphere, Surface Water, and Ground* (1996)
124 *Sources and Magnitude of Occupational and Public Exposures from Nuclear Medicine Procedures* (1996)
125 *Deposition, Retention and Dosimetry of Inhaled Radioactive Substances* (1997)
126 *Uncertainties in Fatal Cancer Risk Estimates Used in Radiation Protection* (1997)
127 *Operational Radiation Safety Program* (1998)
128 *Radionuclide Exposure of the Embryo/Fetus* (1998)
129 *Recommended Screening Limits for Contaminated Surface Soil and Review of Factors Relevant to Site-Specific Studies* (1999)
130 *Biological Effects and Exposure Limits for "Hot Particles"* (1999)
131 *Scientific Basis for Evaluating the Risks to Populations from Space Applications of Plutonium* (2001)
132 *Radiation Protection Guidance for Activities in Low-Earth Orbit* (2000)
133 *Radiation Protection for Procedures Performed Outside the Radiology Department* (2000)
134 *Operational Radiation Safety Training* (2000)
135 *Liver Cancer Risk from Internally-Deposited Radionuclides* (2001)
136 *Evaluation of the Linear-Nonthreshold Dose-Response Model for Ionizing Radiation* (2001)
137 *Fluence-Based and Microdosimetric Event-Based Methods for Radiation Protection in Space* (2001)
138 *Management of Terrorist Events Involving Radioactive Material* (2001)
139 *Risk-Based Classification of Radioactive and Hazardous Chemical Wastes* (2002)
140 *Exposure Criteria for Medical Diagnostic Ultrasound: II. Criteria Based on all Known Mechanisms* (2002)
141 *Managing Potentially Radioactive Scrap Metal* (2002)
142 *Operational Radiation Safety Program for Astronauts in Low-Earth Orbit: A Basic Framework* (2002)
143 *Management Techniques for Laboratories and Other Small Institutional Generators to Minimize Off-Site Disposal of Low-Level Radioactive Waste* (2003)
144 *Radiation Protection for Particle Accelerator Facilities* (2003)
145 *Radiation Protection in Dentistry* (2003)

146 *Approaches to Risk Management in Remediation of Radioactively Contaminated Sites* (2004)

147 *Structural Shielding Design for Medical X-Ray Imaging Facilities* (2004)

148 *Radiation Protection in Veterinary Medicine* (2004)

149 *A Guide to Mammography and Other Breast Imaging Procedures* (2004)

150 *Extrapolation of Radiation-Induced Cancer Risks from Nonhuman Experimental Systems to Humans* (2005)

151 *Structural Shielding Design and Evaluation for Megavoltage X- and Gamma-Ray Radiotherapy Facilities* (2005)

152 *Performance Assessment of Near-Surface Facilities for Disposal of Low-Level Radioactive Waste* (2005)

153 *Information Needed to Make Radiation Protection Recommendations for Space Missions Beyond Low-Earth Orbit* (2006)

154 *Cesium-137 in the Environment: Radioecology and Approaches to Assessment and Management* (2006)

155 *Management of Radionuclide Therapy Patients* (2006)

156 *Development of a Biokinetic Model for Radionuclide-Contaminated Wounds and Procedures for Their Assessment, Dosimetry and Treatment* (2006)

Binders for NCRP reports are available. Two sizes make it possible to collect into small binders the "old series" of reports (NCRP Reports Nos. 8–30) and into large binders the more recent publications (NCRP Reports Nos. 32–156). Each binder will accommodate from five to seven reports. The binders carry the identification "NCRP Reports" and come with label holders which permit the user to attach labels showing the reports contained in each binder.

The following bound sets of NCRP reports are also available:

Volume I. NCRP Reports Nos. 8, 22
Volume II. NCRP Reports Nos. 23, 25, 27, 30
Volume III. NCRP Reports Nos. 32, 35, 36, 37
Volume IV. NCRP Reports Nos. 38, 40, 41
Volume V. NCRP Reports Nos. 42, 44, 46
Volume VI. NCRP Reports Nos. 47, 49, 50, 51
Volume VII. NCRP Reports Nos. 52, 53, 54, 55, 57
Volume VIII. NCRP Report No. 58
Volume IX. NCRP Reports Nos. 59, 60, 61, 62, 63
Volume X. NCRP Reports Nos. 64, 65, 66, 67
Volume XI. NCRP Reports Nos. 68, 69, 70, 71, 72
Volume XII. NCRP Reports Nos. 73, 74, 75, 76
Volume XIII. NCRP Reports Nos. 77, 78, 79, 80
Volume XIV. NCRP Reports Nos. 81, 82, 83, 84, 85
Volume XV. NCRP Reports Nos. 86, 87, 88, 89
Volume XVI. NCRP Reports Nos. 90, 91, 92, 93
Volume XVII. NCRP Reports Nos. 94, 95, 96, 97
Volume XVIII. NCRP Reports Nos. 98, 99, 100
Volume XIX. NCRP Reports Nos. 101, 102, 103, 104
Volume XX. NCRP Reports Nos. 105, 106, 107, 108

Volume XXI. NCRP Reports Nos. 109, 110, 111
Volume XXII. NCRP Reports Nos. 112, 113, 114
Volume XXIII. NCRP Reports Nos. 115, 116, 117, 118
Volume XXIV. NCRP Reports Nos. 119, 120, 121, 122
Volume XXV. NCRP Report No. 123I and 123II
Volume XXVI. NCRP Reports Nos. 124, 125, 126, 127
Volume XXVII. NCRP Reports Nos. 128, 129, 130
Volume XXVIII. NCRP Reports Nos. 131, 132, 133
Volume XXIX. NCRP Reports Nos. 134, 135, 136, 137
Volume XXX. NCRP Reports Nos. 138, 139
Volume XXXI. NCRP Report No. 140
Volume XXXII. NCRP Reports Nos. 141, 142, 143
Volume XXXIII. NCRP Report No. 144
Volume XXXIV. NCRP Reports Nos. 145, 146, 147
Volume XXXV. NCRP Reports Nos. 148, 149
Volume XXXVI. NCRP Reports Nos. 150, 151, 152

(Titles of the individual reports contained in each volume are given previously.)

NCRP Commentaries

No.   Title

1   Krypton-85 in the Atmosphere—With Specific Reference to the Public
    Health Significance of the Proposed Controlled Release at Three Mile
    Island (1980)

4   Guidelines for the Release of Waste Water from Nuclear Facilities with
    Special Reference to the Public Health Significance of the Proposed
    Release of Treated Waste Waters at Three Mile Island (1987)

5   Review of the Publication, Living Without Landfills (1989)

6   Radon Exposure of the U.S. Population—Status of the Problem (1991)

7   Misadministration of Radioactive Material in Medicine—Scientific
    Background (1991)

8   Uncertainty in NCRP Screening Models Relating to Atmospheric
    Transport, Deposition and Uptake by Humans (1993)

9   Considerations Regarding the Unintended Radiation Exposure of the
    Embryo, Fetus or Nursing Child (1994)

10 Advising the Public about Radiation Emergencies: A Document for
    Public Comment (1994)

11 Dose Limits for Individuals Who Receive Exposure from Radionuclide
    Therapy Patients (1995)

12 Radiation Exposure and High-Altitude Flight (1995)

13 An Introduction to Efficacy in Diagnostic Radiology and Nuclear
    Medicine (Justification of Medical Radiation Exposure) (1995)

14 A Guide for Uncertainty Analysis in Dose and Risk Assessments
    Related to Environmental Contamination (1996)

15 Evaluating the Reliability of Biokinetic and Dosimetric Models and
    Parameters Used to Assess Individual Doses for Risk Assessment
    Purposes (1998)

16 *Screening of Humans for Security Purposes Using Ionizing Radiation Scanning Systems* (2003)
17 *Pulsed Fast Neutron Analysis System Used in Security Surveillance* (2003)
18 *Biological Effects of Modulated Radiofrequency Fields* (2003)
19 *Key Elements of Preparing Emergency Responders for Nuclear and Radiological Terrorism* (2005)

Proceedings of the Annual Meeting

No.   Title

1 *Perceptions of Risk,* Proceedings of the Fifteenth Annual Meeting held on March 14-15, 1979 (including Taylor Lecture No. 3) (1980)
3 *Critical Issues in Setting Radiation Dose Limits*, Proceedings of the Seventeenth Annual Meeting held on April 8-9, 1981 (including Taylor Lecture No. 5) (1982)
4 *Radiation Protection and New Medical Diagnostic Approaches,* Proceedings of the Eighteenth Annual Meeting held on April 6-7, 1982 (including Taylor Lecture No. 6) (1983)
5 *Environmental Radioactivity,* Proceedings of the Nineteenth Annual Meeting held on April 6-7, 1983 (including Taylor Lecture No. 7) (1983)
6 *Some Issues Important in Developing Basic Radiation Protection Recommendations*, Proceedings of the Twentieth Annual Meeting held on April 4-5, 1984 (including Taylor Lecture No. 8) (1985)
7 *Radioactive Waste*, Proceedings of the Twenty-first Annual Meeting held on April 3-4, 1985 (including Taylor Lecture No. 9)(1986)
8 *Nonionizing Electromagnetic Radiations and Ultrasound,* Proceedings of the Twenty-second Annual Meeting held on April 2-3, 1986 (including Taylor Lecture No. 10) (1988)
9 *New Dosimetry at Hiroshima and Nagasaki and Its Implications for Risk Estimates*, Proceedings of the Twenty-third Annual Meeting held on April 8-9, 1987 (including Taylor Lecture No. 11) (1988)
10 *Radon*, Proceedings of the Twenty-fourth Annual Meeting held on March 30-31, 1988 (including Taylor Lecture No. 12) (1989)
11 *Radiation Protection Today—The NCRP at Sixty Years*, Proceedings of the Twenty-fifth Annual Meeting held on April 5-6, 1989 (including Taylor Lecture No. 13) (1990)
12 *Health and Ecological Implications of Radioactively Contaminated Environments*, Proceedings of the Twenty-sixth Annual Meeting held on April 4-5, 1990 (including Taylor Lecture No. 14) (1991)
13 *Genes, Cancer and Radiation Protection,* Proceedings of the Twenty-seventh Annual Meeting held on April 3-4, 1991 (including Taylor Lecture No. 15) (1992)
14 *Radiation Protection in Medicine,* Proceedings of the Twenty-eighth Annual Meeting held on April 1-2, 1992 (including Taylor Lecture No. 16) (1993)
15 *Radiation Science and Societal Decision Making,* Proceedings of the Twenty-ninth Annual Meeting held on April 7-8, 1993 (including Taylor Lecture No. 17) (1994)

16   *Extremely-Low-Frequency Electromagnetic Fields: Issues in Biological Effects and Public Health*, Proceedings of the Thirtieth Annual Meeting held on April 6-7, 1994 (not published).

17   *Environmental Dose Reconstruction and Risk Implications,* Proceedings of the Thirty-first Annual Meeting held on April 12-13, 1995 (including Taylor Lecture No. 19) (1996)

18   *Implications of New Data on Radiation Cancer Risk*, Proceedings of the Thirty-second Annual Meeting held on April 3-4, 1996 (including Taylor Lecture No. 20) (1997)

19   *The Effects of Pre- and Postconception Exposure to Radiation,* Proceedings of the Thirty-third Annual Meeting held on April 2-3, 1997, Teratology **59**, 181–317 (1999)

20   *Cosmic Radiation Exposure of Airline Crews, Passengers and Astronauts*, Proceedings of the Thirty-fourth Annual Meeting held on April 1-2, 1998, Health Phys. **79**, 466–613 (2000)

21   *Radiation Protection in Medicine: Contemporary Issues*, Proceedings of the Thirty-fifth Annual Meeting held on April 7-8, 1999 (including Taylor Lecture No. 23) (1999)

22   *Ionizing Radiation Science and Protection in the 21st Century,* Proceedings of the Thirty-sixth Annual Meeting held on April 5-6, 2000, Health Phys. **80**, 317–402 (2001)

23   *Fallout from Atmospheric Nuclear Tests—Impact on Science and Society*, Proceedings of the Thirty-seventh Annual Meeting held on April 4-5, 2001, Health Phys. **82**, 573–748 (2002)

24   *Where the New Biology Meets Epidemiology: Impact on Radiation Risk Estimates*, Proceedings of the Thirty-eighth Annual Meeting held on April 10-11, 2002, Health Phys. **85**, 1–108 (2003)

25   *Radiation Protection at the Beginning of the 21st Century–A Look Forward*, Proceedings of the Thirty-ninth Annual Meeting held on April 9–10, 2003, Health Phys. **87**, 237–319 (2004)

26   *Advances in Consequence Management for Radiological Terrorism Events*, Proceedings of the Fortieth Annual Meeting held on April 14–15, 2004, Health Phys. **89**, 415–588 (2005)

27   *Managing the Disposition of Low-Activity Radioactive Materials*, Proceedings of the Forty-first Annual Meeting held on March 30–31, 2005, Health Phys. **91**, 413–536 (2006)

Lauriston S. Taylor Lectures

No.   Title

1   *The Squares of the Natural Numbers in Radiation Protection by* Herbert M. Parker (1977)

2   *Why be Quantitative about Radiation Risk Estimates?* by Sir Edward Pochin (1978)

3   *Radiation Protection—Concepts and Trade Offs* by Hymer L. Friedell (1979) [available also in *Perceptions of Risk*, see above]

4   *From "Quantity of Radiation" and "Dose" to "Exposure" and "Absorbed Dose"—An Historical Review* by Harold O. Wyckoff (1980)

5   *How Well Can We Assess Genetic Risk? Not Very* by James F. Crow
    (1981) [available also in *Critical Issues in Setting Radiation Dose
    Limits*, see above]

6   *Ethics, Trade-offs and Medical Radiation* by Eugene L. Saenger
    (1982) [available also in *Radiation Protection and New Medical
    Diagnostic Approaches*, see above]

7   *The Human Environment—Past, Present and Future* by Merril
    Eisenbud (1983) [available also in *Environmental Radioactivity*, see
    above]

8   *Limitation and Assessment in Radiation Protection* by Harald H.
    Rossi (1984) [available also in *Some Issues Important in Developing
    Basic Radiation Protection Recommendations*, see above]

9   *Truth (and Beauty) in Radiation Measurement* by John H. Harley
    (1985) [available also in *Radioactive Waste*, see above]

10 *Biological Effects of Non-ionizing Radiations: Cellular Properties and
    Interactions* by Herman P. Schwan (1987) [available also in
    Nonionizing Electromagnetic Radiations and Ultrasound, see above]

11 *How to be Quantitative about Radiation Risk Estimates* by Seymour
    Jablon (1988) [available also in *New Dosimetry at Hiroshima and
    Nagasaki and its Implications for Risk Estimates*, see above]

12 *How Safe is Safe Enough?* by Bo Lindell (1988) [available also in
    Radon, see above]

13 *Radiobiology and Radiation Protection: The Past Century and
    Prospects for the Future* by Arthur C. Upton (1989) [available also in
    Radiation Protection Today, see above]

14 *Radiation Protection and the Internal Emitter Saga* by J. Newell
    Stannard (1990) [available also in *Health and Ecological Implications
    of Radioactively Contaminated Environments*, see above]

15 *When is a Dose Not a Dose?* by Victor P. Bond (1992) [available also in
    Genes, Cancer and Radiation Protection, see above]

16 *Dose and Risk in Diagnostic Radiology: How Big? How Little?* by
    Edward W. Webster (1992) [available also in *Radiation Protection in
    Medicine*, see above]

17 *Science, Radiation Protection and the NCRP* by Warren K. Sinclair
    (1993) [available also in *Radiation Science and Societal Decision
    Making*, see above]

18 *Mice, Myths and Men* by R.J. Michael Fry (1995)

19 *Certainty and Uncertainty in Radiation Research* by Albrecht M.
    Kellerer. Health Phys. **69**, 446–453 (1995)

20 *70 Years of Radiation Genetics: Fruit Flies, Mice and Humans* by
    Seymour Abrahamson. Health Phys. **71**, 624–633 (1996)

21 *Radionuclides in the Body: Meeting the Challenge* by William J. Bair.
    Health Phys. **73**, 423–432 (1997)

22 *From Chimney Sweeps to Astronauts: Cancer Risks in the Work Place*
    by Eric J. Hall. Health Phys. **75**, 357–366 (1998)

23 *Back to Background: Natural Radiation and Radioactivity Exposed*
    by Naomi H. Harley. Health Phys. **79**, 121–128 (2000)

24 *Administered Radioactivity: Unde Venimus Quoque Imus* by S. James
    Adelstein. Health Phys. **80**, 317–324 (2001)

25 *Assuring the Safety of Medical Diagnostic Ultrasound* by Wesley L. Nyborg. Health Phys. **82**, 578–587 (2002)

26 *Developing Mechanistic Data for Incorporation into Cancer and Genetic Risk Assessments: Old Problems and New Approaches* by R. Julian Preston. Health Phys. **85**, 4–12 (2003)

27 *The Evolution of Radiation Protection–From Erythema to Genetic Risks to Risks of Cancer to ?* by Charles B. Meinhold, Health Phys. **87**, 240–248 (2004)

28 *Radiation Protection in the Aftermath of a Terrorist Attack Involving Exposure to Ionizing Radiation* by Abel J. Gonzalez, Health Phys. **89**, 418–446 (2005)

29 *Nontargeted Effects of Radiation: Implications for Low Dose Exposures* by John B. Little, Health Phys. **91**, 416–426 (2006)

Symposium Proceedings

No.   Title

1 *The Control of Exposure of the Public to Ionizing Radiation in the Event of Accident or Attack*, Proceedings of a Symposium held April 27-29, 1981 (1982)

2 *Radioactive and Mixed Waste—Risk as a Basis for Waste Classification,* Proceedings of a Symposium held November 9, 1994 (1995)

3 *Acceptability of Risk from Radiation—Application to Human Space Flight,* Proceedings of a Symposium held May 29, 1996 (1997)

4 *21st Century Biodosimetry: Quantifying the Past and Predicting the Future*, Proceedings of a Symposium held February 22, 2001, Radiat. Prot. Dosim. **97**(1), (2001)

5 *National Conference on Dose Reduction in CT, with an Emphasis on Pediatric Patients*, Summary of a Symposium held November 6-7, 2002, Am. J. Roentgenol. **181**(2), 321–339 (2003)

NCRP Statements

No.   Title

1 "Blood Counts, Statement of the National Committee on Radiation Protection," Radiology **63**, 428 (1954)

2 "Statements on Maximum Permissible Dose from Television Receivers and Maximum Permissible Dose to the Skin of the Whole Body," Am. J. Roentgenol., Radium Ther. and Nucl. Med. **84**, 152 (1960) and Radiology **75**, 122 (1960)

3 *X-Ray Protection Standards for Home Television Receivers, Interim Statement of the National Council on Radiation Protection and Measurements* (1968)

4 *Specification of Units of Natural Uranium and Natural Thorium, Statement of the National Council on Radiation Protection and Measurements* (1973)

5 *NCRP Statement on Dose Limit for Neutrons* (1980)

6 *Control of Air Emissions of Radionuclides* (1984)

7   *The Probability That a Particular Malignancy May Have Been Caused by a Specified Irradiation* (1992)
8   *The Application of ALARA for Occupational Exposures* (1999)
9   *Extension of the Skin Dose Limit for Hot Particles to Other External Sources of Skin Irradiation* (2001)
10 *Recent Applications of the NCRP Public Dose Limit Recommendation for Ionizing Radiation* (2004)

Other Documents

The following documents were published outside of the NCRP report, commentary and statement series:

Somatic Radiation Dose for the General Population, Report of the Ad Hoc Committee of the National Council on Radiation Protection and Measurements, 6 May 1959, Science **131** (3399), February 19, 482–486 (1960)
Dose Effect Modifying Factors in Radiation Protection, Report of Subcommittee M-4 (Relative Biological Effectiveness) of the National Council on Radiation Protection and Measurements, Report BNL 50073 (T-471) (1967) Brookhaven National Laboratory (National Technical Information Service, Springfield, Virginia)
Residential Radon Exposure and Lung Cancer Risk: Commentary on Cohen's County-Based Study, Health Phys. **87**(6), 656–658 (2004)

Index